Ultrastructure of Bacterial Viruses

AF786156

Ultrastructure of Bacterial Viruses

Anna S. Tikhonenko
Institute of Molecular Biology
Academy of Sciences of the USSR
Moscow, USSR

Translated from Russian by
Basil Haigh
Cambridge, England

PLENUM PRESS • NEW YORK–LONDON • 1970

Library of Congress Catalog Card Number 69-17902

ISBN-13: 978-1-4684-1781-4 e-ISBN-13: 978-1-4684-1779-1
DOI: 10.1007/978-1-4684-1779-1

The original Russian text, published for the Scientific Committee on Problems in Molecular Biology of the Academy of Sciences of the USSR by Nauka Press in Moscow in 1968, has been corrected by the author for this edition. The translation is published under an agreement with Mezhdunarodnaya Kniga, the Soviet book export agency.

Анна Сергеевна Тихоненко
УЛЬТРАСТРУКТУРА ВИРУСОВ БАКТЕРИЙ
UL'TRASTRUKTURA VIRUSOV BAKTERII
ULTRASTRUCTURE OF BACTERIAL VIRUSES

© 1970 Plenum Press
Softcover reprint of the hardcover 1st edition 1970
A Division of Plenum Publishing Corporation
227 West 17th Street, New York, N. Y. 10011

United Kingdom edition published by Plenum Press, London
A Division of Plenum Publishing Corporation, Ltd.
Donington House, 30 Norfolk Street, London W.C.2, England

All rights reserved

No part of this publication may be reproduced in any form
without written permission from the publisher

This book is
dedicated to my mother
Aleksandra Davydovna Sheinina

Introduction

After the discovery of the tobacco mosaic virus by D. I. Ivanovskii in 1892 [14], the new science of virology was born and began to develop rapidly.

The number of viruses now known is enormous and they can infect nearly all animal and plant organisms. Microorganisms themselves are no exception to this rule.

Despite intensive study of viruses, their origin and nature are still a subject for speculation and hypothesis.

The general concept of viruses embraces a wide group of biologically active structures occupying an intermediate position between living and nonliving matter. The dual character of viruses is determined by the fact that, while they do not possess an independent system of metabolism, which is a characteristic feature of every living being, they nevertheless carry within themselves all the necessary information for autoreproduction.

A striking feature of the virus is that it consists essentially of two components: a protein envelope and the nucleic acid contained within it.

In contrast to the elementary structural unit of the living organism, the cell, which contains two types of nucleic acid (DNA and RNA), the virus particle contains only one type of nucleic acid – either DNA or RNA. It is perhaps this which is responsible for the imperfection of the virus as a living organism.

Unlike living cells, viruses cannot reproduce by any way known for cellular organisms (by division or gemmation). For their reproduction they utilize the energy resources of another, more highly organized, living system. After infecting the host cell, viruses lose their morphological individuality, and they do not persist as specific structures throughout their cycle of development. The formation of individual structural components of the virus takes place separately within the cell, and it is only at the final stage of intracellular development that they come together to form the mature virus particle.

An extremely characteristic feature of viruses is the strict consistency of their shape and size.

Early electron-microscopic investigations established that most viruses of animals and plants are either rod-shaped or spherical.

In 1941, Ruska [320] showed for the first time that the viruses of bacteria, or bacteriophages, as a rule, are particles of characteristic shape resembling spermatozoa.

The relatively simple organization of viruses, carrying their own genetic system providing for autoreproduction and variation, has attracted the attention of investigators seeking to solve fundamental biological problems.

Bacterial viruses, because of their comparative accessibility and the simplicity of working with them, have proved to be the most convenient viruses for analysis of major virological and general biological problems.

Bacteriophagy as a general biological problem has developed rapidly in the last 20-25 years and has attracted specialists in different fields of science. It should be pointed out that the progress made in many of the fundamental theoretical problems in modern biology is largely bound up with the study of phages. In recent years, phages have occupied the center of the stage as a model for the study of the basic problems in molecular biology. It was this model which was used for classical investigations to study the fine structure of the gene, to decipher the genetic code, to study the mechanism of transmission of information for protein synthesis and so on.

The study of the macromolecular structure of phages is accordingly of considerable interest. It forms the subject of this monograph, which is based largely on the results of investigations carried out by the author and her collaborators.

Contents

Chapter 1

Electron-Microscopic Methods of Investigation of Bacteriophages

The study of biological objects in the electron microscope requires special techniques. The basic electron-microscopic methods used to investigate biological objects have been fully described elsewhere [7].

Since this monograph is concerned with the study of the structure of bacterial viruses, a brief account of electron-microscopic methods used for this purpose must first be given.

THE SUPPORTING GRIDS

Objects to be examined in the electron microscope are held on special grids covered by a thin mounting film.

Usually copper electrolytic grids with between 4 and 10 meshes per millimeter are used for practical work with the electron microscope. Electrolytic meshes are available either ready made or as a metal strip from which grids of specified diameter can be cut with a special punch. The diameter of the grids depends on the type of electron microscope used.

The grids must be clean and even, and before use they must therefore be washed for 2–3 min in weak hydrochloric acid, then in water, alcohol, and acetone, and kept either in alcohol or in dichloroethane. A method of washing grids which can be well recommended is by boiling them for 5 min in concentrated ammonia solution and then washing them carefully in distilled water. Such grids should be kept in alcohol.

The methods described above are also used for cleaning grids to remove badly applied film or films which have previously been in the electron microscope.

PREPARATION OF THE MOUNTING FILM

The role of the slide in the case of the electron microscope is performed by transparent films fixed to the grids. These films must not exceed 200 Å in thickness. Thicker films increase the angular scatter of electrons, thereby reducing very considerably the contrast of the image and resolution of the structures forming the object.

For electron-microscopic examination of biological objects, films made of nitrocellulose, ethylene cellulose, and Formvar, and also films obtained by pulverizing carbon *in vacuo* (carbon films) are mainly used. The principal requirements of these films are transparency, mechanical strength; a lack of structure, and resistance to electron bombardment.

Nitrocellulose Film

To obtain nitrocellulose films, solutions of collodion in amyl acetate are used (instead of collodion, motion picture film, well washed in hot water, may be used). Pure collodion is readily obtained from pharmaceutical solutions of collodion in ether. The pharmaceutical solution of collodion is poured as a thin layer into a clean Petri dish and dried in a fume hood. A transparent film is formed on the floor of the Petri dish. Before a solution is prepared from this film, it should be kept for 24-48 h in a vacuum of the order of 10^{-4}-10^{-5} mm Hg in order to remove residues of solvent which are firmly bound to the nitrocellulose molecules (clean motion picture film must also be kept for a time *in vacuo*). From nitrocellulose prepared in this manner, homogeneous, absolutely transparent, and strong films can subsequently be obtained. Films prepared from nitrocellulose which have not been kept *in vacuo* are less strong. A solution of nitrocellulose in amyl acetate is next prepared. Depending on the size and density of the object to be examined, solutions of different concentrations are used (from 0.5 to 2%). The smaller the object, the less concentrated the solutions which can be used to prepare the films. Usually, films made from 0.5–1% solutions are used for investigation of biological objects. From 18 to 24 h is necessary for the nitrocellulose to dissolve. The solution should be kept in darkness, for in light insoluble substances form in it and the film obtained from it is not very strong. It is better to make small quantities of solution, because it quickly deteriorates.

To prepare the film, distilled water is poured into a Petri dish and one drop of collodion solution is carefully placed on its surface by means of a Pasteur pipet. The drop spreads over the surface of the water, and after evaporation of the amyl acetate a thin film is formed. Usually the first film is not strong and is contaminated with dust floating on the surface of the water. This film is removed with forceps. Films obtained from the second, third, and subsequent drops can be used for work with the electron microscope.

This method has several modifications. Drummond [153], for instance, recommends applying a drop of the solution of nitrocellulose in amyl acetate to the surface of the convex meniscus of water poured into a dish 20 cm in diameter as far as its edge. In this way a film of more uniform thickness is obtained.

Ruska [321] suggested using water saturated with amyl acetate vapor for preparing the films. A small quantity of amyl acetate is poured into the water 24 h before the films are made, and the mixture is vigorously shaken and allowed to stand. The film obtained on the surface of such water is stronger and more homogeneous.

Formvar Films

Films made from Formvar (polyvinylformaldehyde) are stronger than those made from nitrocellulose. However, it is more difficult to make a film of uniform thickness from Formvar, because solvents of Formvar (dioxane, dichloroethane) do not flow as uniformly as amyl acetate over the surface of water.

Formvar films are prepared on the surface of a well-polished glass slide, which is first thoroughly washed with soap solution, and then, before the slide has dried, it is rubbed with cotton-wool pads soaked successively with distilled water, acetone, and water again, and then wiped dry. To remove particles of dust from the surface of the glass, air from a rubber bulb is blown over it.

To prepare the Formvar film, a large drop of 0.1-0.2% Formvar solution in dichloroethane is placed on one edge of the surface of a clean slide. The drop is distributed over the surface of the glass by rapid shaking in a horizontal direction, and the slide is then immediately placed vertically. The remains of the Formvar solution thereupon flow toward the lower edge. After evaporation of the solvent a thin film is formed on the slide. A U-shaped incision is made on the film at the edge of the slide with a razor or scalpel (Fig. 1a) and the slide is immersed at an angle of 45° in distilled water, as shown in Fig. 1b. In this way the film separates from the slide and floats on the surface of the water. It must be noted that in this case only a small area of the upper part of the film (about one-third of its surface) can be used, because the thickness of the remainder is very irregular.

More homogeneous films, without internal stresses, can be obtained by drying them in vapor of the solvent.

To obtain such a film the following method is used. A slide is immersed to four-fifths of its area in a 0.1-0.2% solution of Formvar contained in a tall cylinder with a lid (Fig. 2a), and it is held in this position for 10 min. During this time the upper part of the cylinder becomes saturated with vapor of the solvent, and as a result a film of more uniform thickness can be obtained on the slide. The slide is then lifted above the surface of the solution and held in that position for 5-10 min (Fig. 2b). Excess of solution runs off the slide, and after evaporation of the solvent, a film is formed. The slide is then taken from the cylinder and held in air for 5-10 min to allow the film to finish drying. Next, a U-shaped incision is made on one surface of the slide (Fig. 2c) and the film removed from the slide as described above. By this method a thin homogeneous film can be obtained, especially in the upper part of the slide.

Carbon Films

Carbon-collodion films are frequently used in practical electron microscopy. They are made as follows. Graphite rods are evaporated on grids with a thin collodion film in a high vacuum, as a result of which the film is covered with a thin layer of carbon.

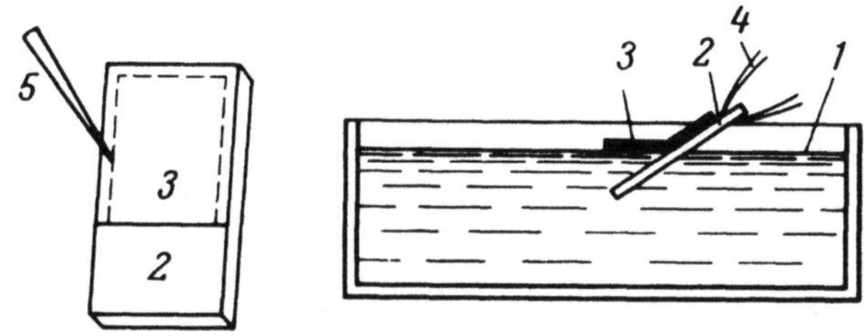

a b

Fig. 1. Preparation of Formvar film: a) cutting the film on the slide; b) separating the film from the slide on the water surface. 1) Surface of water; 2) glass slide; 3) Formvar film; 4) forceps; 5) point of scalpel.

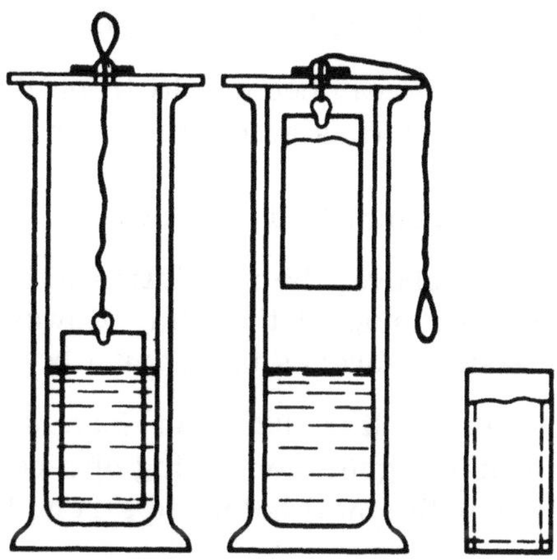

a b c

Fig. 2. Preparation of Formvar film on a glass slide by immersion in a solution of Formvar in dichloroethane (dioxane): a) immersing the slide in the solution; b) holding the slide in dioxane vapor; c) slide ready for separation of the film on a water surface.

Full details of the method of graphite evaporation can be found in the paper by Biryuzova and co-workers [7].

The thin carbon covering protects the film against mechanical breakage and makes it more resistant to electron bombardment. To reduce the thickness of the film, the collodion layer underneath can be dissolved, leaving only the thin covering layer of carbon.

Carbon films are more hydrophobic than collodion, thus interfering with the uniform distribution of a suspension of the test object on it.

Carbon films are made less hydrophobic by the following methods. 1) The grids with the film are placed on filter paper soaked in amyl acetate for 18 h and covered by a Petri dish. The collodion film thereupon dissolves and the remaining carbon film becomes less hydrophobic because amyl acetate, together with the collodion, removes impurities from the oily vapor appearing when graphite is evaporated in a vacuum apparatus. 2) Grids with carbon — collodion films are ionized in a low vacuum.

Films treated in this way become hydrophilic, and the liquid applied to them is distributed as a uniform layer.

Preparation of Perforated Films

As was mentioned above, the resolution in the electron microscope depends on the thickness of the film. However, the thinner the film, the more easily it breaks up under a beam of electrons.

Several investigators [218, 323, 344] have suggested the use of an additional supporting grid, consisting of a perforated film of collodion or Formvar with small holes, to strengthen very thin films.

To prepare perforated films, Sacata [323] suggested using a 3% collodion solution in amyl acetate, one drop of which is applied to the surface of ice-cold water. By breathing on the film before it is completely formed, drops of moisture condense on it and make holes in the film. Such a film is mounted on the grid and the very thin membranes left over the interstices of the grid are removed by gentle flaming. To attach the perforated membrane it is covered with a layer of carbon in a vacuum apparatus.

Huxley's method [218], as modified by Marikhin and Romankova [26], is a simple method of preparing perforated films. It consists essentially as follows. A well-cleaned glass slide is half immersed in a vessel containing a solution of collodion in acetone; the slide is then removed and dried in a vertical position on filter paper. After evaporation of the solvent an opaque bluish-white collodion film is left on the slide. This is cut into squares of the required size and removed from the slide by immersion in water at an acute angle. The film taken from the slide is mounted on grids, dried, and fixed with carbon. Such a film has perforations running completely through it and it is therefore unnecessary to flame it to remove the membranes.

Other methods can be used to prepare perforated film. By the method of Stefanov and Graf [38] perforated films can be made with a stipulated mesh size. For this purpose a drop of 2.0-2.5% collodion solution in amyl acetate is placed on the surface of cold water (+1°). After 5-7 sec the dish containing the incompletely formed film is covered by a glass lid, which is heated above the vessel with boiling water and filled with vapor. Vapor in the form of tiny droplets condenses on the cold film, forming pits in it. The film is thereby made opaque, and is tinted different colors: areas with a reddish green tint give a mesh of 4-7 mμ, bluish areas a mesh of 25-40 mμ. This film is mounted on grids. The thin membranes covering the mesh are melted by means of a hot metal plate.

One other method of obtaining films with holes of a certain diameter has been described, using a mixture of glycerol with 0.2% Formvar solution [194]. A drop of this mixture is spread over the surface of a slide and after 10 min the slide is placed in a jet of steam. The film is then separated from the slide onto the surface of water, a grid is mounted on it, and it is covered with a layer of carbon. The size of the holes in the film depends on the ratio between the glycerol and the Formvar solution in the mixture.

0.25% Formvar solution	Glycerol	Maximal diameter of holes, μ
8 parts	1 part	25
16 parts	1 part	14
32 parts	1 part	7
120 parts	1 part	4

As these figures show, the more Formvar present in the mixture, the smaller the holes in the microgrid thus formed.

The microgrids made in this manner are covered with a thin film prepared from 0.1% collodion solution.

Mounting the Film onto the Grid

A very convenient way of obtaining large numbers of grids with films is as follows. Clean grids are placed accurately on a film floating on the surface of water, choosing the most even areas of the film. They are covered on top with a piece of filter paper, which at once becomes soaked and comes into close contact with the collodion film. By a sliding movement the filter paper, together with the grids and film, is removed with forceps from the surface of the water and dried.

If only slight contact is made between the interlacing of the grid and the film, drifting of the film may take place under an electron beam. To avoid this, it is recommended that the grid be immersed in the original collodion or Formvar solution, diluted 1:1 with the appropriate solvent, before application to the film. This operation is performed as follows: the grid is seized with forceps and immersed for 1 sec in this solution, after which it is transferred to filter paper, which quickly soaks up excess of solution. The interlacing of the grid thus becomes coated with a thin layer of collodion or Formvar solution, enabling closer contact to be made between it and the film.

In cases when the test object is already placed on the film, it can be mounted on grids by a different method. A porcelain Bunsen funnel with holes is used for this purpose. The grids are placed on the bottom of this funnel which is then filled with water, having first closed the outlet of the funnel with a clip. The film is separated from the slide or agar block on the surface of the water and the water is allowed to drain slowly out of the funnel. As the water level falls, so also does the film until it reaches the bottom of the funnel where it covers the grids.

METHODS OF PREPARING SUSPENSIONS OF BACTERIOPHAGES

A simple method of preparing suspensions of phages [53] for studying their morphology is by washing phage particles from the surface of a plaque formed after lysis of bacteria on a solid medium. This method uses up the minimum quantity of material and is particularly convenient when the particle morphology of a phage, forming an individual plaque, has to be studied. For this purpose, a single plaque is cut out of the surface of an agar plate with a platinum needle and transferred into a small volume (up to 0.1 ml) of water or physiological saline or 1% ammonium acetate. After vigorous shaking the phage particles go into suspension, which is then used for obtaining electron-microscopic specimens without further purification.

Another advantage of this method is that a phage suspension can be made from a strictly specified area of a plaque. Often plaques formed at the place of lysis of bacteria by certain phages are heterogeneous in structure. In the course of investigations, it is sometimes necessary to study material from a particular part of one plaque. This part can be cut out of the agar with a glass capillary tube of suitable size, used as a drill. The piece of agar cut out by the capillary tube is pushed along by a needle toward the other end of the capillary tube so that agar from the area of the plaque projects beyond the walls of the capillary tube to a distance not exceeding 1 mm. With this end of the capillary tube, the phage particles are then either carefully applied to the grid covered with the film to which they adhere or they are suspended in a small drop of water or volatile buffer. In the case of suspension, the end of the capillary tube with the test material is immersed in a drop of the liquid and smeared gently over the surface of a slide. This method is also suitable for obtaining suspensions of phages forming very small plaques.

METHODS OF OBTAINING CONCENTRATED SUSPENSIONS OF PHAGES

Concentrated suspensions are used to study the morphology of bacteriophages and also for certain biochemical and physicochemical investigations.

Each particular phage — bacterium system requires specific conditions for the production of high titers. Accordingly, a description of methods of obtaining concentrated suspensions of those phages used in my more important investigations is given below.

Phage No. 1. Preparations of phage No. 1 of *Bacillus mycoides* were concentrated and purified as follows. Confluent lysis of a plate culture was obtained in Petri dishes by the agar layer method [352] after 48 h at 27°C. This method provides the largest quantity of phage per area of lysed culture. The top layer of agar was removed with a spatula and suspended in a small volume of 0.9% NaCl in the proportion of 5 ml per Petri dish. Further concentration and purification were carried out by differential centrifugation. The agar suspension and remnants of the bacterial cells were sedimented by spinning at 6000 g for 30 min. Phage was sedimented at 20,000 g for 1 h. The residue was suspended in 5 ml 0.9% NaCl and mixed with a magnetic stirrer for 1 h at 4°C. The resulting phage suspension was again centrifuged at 6000 g for 30 min to remove remnants of bacterial cells and other impurities, and the supernatant was used for work. Purified preparation of phage No. 1 contained 10^{12} or more phage particles per ml [60].

This method is also suitable for obtaining concentrated suspensions of other phages growing poorly on synthetic media.

Phage T2. A high-titer suspension of phage T2 was obtained as follows. A culture of *Escherichia coli* B was grown in 5-liter flasks with aeration at 37°C to a concentration of 10^8–$2 \cdot 10^8$ cells/ml in a medium of the following composition: solution I – 35 g Na_2HPO_4, 15 g KH_2PO_4, 2.5 g NaCl; solution II – 20 g glucose, 5 g NH_4Cl, 0.125 g $MgSO_4 \cdot 7H_2O$, 0.1 g $CaCl_2$. The salts were dissolved in 250 ml of distilled water separately for each solution and sterilized at 0.4 atm for 15 min. Solutions I and II were added to 4500 ml of sterile distilled water.

The culture was grown for 3–4 h and then infected with phage T2 at the rate of one phage particle per bacterial cell. Lysis with aeration continued for 4 h, after which time the flask was left overnight without aeration at room temperature. The resulting lysate had a titer of $5 \cdot 10^{10}$–10^{11} phage particles/ml.

Next morning, the flask with lysate was cooled to 5–8°C and the phage precipitated at the isoelectric point at pH 3.9–4.0 with glacial acetic acid diluted 1:5. The precipitate thus formed was collected by centrifugation at 3000 rpm for 30 min and suspended in borate buffer (pH 7.2) until the pH of the phage suspension reached 7.0. The suspension thus obtained was centrifuged at 5000 rpm for 30 min to remove impurities and large clumps. Further purification of the phage suspension was carried out on a DEAE column. The column, with phage applied to it, was washed with 0.05 M borate buffer, pH 7.1. Phage was eluted with NaCl solution. The most suitable concentration of NaCl solution used for the surfaces was found to be 0.18 M. Purified suspensions of phage obtained from the column were centrifuged at 20,000 rpm for 1 h and the residue suspended in a small volume (up to 20 ml) of physiological saline. A purified phage suspension of this type with a titer of $5 \cdot 10^{12}$–10^{13} phage particles/ml was used as material for several different investigations.

Phage s_d. A concentrated suspension of phage s_d was prepared in 20-liter flasks in the synthetic medium used for cultivation of phage T2, with initial titers of 5–$8 \cdot 10^{10}$ phage particles/ml on a culture of *E. coli* CK. The phage was concentrated and purified by the method described by Tikhonenko and co-workers [63, 66]. The concentrated suspension of phage s_d had a titer of 3–$5 \cdot 10^{12}$ phage particles/ml.

The titer of the phages was determined by counting plaques on a bacterial plate culture by the agar layer method as described by Adams [1].

PURIFICATION OF BIOLOGICAL PREPARATIONS

Before biological objects can be investigated in the electron microscope they must first be purified to remove the medium.

The most convenient methods of purifying bacteriophages are differential centrifugation, drop dialysis, and filtration in agar.

Centrifugation

A suspension of phage in a medium containing large quantities of salts and other admixtures can be purified by differential centrifugation, first at low speeds to remove large particles and then by ultracentrifugation at 20,000–40,000 g. The residue obtained after ultracentrifugation, consisting largely of phage particles, is suspended in a small volume of water, physiological saline, or buffered solution. If salt solutions are used for suspension, purification is carried out in combination with other methods such as dialysis in collodion bags.

Drop Dialysis

The most effective method of purifying small quantities of a test object is drop dialysis, and I have used it frequently. This method was developed in 1948 by Kriss, Biryuzova, and Zolkover [23], and it is based on the use of the collodion supporting film as dialysis membrane.

The method is essentially as follows. A drop of 1-2% solution of collodion in amyl acetate is placed on the surface of distilled water in a sterile Petri dish. The drop spreads over the surface of the water and, after evaporation of the amyl acetate, forms a thin film. Drops of the phage suspension to be tested, 0.1-0.2 ml in volume, are placed on it (Fig. 3). The covered Petri dish is incubated at 26-30°C. Dialysis continues for between 3 and 24 h depending on the composition of the medium in which the object is placed. Broth suspensions are usually dialyzed for 20-24 h.

In the course of this time salts and other soluble substances in the medium pass into the distilled water. The object, purified from the medium, remains on the collodion film from which it is transferred by means of a microbiological loop to electron-microscopic grids covered with collodion or carbon — collodion film. The test suspension can also be dialyzed against 4% formalin solution in distilled water. Electron-microscopic preparations thus obtained are then contrasted in various ways as will be described below.

Purification of a test object by dialysis can be carried out by a somewhat different method [53]. An electron-microscopic grid, covered with sterile filter paper, is placed on a collodion film obtained in a Petri dish from the surface of sterile distilled water. With a sliding movement the filter paper, together with the grid and film, is removed with forceps from the surface of the water and dried in a sterile Petri dish. After drying, small drops of phage suspension are placed on the grid. The filter paper, with drops of the object placed on the grid, is transferred to the surface of distilled water. Dialysis takes place through the collodion film covering the grid and through the filter paper (Fig. 4) and continues for 18-20 h. At the end of dialysis, the paper with the grid is taken from the surface of the water, the object is contrasted, and dried. This method enables one to use small amounts of material. It is also suitable for labeling preparations (the necessary inscriptions are made on the same filter paper).

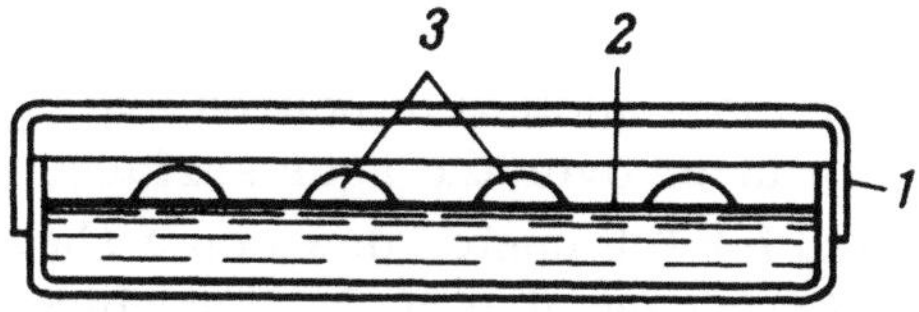

Fig. 3. Dialysis of drops placed on a collodion film resting on the surface of sterile distilled water: 1) Petri dish; 2) film; 3) drops of suspension to be dialyzed.

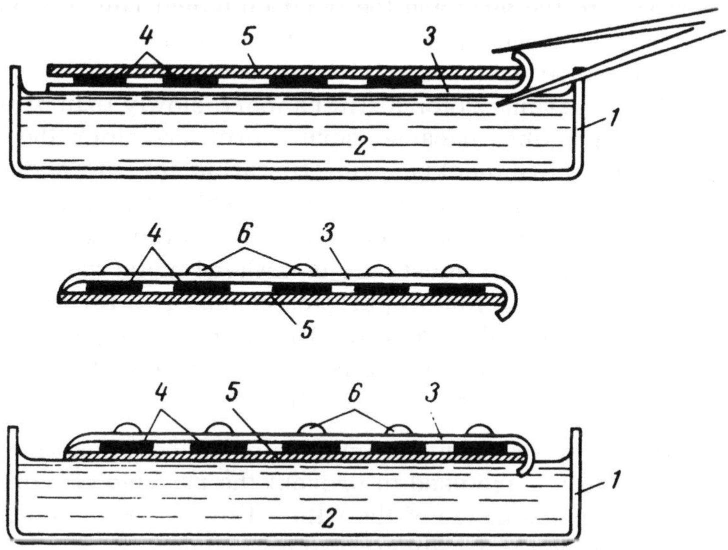

Fig. 4. Modification of drop dialysis: 1) Petri dish; 2) water; 3) film; 4) grids; 5) filter paper; 6) drops of suspension to be tested.

Purification by Filtration in Agar

The method of purification by filtration in agar [232] is as follows. Into a Petri dish is poured 20 ml of 1.5-3% agar with the addition of salts contained in the suspending fluid for the object. After the agar has solidified, its surface is washed with purified petroleum ether to remove grease marks and other impurities that may be present. The surface of the agar is then dried in front of a fan until all moisture has evaporated, after which a 0.2-0.4% solution of collodion in amyl acetate is poured over it and spread quickly as a uniform layer over the agar surface. Dishes prepared in this way are dried for 6 h upside down on a sheet of clean paper. Next, 2-4 drops of the suspension of the test object in its usual nutrient medium are applied to the film thus obtained, covering the agar, and by means of a sterile spatula they are carefully spread over the surface of the film taking care not to damage it. The Petri dish is then immediately covered to prevent evaporation of the moisture. The liquid applied filters for 10-20 min through the collodion film into the agar and the purified object remains on the surface of the film. The speed of filtration depends on the organic components of the filtered suspension. A suspension containing a large quantity of serum proteins filters more slowly than ordinary nutrient broth, possibly because serum proteins block the pores in the film more quickly. After filtration, the agar plates are fixed in formalin vapor for 7-10 min, after which a small block is cut out of the agar and transferred into a 2% solution of lanthanum nitrate with the film uppermost. Places where moist areas have remained are unsuitable for preparation of material for examination. On the surface of the liquid the film is easily separated from the agar block and floats. An electron-microscopic grid is placed under the film and they are dried on filter paper.

Fixation with formalin and immersion of the block in lanthanum nitrate solution are used to prevent the passage of moisture through to the upper surface of the film. The object is then contrasted and examined in the electron microscope.

Method of Cultivation of Microorganisms and Their Lysis by Bacteriophage on Film Mounts

Hillier and Baker [202] suggested a method of cultivating microorganisms on collodion film which is then used as mounting film for the test object. The main advantage of this method is that the investigator can study an object without changing its natural position during growth and development, and in the case of phagolysis, without disturbing the topographic arrangement of the lysed cells.

In Hillier's method sterile distilled water is poured onto the surface of nutrient agar in a Petri dish and run off twice or three times to wash the surface of the agar. Sterile distilled water is again poured on, and a drop of 0.5-1% collodion solution in amyl acetate placed on its surface. After evaporation of the amyl acetate, a thin collodion film is formed on the surface of the water. The distilled water is withdrawn from under the film by means of a pipet, after which the film rests firmly on the surface of the agar. With a pipet, bacteria infected with phage and suspended in water or physiological saline are placed on the film and the excess of moisture is removed with the same pipet. The height of the drop left on the film must not exceed 1 mm and its diameter 1-2 mm. The Petri dish is then incubated at a suitable temperature for the required time. If it is desired to localize the position of a colony of microorganisms the film surface must be slightly dried. When growth of the bacteria has reached the desired stage (verified with the optical microscope), the selected area of agar together with the film is cut out with a pointed scalpel and the piece is transferred to a dish containing water. The film is easily separated from the agar and floats on the surface of the water. The film thus obtained is mounted on a grid.

Microorganisms can also be cultivated on a film in a liquid medium. In this case an empty Petri dish is filled with sterile distilled water on the surface of which a collodion film is made as described above. The water from under the film is removed with a pipet and replaced by liquid nutrient medium. A suspension of bacteria is applied to the film and they are incubated for a stipulated time. The nutrient medium is then twice replaced with distilled water to remove impurities left behind from the liquid nutrient medium from the under surface of the film. Selected areas of the film are mounted on grids.

A slightly modified method of cultivating microorganisms directly on a grid covered by a film was suggested by Pokotinskii and co-workers [34]. Pieces of filter paper or membrane ultrafilters are first boiled three times in distilled water to sterilize them. A drop of 1% collodion solution in amyl acetate is placed on the surface of sterile distilled water in a Petri dish. The grid is placed on the film thus formed and covered by the membrane ultrafilter or sterile filter paper. The edges of the film are curled over the ultrafilter which is then taken from the water with forceps. The ultrafilter with the grid covered by collodion film is placed on the surface of a solid nutrient medium in a Petri dish with the film above so that the filter is in firm contact with the agar surface. The filter with the grid and film is then dried in an incubator. A small drop of aqueous suspension of microorganisms or of a mixture of bacteria with phage is placed on the edge of the grid. After stipulated time intervals, during which either growth or lysis of the microorganisms takes place, the grid with the film is taken from the filter and dried. In this way the microorganisms on the surface of the film are completely isolated by the filter from contamination with nutrient medium. Nutrient substances, however, reach the microorganisms by diffusion from the agar through the filter and film. By means of this method microorganisms can be grown while maintaining their natural position on the film. A disadvantage of the method is that the supply of nutrient substances is considerably interfered with, so that some microorganisms sensitive to changes in conditions of nutrition develop very slowly or do not grow at all.

To study the process of phagolysis this method is best used in my modification [7]. A boiled ultrafilter or piece of sterile filter paper is placed on a collodion film formed on the surface of distilled water. The edges of the film are curled over the filter and the film together with the filter is taken from the surface of the water. The filter, covered by the film, is placed on solid nutrient medium with the film uppermost. Several filters covered by a film can be placed on the surface of agar in a single Petri dish. The film on the filter is dried and infected with a drop of a mixture of bacterial cells with phage, and this is carefully spread with a spatula over the surface of the film. After certain time intervals, depending on the experimental conditions, the filters are removed with forcepts from the agar surface, cut off at the edges with scissors, and placed in water. On the surface of the water the film readily separates from the filter or paper. A piece of film with easily distinguishable plaques formed by lysis of the bacteria by the phage is mounted on films.

The method of cultivation of microorganisms on films is very convenient for studying their development over a period of time and the process of phagolysis of bacteria.

CONTRASTING OF OBJECTS

To detect the structural details of biological objects during their examination in the electron microscope, methods of increasing contrast are of considerable importance.

Contrast is determined principally by two factors: the scattering power of the object and its thickness. The low scattering power of atoms composing biological objects (carbon, oxygen, hydrogen, nitrogen) does not give them adequate contrast, and the structural details of the objects are difficult to distinguish on a mounting film having almost the same ability to scatter electrons. The contrast of small biological objects such as viruses, phages, and biopolymers, which are of comparatively small thickness, is particularly low. This was one of the first difficulties encountered by investigators seeking to apply electron microscopy to biology, and their efforts were thus largely concentrated on finding methods for increasing contrast.

One of the first methods of contrasting to be used was that of, oblique shadowing of objects with a metal. This method, suggested in 1946 by Williams and Wyckoff [391], and called metallic shadow-casting is still used in electron microscopy. Contrast is achieved in this method by a difference in thickness of a film of metal covering the object. With oblique shadowing, areas of an object lying nearer to the source of metal dust are covered much less thickly than areas further away from the source and protected from it by the height of the object (for further details, see [7]).

By the use of this method the investigator can distinguish the shape and some details of the surface of the object examined; he can also form an idea of its height. However, the method of shadow-casting has several disadvantages which do not allow full use to be made of the high resolving power of modern microscopes. Granularity of the layer of metal dust reduces the possibility of distinguishing structural details of the object. In addition, the metal film may hide the internal, and sometimes external, structural details of the object examined. A further important disadvantage of this method is that, as a rule, it is used with objects dried in the air. Practical experience with electron microscopy has shown that biological objects, when dried in the air, undergo flattening, deformation, and even destruction by the action

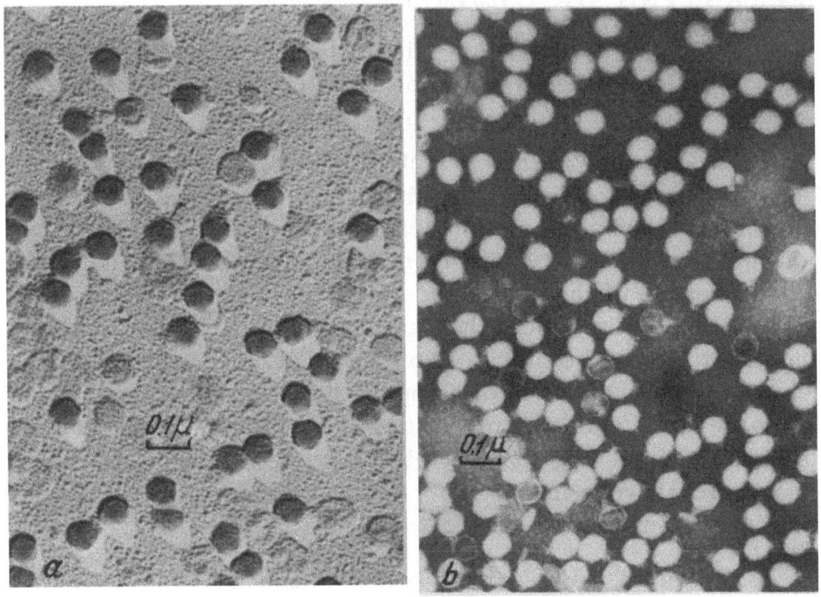

Fig. 5. Particles of phage s_d of *Escherichia coli* CK: a) shadowed with chromium; b) negative contrasting with PTA. 50,000×.

of forces of surface tension. For that reason, there is often the risk that distorted information is obtained regarding the shape, size, and structure of an object. For instance, the dimensions of phage particles obtained by the shadow-casting method are considerably greater than the dimensions of the same particles obtained by the use of negative contrasting [43].

Negative Contrasting

Nowadays another method of contrasting is widely used, enabling the finest details of the structure of small biological objects to be revealed. To increase contrast, various workers [162, 190, 215] have used solutions of salts of heavy metals as "filling" material in which the object is sealed. Light particles of the object to be examined are arranged against the dark background of the contrasting material, and its structural details can be clearly seen. This method came to be known as negative contrasting.

The most widely used method of negative contrasting is by means of an aqueous solution of phosphotungstic acid (PTA) [109]. An aqueous solution of uranyl acetate has also been used successfully for the same purpose [292].

The superiority of the negative contrasting method over the method of shadow-casting with metal becomes obvious when the structure of the same object is studied. For example, particles of phage s_d applied to collodion film as an aqueous suspension, and then dried on it and shadowed with metal, appear round without any projections (Fig. 5a). Particles of the same phage, applied to a collodion film mixed with PTA, are hexagonal in shape in cross section and a short projection can be clearly distinguished on them (Fig. 5b); being masked in the first case by the greatly flattened head, its mass is large in comparison to that of the projection.

The example given clearly demonstrates the superiority of the method of negative contrasting over that of shadow-casting with metal.

The principle of negative contrasting also favors the more reliable preservation of the shape and structure of an object, because, while it dries, the object is protected from the forces of surface tension by the material surrounding it.

Negative contrasting of preparations is carried out as follows: small drops of the purified phage preparations are placed on an electron-microscopic grid covered with collodion or carbon-collodion film. To the drop of phage suspension is added either a similar drop of 2% PTA solution in distilled water, with its pH adjusted to 7.2 with 1 *N* KOH or NaOH, or a drop of 2% aqueous solution of uranyl acetate (pH about 4.5). The excess of liquid is removed with filter paper and the preparation dried.

Optimal density of the film of contrast substance with the more electron-transparent object sealed in it provides an electron-microscopic picture of high resolution.

It must be remembered that negative contrasting with substances containing atoms of heavy metals in some cases leads to fragmentation of individual structures in biological objects examined. Different contrasting materials, moreover, destroy particular biological structures. For example, Huxley [216] observed that during negative contrasting of artificial myosin and actin fibers the PTA destroys the structure of the contractile fibers of muscles, whereas, if uranyl acetate is used they are completely preserved. I have also noted that during negative contrasting of phage No. 1 of *B. mycoides* with PTA (pH 7.2), more particles are found with an intact pale sheath than if uranyl acetate is used for contrasting. This distinction was not observed with phage T2.

It was originally thought that differences between the action of these agents depend on pH, because the pH of uranyl acetate solution is about 4.5, compared with 7.0–7.4 for PTA. However, the use of PTA at pH 4.5 causes greater destruction of the object than its use at neutral pH. This must be borne in mind when the choice of substance for contrasting is made in accordance with the purpose of the investigation.

Positive Contrasting

The salts of heavy metals can react specifically with certain biological substances. When they combine with certain substances the atoms and molecules of heavy metals accumulate at particular sites on the biological object, increasing the contrast of the corresponding structures. This property can be used as a specific "staining method" or to increase the contrast of low-contrast structures of a test object. For example, osmium reacts readily with lipids, while lanthanum nitrate and uranyl acetate combined with nucleic acids, and the salts of phosphotungstic and phosphomolybdic acids and lead salts react with the protein components of cells and viruses.

The increase in contrast of structures resulting from their interaction with salts of heavy metals brings about positive contrasting of the object, because, as a result of "staining," the structures become less permeable to electrons and appear dark against the light background of the preparation.

Positive contrasting of objects is carried out as follows: a drop of suspension of the purified object, either unfixed or preliminarily fixed with formalin, is placed on a grid with a collodion film, and a short time later it is washed either with water or with suspending solution. The grid with the object is then immersed in contrasting solution, then washed with distilled water and placed on filter paper to remove excess of liquid [217]. In preparations obtained in this way, the scattering power relative to electrons is increased because of the specific reaction between the solution containing atoms of heavy metals and a particular substance present in the object.

As contrasting substances producing negative and positive contrast, the following solutions (in distilled water) can be used: 1-2% phosphotungstic acid (pH 7-7.4); 2% osmic acid; 1-2% phosphomolybdic acid; 2% uranyl acetate or uranyl formate; 2% lanthanum nitrate; 0.59 *M* lead acetate.

Depending on the experimental conditions and the nature of the object, solutions with higher or lower pH values can be used.

By the use of negative and positive contrasting methods, the finest structural details of small biological objects can be detected. For example, it has been shown in this way that the protein sheath of virus particles is built up of small subunits arranged in a strict order.

Recent progress in the field of virus architectonics achieved by the use of new contrasting methods is obvious. However, it should not be forgotten that, despite their undoubted advantages over other methods of contrasting, these methods also have their disadvantages associated with possible distortion of the true structure of the object.

The problem of veracity of structures observed in the electron microscope is highly complex. In particular, care must be taken when the reality of structures is assessed by the use of a new method.

It is essential to know the effect of the contrasting substances used on the structure of biological objects.

The work of Sanyal and co-workers [327] has shown that salts of PTA, at different pH values, may interact with hemoglobin. Investigations showed that at pH values of the order of 5.0-7.0, the sedimentation coefficient is increased while the optical absorption falls sharply. At pH 7.0-9.0, this interaction is less marked, but the molecules have an increased tendency toward aggregation. These workers postulate that the changes observed can be due either to a change in the architectonics of the hemoglobin molecule itself or to the formation of a selective bond with macroions.

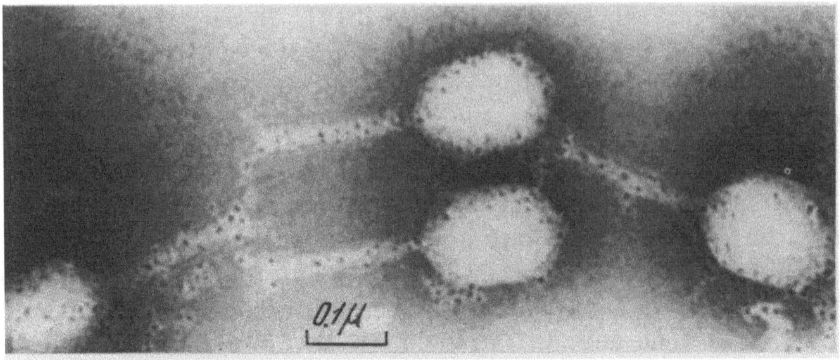

Fig. 6. Phage T2 of *Escherichia coli* B treated with 2% $HgCl_2$ solution. PTA, 100,000×.

Despite these warnings, it can be claimed that the use of this power of atoms of heavy metals to react with certain biological structures is potentially extremely valuable for the development of new electron-microscopic methods of investigation.

An attempt to use mercury salts ($HgCl_2$) as a contrasting agent showed that mercury atoms or molecules form stable bonds with certain protein groups of phage T2 of *E. coli* B (Fig. 6) and phage No. 1 of *B. mycoides* [46]. The mercury molecules then appear as dots, impervious to electrons, lying on the surface of the protein membrane of the head and tail of the phage particles, not disappearing after repeated washing with water. This fact indicates that salts of the heavy metals can be used for detecting the specific localization of particular chemical groups in biological objects.

As a result of recent improvements in the method of preparation of specimens for electron microscopy it has thus become possible to take advantage of the high resolution of modern instruments and to investigate the detailed macromolecular organization of biological structures.

METHODS OF FIXATION OF BACTERIA FOR PREPARATION OF ULTRATHIN SECTIONS

To study the structure of biological tissues and cells in ultrathin sections, it is first necessary to fix and dehydrate the preparation before it can be embedded in special media which are insoluble in water, and solidify after polymerization.

Particular types of plant and animal tissue require specific fixation depending on the density of the tissue, its water content, the degree of permeability of its cell membranes, etc.

The most suitable method for studying the fine structure of bacteria in ultrathin sections is that developed by Ryter, Kellenberger, and co-workers [322]. This method allows adequate preservation of the cell structure and, what is particularly important, of the fine structure of the strongly hydrated nucleoid of bacteria, which is easily injured during fixation by the usual methods developed for other biological objects [126, 141, 266, 294, 343].

For fixing bacterial cells by the method of Ryter and co-workers [322], the following standard solution is prepared: sodium acetate, 19.428 g; veronal sodium, 29.428 g; sodium chloride, 34 g; distilled water, 1 liter.

To 5 ml of the solution thus prepared, 7 ml 0.1-N HCl, 13 ml of distilled water, and 0.25 ml 1 *M* $CaCl_2$ solution (pH of buffer 6.0) are added. The fixing agent is 1% OsO_4 in acetate — veronal buffer, pH 6.0.

The first step to be carried out is preliminary fixation. To a culture of bacteria in a liquid medium (one part) a 0.5-1% solution of OsO_4 in acetate — veronal buffer, pH 6, is added (10 parts), after which the suspension is centrifuged for 5 min at 4000 rpm. The main fixation is then carried out. The residue is suspended in 0.1 ml of nutrient medium, 1 ml of 1-3% OsO_4 in acetate — veronal buffer with 10% tryptone is added, and the mixture is allowed to stand overnight at room temperature. This small volume of mixture is then diluted with 8-10 ml buffer and centrifuged for 4 min at 4000 rpm. The residue is then mixed with 0.03 ml 2% agar, well mixed, and a drop is applied to a slide at 45°C. The solidified drop is cut into small cubes (1 mm^3) and treated with 0.5% uranyl acetate in buffer for 1-2 h. Dehydration is carried out in a series of alcohols or acetone, followed by embedding either in methacrylates or in Vestopal.

However, fixation by this method [322] has proved to be unsuitable for some species of bacteria. For example, after treatment by this method, cells of *B. mycoides* became distorted, their cytoplasm was compressed, and their cell wall partially destroyed.

To obtain reproducible results and to preserve the fine structure of bacterial cells of different species, whether normal or infected with phage, in ultrathin sections, the author and Bespalova [54] modified and simplified Ryter's method as follows. At definite time intervals, bacteria grown in liquid nutrient medium and infected with phage were fixed with 0.1% osmium in acetate — veronal buffer, pH 6.0, and immediately centrifuged at 5000 rpm for 20 min. The residue was suspended in 0.1 ml of nutrient broth, 1 ml of 1% osmium in acetate — veronal buffer was added to the suspension, and the mixture was left overnight at room temperature. The fixed suspension was then diluted 1:10 with acetate — veronal buffer and centrifuged at 5000 rpm for 20 min. A 2% solution of agar, melted and cooled to 40°C, was added to the residue, mixed well, and poured on a slide in a thin layer. The solidified agar was cut into small pieces (2 × 2 mm), transferred quickly into 3% uranyl acetate solution in 30°C ethanol, and allowed to stand for 2 h. By transferring the material fixed in osmium into 3% uranyl acetate quickly, when the process of dehydration was just beginning, it was possible to prevent destruction of the structural elements of the cell, especially its nucleoid. If the uranyl acetate was added in 70°C alcohol, the nucleoid of the bacterial cell was destroyed.

The pieces of agar with bacterial cells embedded in them were taken from the 30°C alcohol with uranyl acetate through a series of alcohols as follows: 15 min in 50°C ethanol, 1 h in 75°C ethanol, 15 min in 96°C, 30 min in 100°C (twice), 30 min in 100°C ethanol + butyl-methacrylate (1:1) and 1 h in butyl- + methylmethacrylate (4:1). The dehydrated material was placed in gelatin capsules, into which a mixture of butyl- and methyl-methacrylates (4:1) with the addition of 0.5% benzoyl peroxide was poured. Polymerization took place at 60°C for 24 h.

In sections of bacteria prepared by this method, the fine structural details of all elements of the bacterial cell are well preserved. The photomicrographs illustrating this book were produced with a JEM-5Y electron microscope (voltage 80 kV).

TERMINOLOGY

The use of electron microscopes with high resolving power and recently introduced improvements in methods of preparing specimens for electron microscopy have led to the discovery of the fine organization of viruses, and this has led, in turn, to the need for a special terminology to describe their structural components.

Lwoff and co-workers [267] proposed the terms "capsid" and "capsomeres" to describe the protein membrane of viruses and the units composing it, and the term "virion" to describe the infective particle as a whole, i.e., the capsid filled with nucleic acid. However, this terminology is more appropriate for simply organized virus particles and is difficult to apply to complex viruses.

Caspar and co-workers [125] later proposed a number of amendments to the terminology, as follows: 1) the virion is regarded as the infective virus particle; 2) the capsid, as before, is the name given to the symmetrical protein membrane of the virus; 3) the capsid, together with the nucleic acid contained in it, is described as the nucleocapsid; if the particle has no other elements this term can apply to the infective virus particle or virion (in myxoviruses the nucleocapsid is further enclosed in a common envelope); 4) capsomeres are morphological units distinguishable in the electron microscope on the surface of the capsid of many viruses; 5) particles forming individual capsomeres are described as structural units.

Advances in the interpretation of the macromolecular structure of bacteriophages have made it necessary to introduce order into the terminology used to describe structural components of the phage particle in accordance with that proposed by Caspar and his collaborators [125] for the viruses of plants and animals. The need for a more precise terminology is due to the fact that most phages, unlike viruses of animals and plants, possess a tail in addition to the head, and a precise terminology is also required for the structural components of the tail. Up to the present, in the scientific literature, different terms have frequently been used to describe the same structural components of the phage particle, for example: the tail, the tail process, or the process.

With these considerations in mind, I propose the following names for the structural components of bacteriophages:

1. The infectious phage particle is to be called the virion, or phage particle.

2. The main parts of the phage to be called the head and tail.

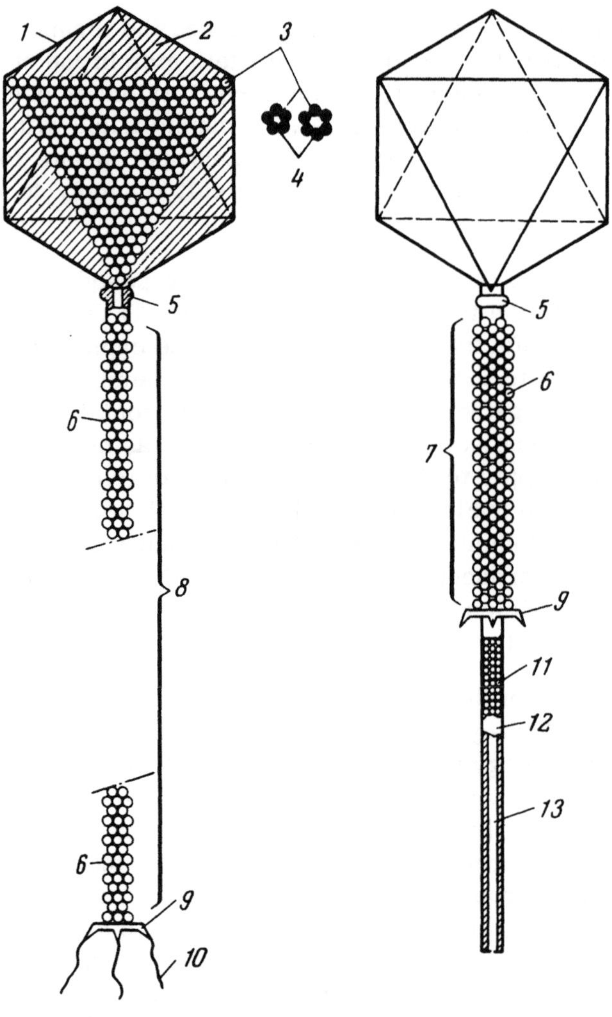

Fig. 7. Diagram of the phage particle with names of individual structural elements: 1) capsid; 2) nucleic acid; 3) capsomeres; 4) structural units of the capsomere; 5) collar; 6) morphological subunits of the sheath; 7) contracted sheath; 8) stretched sheath; 9) end plate; 10) tail fibers; 11) morphological subunits of the rod; 12) rod; 13) rod canal.

3. The phage particle without its nucleic acid, but preserving all other structural elements, to be called the protein envelope or "ghost."

4. The protein membrane of the head to be called the capsid.

5. The morphological subunits of the capsid distinguishable in the electron microscope to be called capsomeres.

6. The structural elements of the tail to be called the outer sheath, or simply the sheath; the inner rod, or simply the rod; the terminal structure of the tail to be called the end plate; the thin fibrils attached to the end plate to be called tail fibers.

7. The separate morphological units of the sheath, distinguishable in the electron microscope, to be called morphological subunits of the sheath.

8. Separate morphological units of the rod distinguishable in the electron microscope to be called morphological subunits of the rod.

9. Protein molecules or groups of them composing the capsomeres of the capsid or morphological subunits of the sheath and rod to be called structural units.

A diagram of the phage particle and its structural elements is given in Fig. 7.

Chapter 2

Classification of Phages Based on Morphological Characteristics

The classification of bacteriophages at the present time is in a most unsatisfactory state for a variety of reasons, the most important being the absence of a single taxonomic criterion.

In the course of studying the bacteriophages, many attempts have been made to classify them on the basis of various characteristics.

Holmes [210] proposed using the binomial system of Linnaeus in order to identify viruses for this purpose. The use of this system, however, implies the existence of adequate criteria for defining the categories of genus and species among the phages. Since no such criteria have yet been found for the phages, workers describing them for the first time have continued to give them highly arbitrary names.

Takahashi [353] proposed a special nomenclature to describe the phages of *Bacillus subtilis*, but no similar nomenclature has been worked out for the other phages.

It would seem to be the best solution to name the phages on the basis of their connection with the particular species of microorganism which they infect. This principle was used by many workers when drawing up their various classifications. However, not even this principle can provide the necessary accuracy, because it is now known that one strain of phage may have a broad lysogenic spectrum, infecting different species of microorganisms.

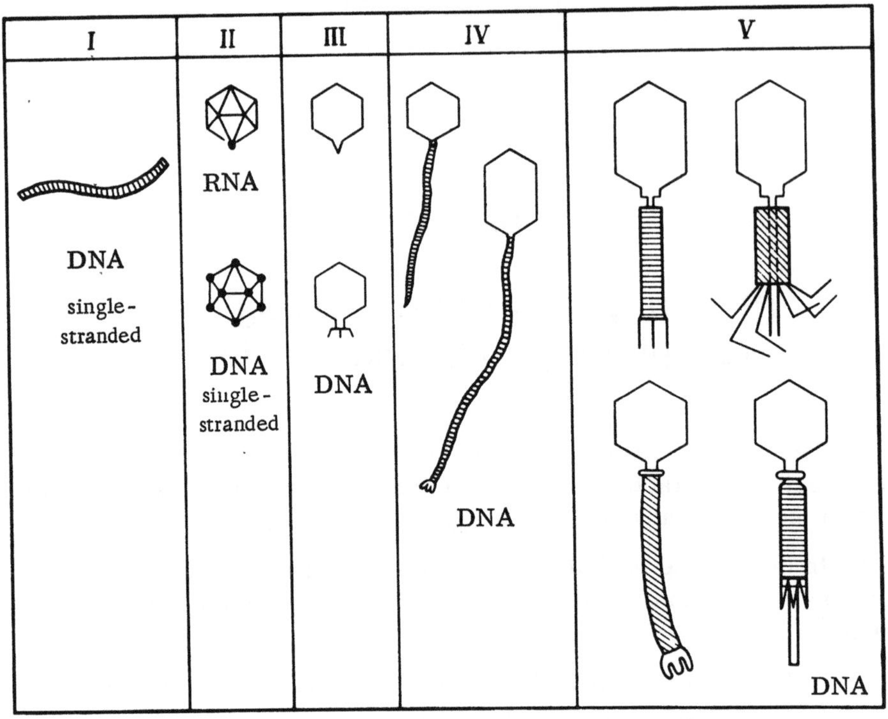

Fig. 8. Scheme illustrating members of different groups of phages.

The same bacterial strain can also be infected by many phages, differing from each other in many of their properties, including morphology, whereas some phages which are active against different species or even genera of microorganisms may appear identical in their morphology. Furthermore, cases have been described when even a mutant differs sharply from the original phage both serologically and morphologically [394]. Usually, mutants are morphologically identical.

Attempts have also been made to classify phages on the basis of a sum of several different characteristics (antigenic, physiological, biochemical, and physicochemical properties, morphology of plaques, spectrum of lysogenic action, etc.). However, all these attempts have so far proved unsuccessful.

I do not propose to dwell at great length on this question in this book, because the classification of phages in accordance with the principles mentioned above, as drawn up by various investigators, has been described adequately in the monographs by Adams [1] and Gol'dfarb [11]. In my opinion, the reason for the failure of all attempts to find a satisfactory classification of phages is that in general, investigations into the nature of viruses and, in particular, into the phylogenetic connection between various groups of phages, between phages and other viruses, and also between phages and the cells acting as their hosts, are still incomplete.

With the development of electron microscopy it became possible to classify phages on the basis of their morphology.

In 1960, Bradley and Kay [108], after studying the morphology and structural properties of 22 different types of phages, subdivided them into three groups on the basis of their tail morphology: 1) phages with a short tail; 2) with a noncontracting tail; and, 3) with a contracting tail.

Later, Almeida [75] suggested more general principles of classification associated with the type of symmetry to which the individual phages conform (cubical or mixed), and the type of nucleic acid contained in them.

Bradley [104], in 1965, proposed dividing the phages into 6 morphological groups: 1) phages with a tail possessing a contractile sheath; 2) phages with a long, noncontracting tail; 3) phages with a short tail; 4) phages with no tail and with large capsomeres; 5) phages with no tail and with small capsomeres; 6) filamentous phages.

However, the view has been expressed that the large capsomeres in phages of group 4 (phages of type ϕX 174) perform the function of a tail; in turn, the "spherical" phages of group 5 (RNA-containing phages), in my opinion, also have a structure which is analogous to the tail. On these grounds I should prefer to combine Bradley's phage groups 4 and 5 into a single group.

It will be realized that morphological criteria do not exhaust all the properties of phages, nor can they provide the means for constructing a precise and universal classification.

Although not claiming that the classification of phages on the basis of their morphology is perfectly satisfactory, I consider that for convenience in describing a wide variety of forms of phages it is logical to divide them into five main morphological groups, based largely on Bradley's classification: (I) filamentous phages; (II) phages with analogs of a tail; (III) phages with a short tail; (IV) phages with a long and noncontractile tail; and, (V) phages with a tail of complex structure with a contractile sheath. Examples of phages belonging to these different groups are illustrated schematically in Fig. 8. As this figure shows, phages vary widely in their morphology. No such variation in morphology is found among the viruses of animals and plants.

All animal viruses presently known are usually polyhedral (polyoma virus adenovirus, poliovirus, etc.) or complex in shape, and at first glance are without any orderly structure. However, the internal components of these viruses possess a definite structure conforming to a helical type of symmetry (the group of myxoviruses). Viruses of plants are either polyhedral (cubical type of symmetry) or cylindrical, composed of tightly packed turns of a helix (helical type of symmetry). The orderly structure of viruses thus conforms to a definite type of symmetry.

So far as the phages are concerned, they include forms with both helical (filamentous phages) and cubical types of symmetry (phages without a well-developed tail). However, many, perhaps the great majority, of the phages which have now been studied combine both types of symmetry in the same particle: cubical in the head and helical in the tail.

The strict orderliness of the morphology of the viruses is determined by the properties of the homogeneous structural units from which their protein envelopes are built.

The simplest shapes, in the form of a tetrahedron, octahedron, and icosahedron, belong to the cubical types of symmetry.

The commonest shape for the head of bacteriophages is an icosahedron (a 20-sided figure with axes of symmetry 5 : 3 : 2), but less frequently they are octahedral in shape (an 8-sided figure with axes of symmetry 4 : 3 : 2). Viruses of tetrahedral shape have not yet been described, and in all probability this type, which would be the least rational for viruses, does not exist.

Since the principles governing symmetry of viruses, including phages, have been fully described elsewhere [9, 19, 124, 212, 244], there is no need to consider this matter further here.

Chapter 3

Filamentous Phages and Phages with Tail Analogs

FILAMENTOUS PHAGES (GROUP I)

The first group includes a number of recently discovered phages which are threadlike in shape. The dimensions of the virion of the various phages of this group are given in Table 1.

Filamentous phages were first discovered in association with bacteria of the enteric group, and were shown to be active only against male forms of these bacteria.

The first to be described was filamentous phage fd, specific in relation to *E. coli* [273, 274]. Later other filamentous phages of the enteric group were studied: f1 [121, 396], M13 [209], ZJ/2 [103], Ec9 [150], and AE2 [295].

Table 1. Dimensions of Virion of Filamentous Phages

Phage	Length, Å	Width, Å	Species of host	Literature
M13	8000	80	*E. coli*	[207]
M13	8000	—	"	[324]
fd	7000	50	"	[273]
fd	7600	50	"	[274]
f1	8500	43—63	"	[396]
f1	8500	60—70	"	[121]
ZJ/2	8300	68	"	[103]
AE2	8000	50	"	[295]
Pf	—	—	*P. aeruginosa*	[355]

Recently, Takeya and Amako [355] have described filamentous phage Pf, which in its morphology and size is similar to the filamentous coliphages, but produces lysis of cells of *Pseudomonas aeruginosa*.

The distinctive shape of the phages of this group (Fig. 9) allies them with the rod-shaped plant viruses. In contrast to the latter, the filamentous phages contain DNA instead of RNA, but their DNA is single-stranded.

According to some investigators [203, 273], the virion of phage fd contains 11.6-12.2% of DNA, the molecular weight of which is $1.37 \cdot 10^6$. According to Zinder and co-workers [396], the DNA content of phage f1 is 11%.

Phage Pf, active against *P. aeruginosa*, also contains single-stranded DNA which constitutes 12% of the virion [355].

Filamentous phages producing lysis of *E. coli* cells are very resistant to heat and other mechanical agents, and also to the action of trypsin and deoxyribonuclease (DNase) [103, 324]. Filamentous phage Pf is resistant to DNase but sensitive to the proteolytic enzyme nagarase and to ultrasound [355].

The capsid of the filamentous phages is constructed from separate capsomeres and conforms to a helical type of symmetry.

X-ray diffraction studies have shown that the capsid of this phage is an α-helix with a turn measuring 56-60 Å and a spacing of 32.2 Å between turns. Each turn contains 6 subunits [273, 275]. Day [148] also considers that the capsid of phage fd is formed by a right-handed α-helix.

Cross striation of the capsid has also been discovered in another filamentous phage ZJ/2 with a period of 20-30 Å, and this also indicates that it is helical in structure [103].

According to Marvin [275, 276], the DNA of phage fd is circular in structure. Within the capsid the DNA ring is twisted into a double helix.

The DNA molecule in phage M13 has also been found to be circular, and its length is $2.19 \pm 0.07\ \mu$ [312].

The distinctive shape of the phages of group I naturally suggest that the mechanism of their interaction with the host cell must

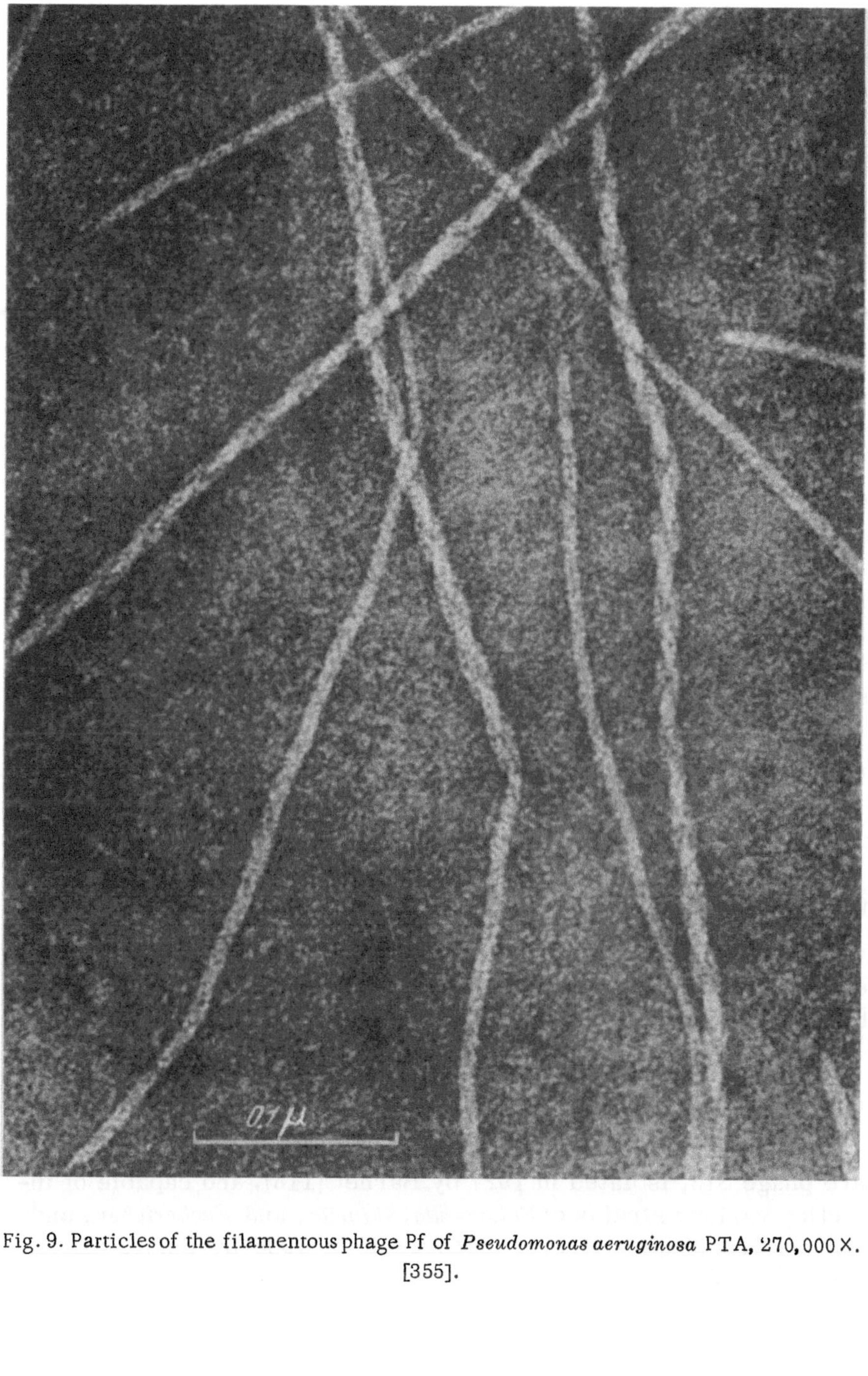

Fig. 9. Particles of the filamentous phage Pf of *Pseudomonas aeruginosa* PTA, 270,000×. [355].

also differ from the mechanism of interaction of phages of different morphology. However, the mode of infection of bacteria by these phages and of their reproduction in the cell is not yet sufficiently clear.

Tzagaloff and Pratt [367] found that on the surface of the host cell there are only a very few places where phage M13 can be adsorbed. The investigations of Caro and Schnös [121] shed some light on the mechanism of interaction between filamentous phages and the cell. They showed that filamentous phage f1 is adsorbed specifically on the pili of male strains of *E. coli*, which are rigid threadlike outgrowths of the cell of different lengths and about 80 Å in diameter. Adsorption of filamentous phages takes place only at the end of the pili, where there are two or more receptor sites. Only one end of the filamentous phage is attached to the pili.

The first investigations showed that filamentous phages do not produce lysis of the cells, and this distinguishes them essentially from other phages. Filamentous phages are liberated from bacteria without destroying them. The bacteria continue to reproduce, liberating fresh phage particles [204, 205, 209, 295]. According to Hoffmann-Berling and co-workers [204], nonlytic infection of this type leads to unstable lysogenization or to a phage carrier state.

PHAGES WITH TAIL ANALOGS (GROUP II)

This group includes small phages with no clearly differentiated tail such as is characteristic of most phages.

It is generally considered that these phages have no tail whatever, but their particles do possess a structure which in all probability is analogous to a tail.

Some phages in this group contain RNA, but others contain DNA, although the DNA is single-stranded.

Typical members of the DNA-containing phages of group II are phage S13, isolated in 1927 by Barnet [116], and capable of infecting various strains of *Salmonella*, *Shigella*, and *Escherichia* , and the related phage ϕX 174, discovered in 1935 by Sertic and Boulgakov [339].

Phages containing RNA were first described for *E. coli*: f2 [262, 263], MS2 [142], R17 [297], fr [273, 274], μ2 [301, 302], M12 [207], ZJK/1, ZJ/1, and ZG/1 [103].

RNA-containing phages were subsequently found also for bacteria of the genus *Pseudomonas*: 7S [165, 166], PP7 [104], and for the stalked bacteria of the genus *Caulobacter*: phages ϕCb23r, ϕCb12r, and ϕCb8r [331].

A characteristic feature of the RNA phages is their specificity for male strains of bacteria.

Both the RNA phages and phages containing single-stranded DNA are icosahedral in shape. However, they differ from each other in certain structural details.

Phages of type ϕX 174 containing single-stranded DNA have a thickening at each apex of the icosahedron which is possibly the analog of a tail. Kay [226], who studied the structure of phage ϕR, similar in its morphology to phage ϕX 174, concluded that only one of these thickenings possesses adsorptive properties and thus performs the function of the tail.

Most workers consider that the RNA phages are particles of icosahedral shape without thickenings on their apices and without a tail. However, the absence of a tail on RNA-containing phages in my opinion is doubtful, as I shall discuss more fully below.

DNA- and RNA-containing phages of this group isolated by different investigators from different habitats are strikingly homogeneous both in the size and in the morphology of their particles.

The molecular weight of RNA isolated from one particle of phage f2 is $1.8 \cdot 10^6$ Dalton [263], compared with $1.1 \cdot 10^6$ for phage MS2 [351], $1.3 \cdot 10^6$ [160] and $1.1 \cdot 10^6$ [170] for phage R17. The single-stranded DNA contained in the particle of phage ϕX 174 [342] and in the morphologically similar phage 1ϕ7 [69] is approximately the same ($1.7 \cdot 10^6$).

The nucleic acid content in these phages is thus 80 times less than in the particle of phage T2, containing double-stranded DNA and a virion of complex structure. The particle of phage T2 (group V) is also much larger in size than the virions of these phages. It is interesting to note in this connection that the phages which I have grouped together on the basis of what is apparently a very formal characteristic, namely the absence of a clearly differentiated tail, exhibit a number of common features: small particle size varying between 230 and 300 Å (Table 2), and a roughly equal and comparatively small content of nucleic acid. In all probability, these two characteristics are interconnected because the small amount of nucleic acid contained in these phages can provide information for building particles with a comparatively simple structural organization.

Virion Structure of RNA-Containing Phages

As Table 2 shows, all RNA-phages which have been studied are highly constant in size. The slight variations in size described by different workers can evidently be attributed to errors of measurement, which are, unfortunately, still unavoidable in electron microscopy.

The particle of these phages is an icosahedron with a hexagonal plane surface. When present in large numbers, they frequently show a tendency to pack closely together, forming small clusters or paracrystals (Fig. 10).

Despite the small size of the virion, the capsid of the RNA phages is built of readily distinguishable capsomeres. Capsomers measuring 45-50 Å have been found in phages ZJK/1, ZJ/1, ZG/1 [103] and in phage $\mu 2$ [301, 302].

In my own studies of the fine structure of RNA phages MS2, f2, B6, and B7, I also found that their capsids are composed of separate capsomeres about 50 Å in diameter (Fig. 11a, b; Fig. 12).

It is generally accepted that the RNA phages do not possess a tail. However, on some particles of phages MS2, f2, B6, and B7, I was able to distinguish a very short tail [49, 56, 362], projecting from one apex of the icosahedron and attaining a length of 60-70 Å and a width of about 50 Å (Fig. 11a, b, c; Fig. 12). This tail is very small and the details of its structure have not yet been distinguished. There are two reasons for the difficulty in detecting the tail on particles of these phages: 1) the small tail may easily be hidden by the relatively massive head of the phage; 2) particles of RNA phages are rarely seen separately.

Table 2. Dimensions of the Virion of Group II Phages

Phage	Size of head, Å	Species of host	Literature citation
		RNA containing	
MS2*	250	*E. coli* K-12 (F^+, Hfr)	[56, 362]
f2, fr, B6, B7†	250	"	[49]
MS2	250	"	[142]
f2	—	"	[263]
R17	like f2	"	[297]
fr	200—220	"	[273]
M12	270	"	[207]
μ2	240	"	[301, 302]
Zj/1	225	*E. coli* C (3000F^+)	[103]
ZJK/1	225	"	[103]
ZG/1	225	"	[103]
7s	250	*Pseudomonas aeruginosa*	[165, 166]
PP7	—	"	[104]
φCb23, φCb8, φCb12	210—230	Caulobacter	[331]
		DNA containing ‡	
φX174	248±10	*E. coli* C	[342]
φX174	243—252	"	[191, 270]
φΦ174	225	"	[366]
φX174	250	"	[49]
φR	300±30	"	[99, 227]
α3, α10, δ1, ζ3, η8, 06, WA/1, WF/1	230—250	*E. coli* C2	[100]
M20	300	*E. coli* C	[207]
S13	256 (233)	"	[270]
1φ1, 1φ3, 1φ7, 1φ9, dφ4, dφ5, dφ3	250±10	"	[18]

* Obtained from A. Clarke (University of California, USA).

† Obtained from I. Schindler (Prague).

‡ All virions have a thickening on apices of the head and single-stranded DNA.

In unpurified lysates the RNA phages are mainly found adsorbed on bacterial pili [27, 154]. They adhere to the pili in clusters, indicating their high affinity for these bacterial structures (Fig. 11a, b, c; Fig. 12).

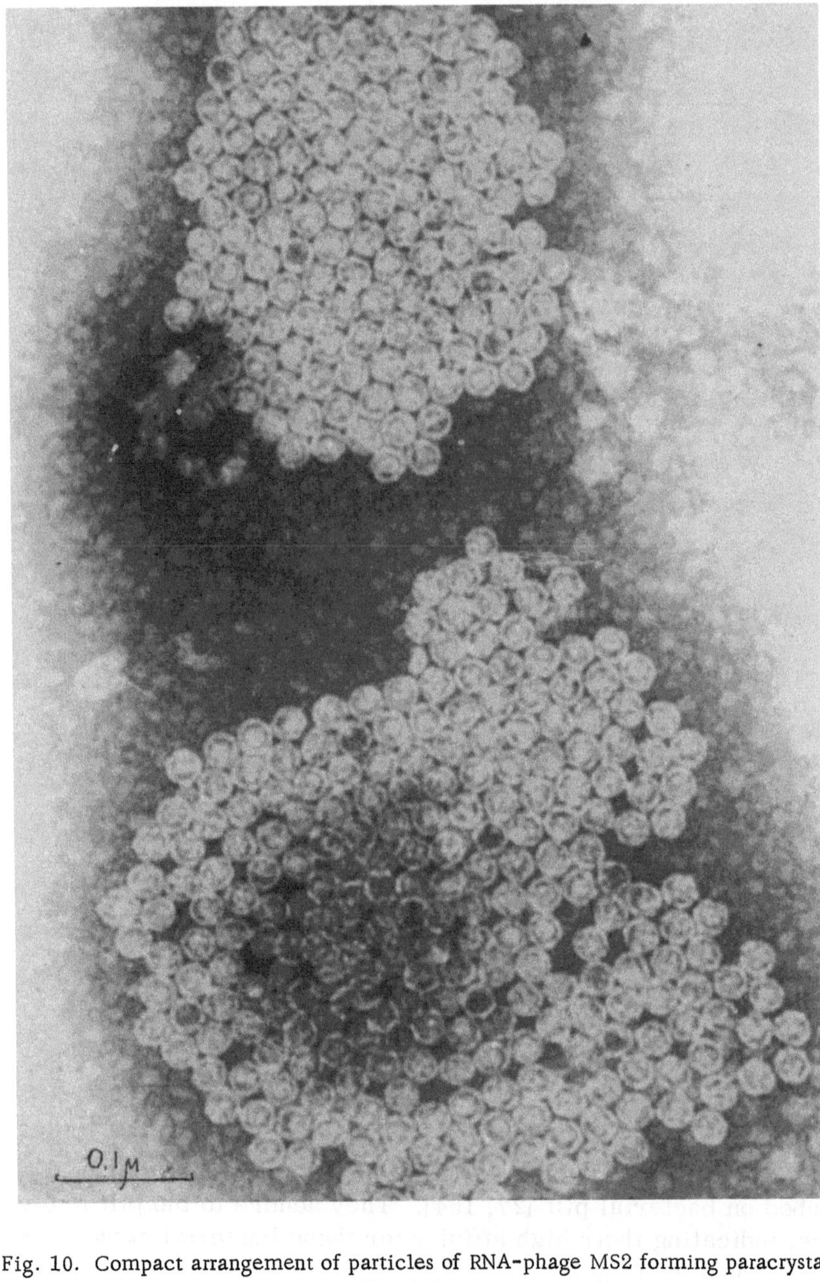

Fig. 10. Compact arrangement of particles of RNA-phage MS2 forming paracrystals. PTA. 180,000×.

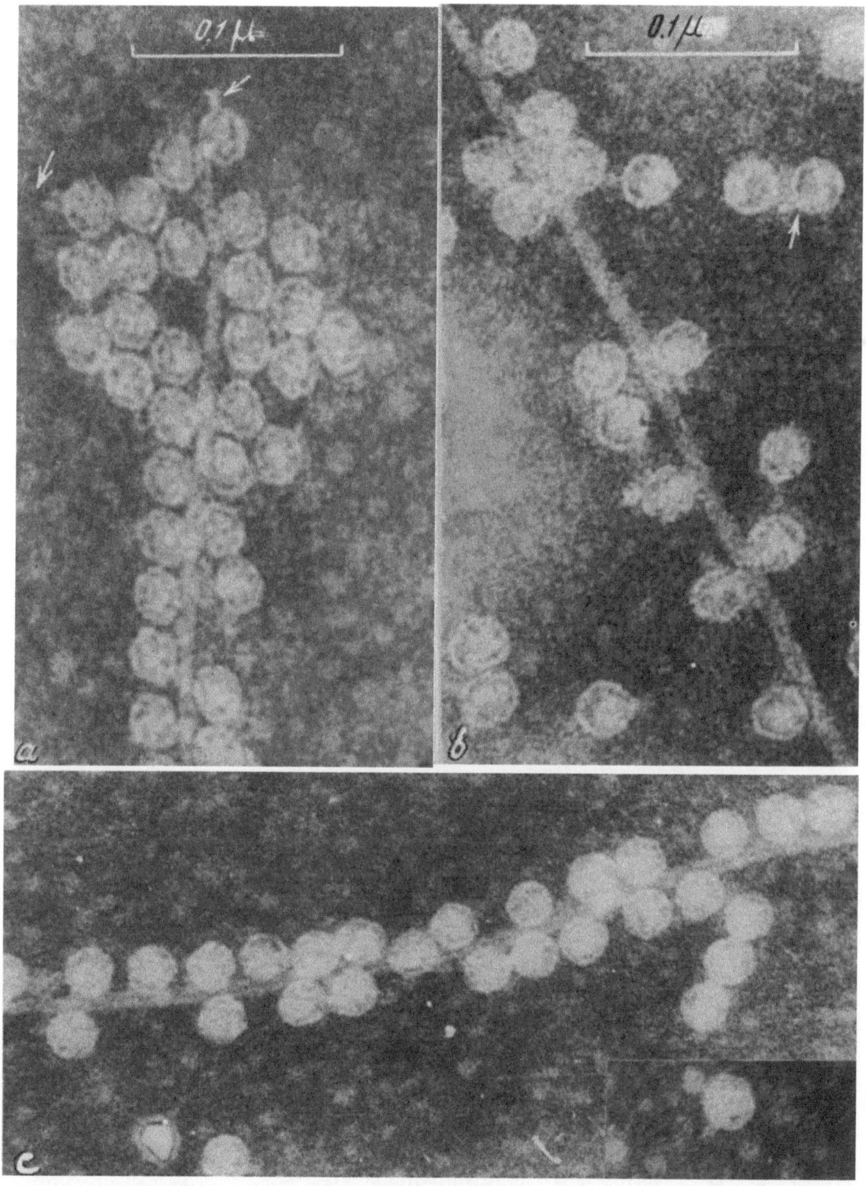

Fig. 11. Particles of RNA-phages with short tail (indicated by arrows). PTA. a) MS2, 280,000×; b) B7, 280,000×; c) f2, 250,000×.

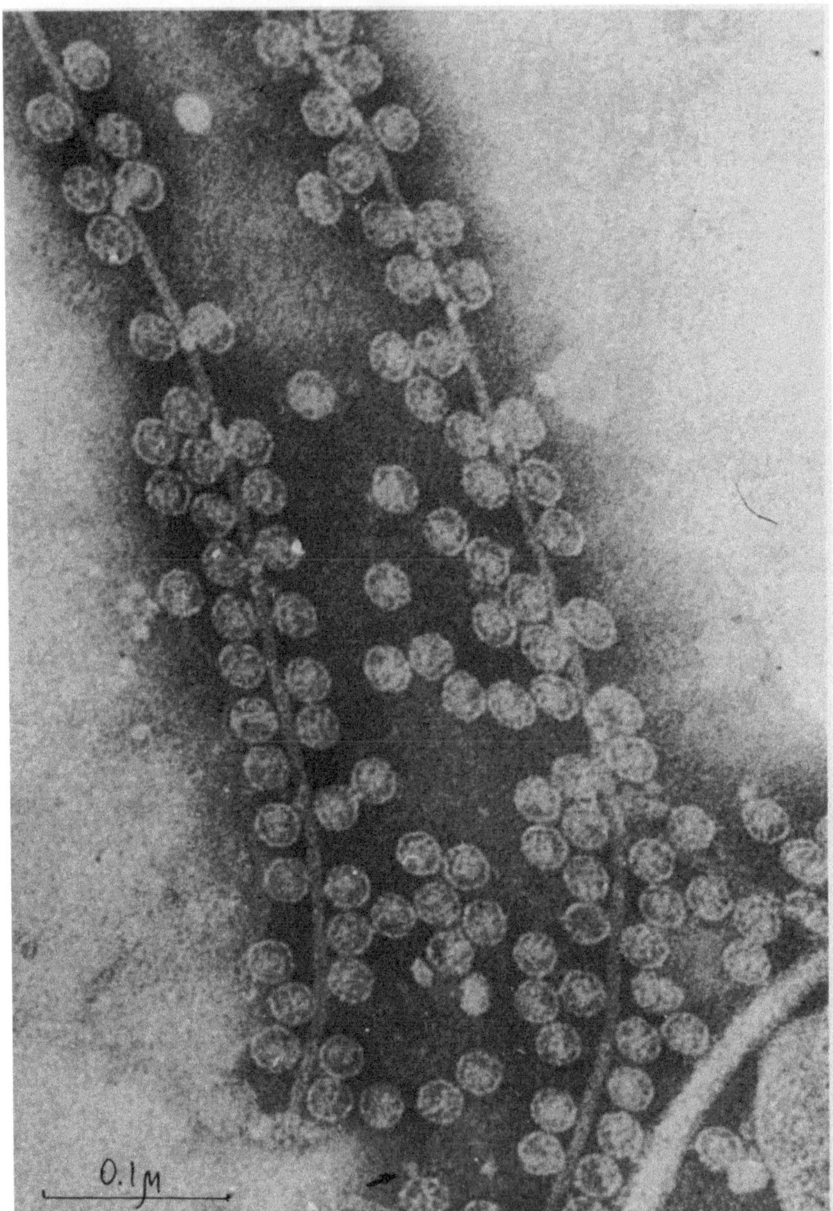

Fig. 12. Particles of RNA-phage B6 adsorbed on fimbriae. Capsomeres of capsid can be distinguished. PTA. 250,000×.

I consider that the particles are attached to the pili by means of the short tail, which cannot be clearly distinguished in this case. However, photographs show that individual phage particles in fact lie a short distance away from the pili, and yet are connected to them, which may serve as evidence in support of the existence of a short tail on RNA phage particles.

However, the possibility cannot yet be ruled out that the structure of the very short tail can be simulated by particles accidentally adherent to the phage head, although the constant size of the structures observed would seem to be evidence against this suggestion.

Reproduction of RNA-Containing Phages in the Bacterial Cell

Phages containing ribonucleic acid are the subject of intensive research at the present time. One feature which distinguishes these phages is that they have a very high average burst size, of the order of several thousands [142, 263, 302].

Because of their importance as a convenient model for studying interactions, between RNA-containing viruses of animals and plants and the host cell, the RNA phages are of considerable interest in relation to the study of several problems in molecular biology, notably the investigation of the simplest mechanism of transmission of the genetic code directly from RNA to protein. As Davis and co-workers [142] and Nathaus and co-workers [290] point out, in the RNA phages all genetic information is contained in the RNA, and the DNA of the cell plays no part in the formation of mature phage particles [151, 152]. The RNA injected by the phage into the infected cell thus plays the role simultaneously of the template for duplication of the phage genome and of the carrier of the program for synthesis of early phage proteins (RNA-synthetase) [385, 386] and capsid proteins of the phage virion [290].

Cooper and Zinder [131] also showed that reproduction of RNA phages, in contrast to virulent DNA phages, does not affect the synthesis of cell DNA and is not disturbed even if this synthesis is completely suppressed. It can thus be postulated that during reproduction of RNA phages the nuclear apparatus of the bacterial cell is not involved in the disintegration process, as happens in infection by virulent DNA-containing T-even phages attacking *E. coli* B [233] or phage No. 1 of *B. mycoides* [361]. Replication of the RNA phages apparently takes place entirely in the cytoplasm, independently of the cell nucleoid. These results have been confirmed by the electron-microscopic study of cells of a male strain of *E. coli* infected with phage MS2 [56, 362].

The use of negative contrasting showed that cells infected with phage contain an enormous number of phage particles. Most of these particles lie at the periphery of the cell, i.e., where the cytoplasm used to be. During formation of the phage particles, the bacterial cell becomes more transparent to electrons. The cytoplasmic membrane and a central portion free from phage particles can be distinguished in the cell. The latter, in all probability, is the nucleoid, whose fine structure is masked by the cell membranes (Fig. 13).

A more complete picture of the intracellular localization of phage was obtained from sections of bacteria infected with phage MS2. In sections made from cells infected with phage it can be seen that the phage particles are adsorbed not only on the pili, but also directly onto the cell wall (Fig. 14; Fig. 15a, b). Possibly, adsorption of virions of the RNA phage on the cell membrane is nonspecific. A more probable explanation, however, is that the RNA phages utilize the receptor apparatus on the pili of the bacterial cell and infect the cell through them, because RNA-containing viruses are mainly found adsorbed on these cell structures. This is confirmed by the work of Crawford and Gesteland [133], who showed that another RNA phage (R17) is specifically adsorbed on the pili of male strains and is not adsorbed on female cells. From this they concluded that RNA-containing phages transmit the infective principle to the infected cell through the pili.

Valentine and co-workers [370] later showed that RNA-containing phage f2 could not be adsorbed on cells not possessing pili. These workers also claim that pili, which are hollow in structure, participate in the transportation of infectious RNA from phage to cell. Valentine and Strand [369] also found that calcium ions are essential for the formation of the complex between the RNA phage and F-pili of F^+ bacteria, and also for adsorption of many other phages onto the bacterial cell wall. Paranchych [296] showed that bivalent ions have an influence on the introduction of phage RNA into the cell.

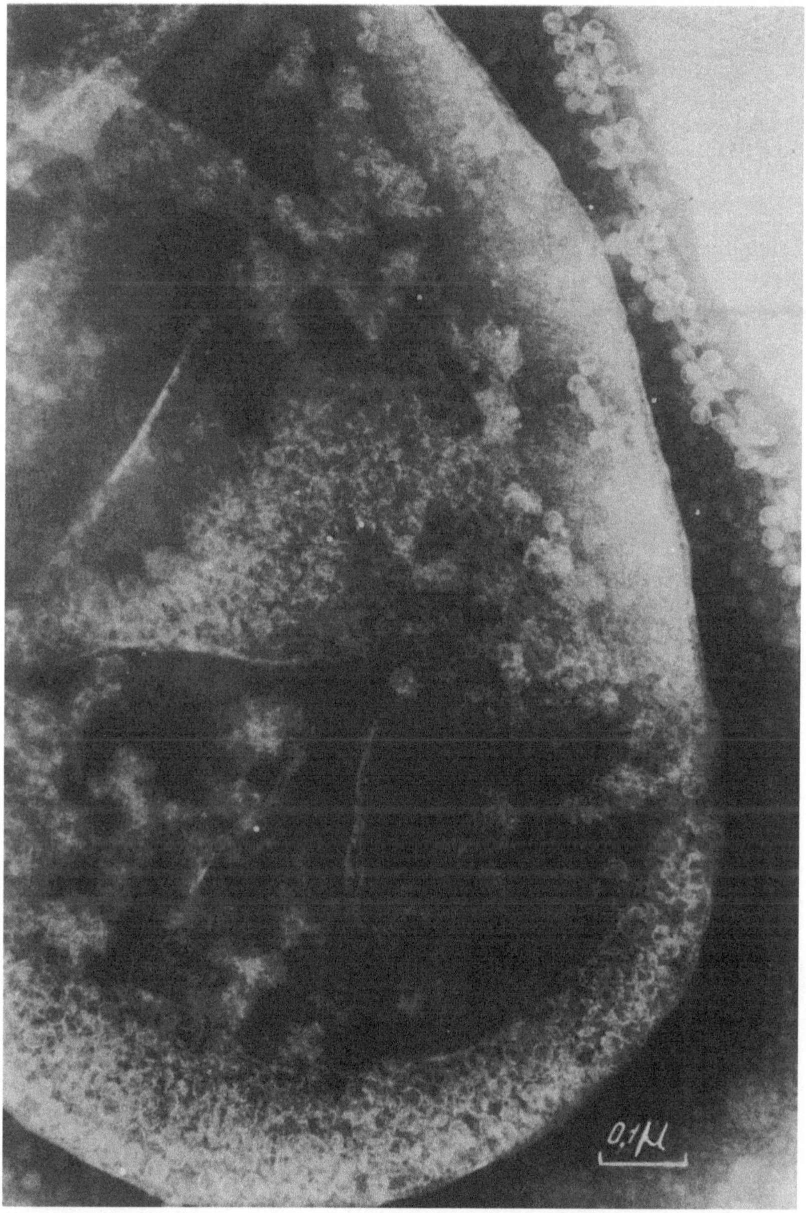

Fig. 13. Bacterial cell with intracellular phage MS2. PTA. 120,000 ×.

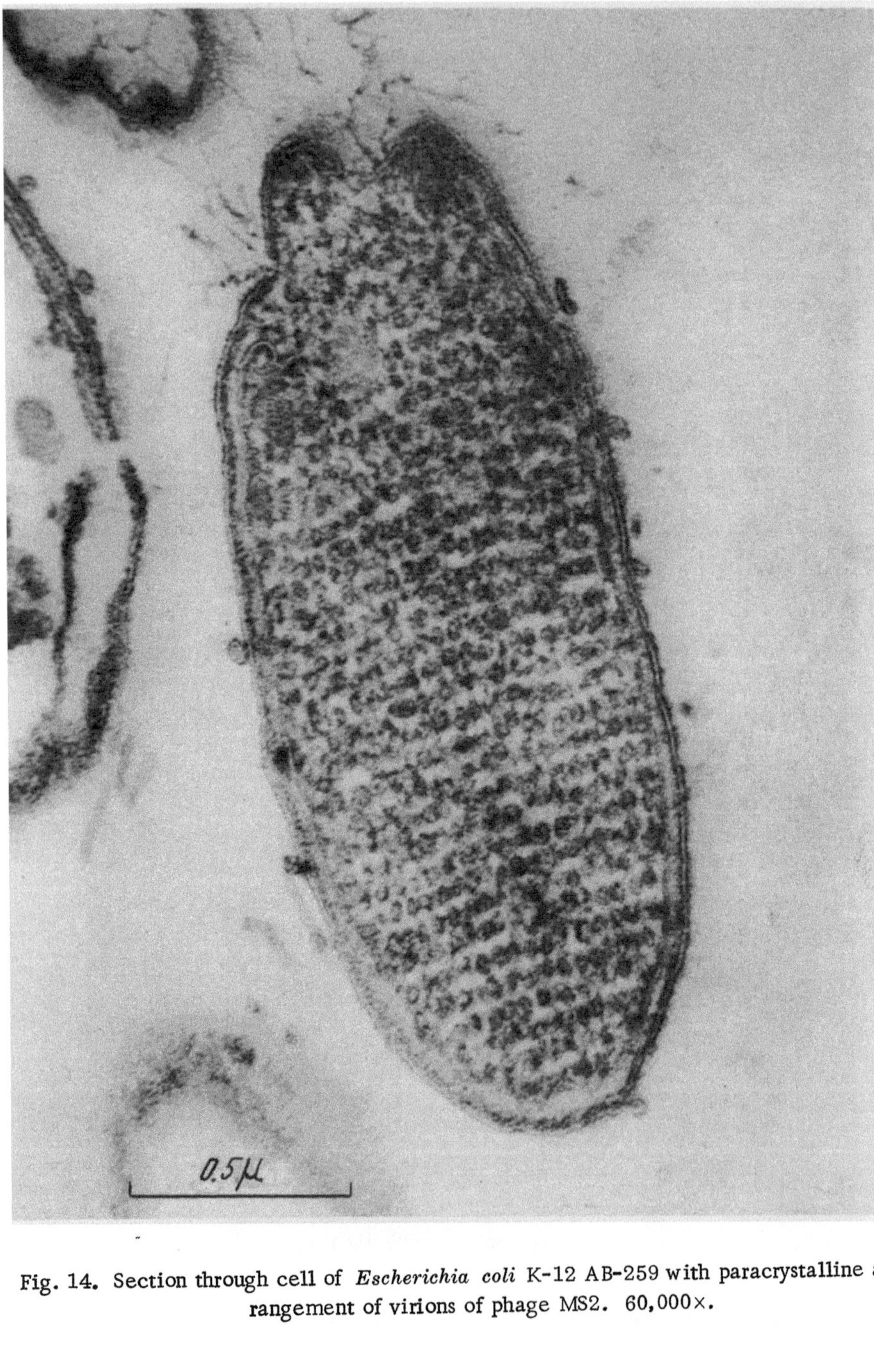

Fig. 14. Section through cell of *Escherichia coli* K-12 AB-259 with paracrystalline arrangement of virions of phage MS2. 60,000×.

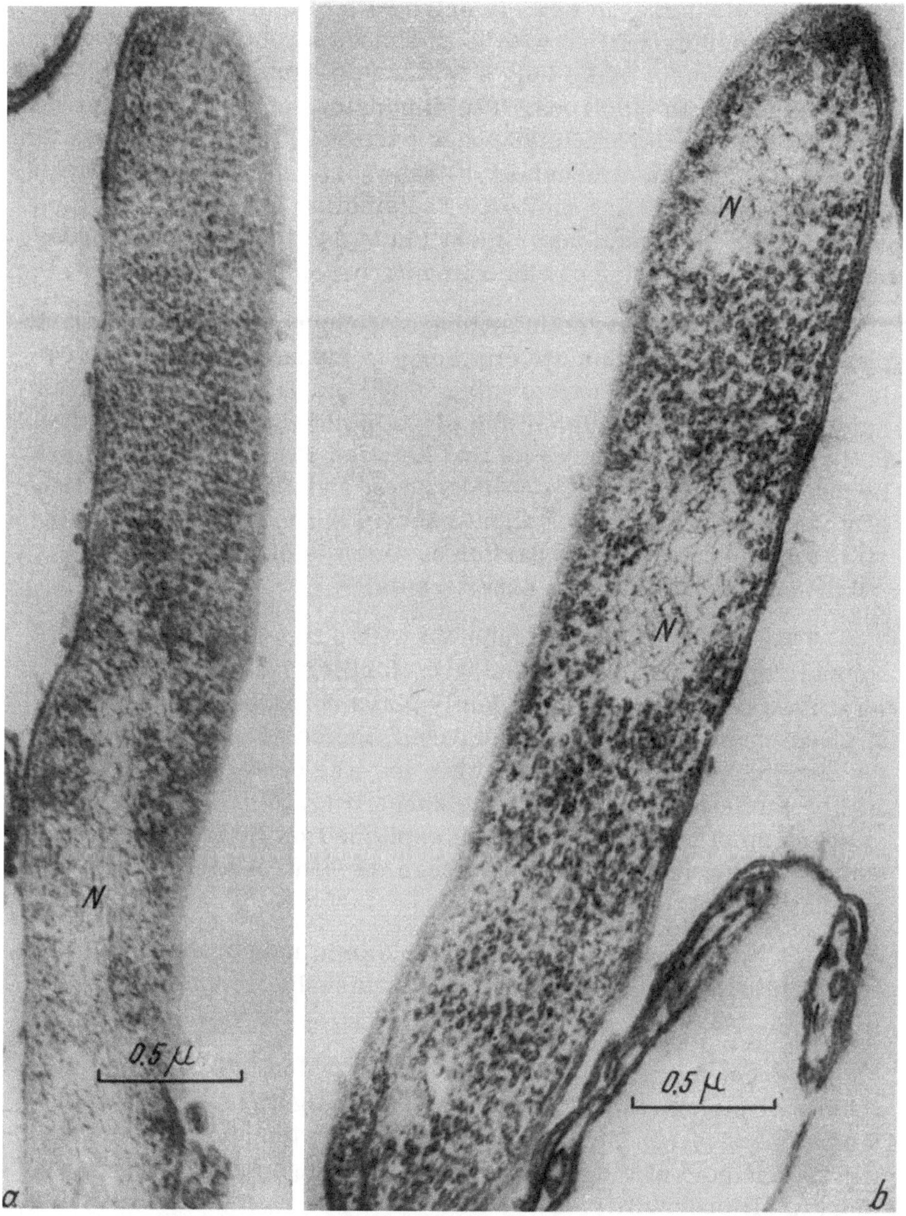

Fig. 15. Sections through cells of ***Escherichia coli*** K-12AB-259 with intracellular phage MS2 (N represents nucleoid). Adsorbed phase particles are visible on the surface of the bacterium. 40,000×. a) Nucleoid occupies central part of cell; b) nucleoid in separate zones.

Tikhonenko, Bespalova, and Kriviskii [56, 362] showed by the study of sections that in cells infected with phage MS2 the cytoplasm is completely filled with ring-shaped structures, most of which appear empty, while only a few have a central zone which is less permeable to electrons. The dimensions of the circular structures, which are intracellular phage particles, are slightly smaller in sections than the dimensions of three virions when studied by the negative contrasting method. The smaller size of intracellular phage particles in sections is most likely due to differences in the methods of preparation of electron-microscopic specimens.

Particles of intracellular phage occupying nearly all the cytoplasm are arranged in a strictly regular manner, as a rule, forming clusters known as paracrystals (Fig. 14; Fig. 15a). The mean number of phage particles in the plane of one section through the cells is 350-400. Considering that between 25 and 30 sections can be cut from a cell 0.75-1 μ in thickness, and assuming conventionally that the cell is rectangular in shape, it can therefore contain up to 10,000-12,000 phage particles, which is of the order of the number found in biological experiments.

The nucleoid of a cell infected with phage MS2, like that of normal cells (Fig. 16), is filled with fibrillar material. It is always free from phage and evidently plays no part in the process of phage reproduction. In some cases, the nucleus is pushed by the developing mass of phage either into the center of the cell (Fig. 17), or into a number of separate zones (Fig. 15b). This apparent splitting up of the nucleoid can be explained on the grounds that the section evidently did not pass through the central part of the nucleoid, but through its ramifications.

The complex structure of cytoplasmic membranes and of the cell membrane becomes clearly distinguishable in infected cells (Figs. 14, 17).

Hence, morphological observations which fully confirm the results of biological and biochemical investigations show that the formation of phage MS2 takes place in the cytoplasm without involving the nucleoid of the bacterial cell. The high burst size of phage MS2, in all probability, is the reason for the formation of extensive clusters of paracrystals, consisting of densely packed, separate virions inside the infected cell.

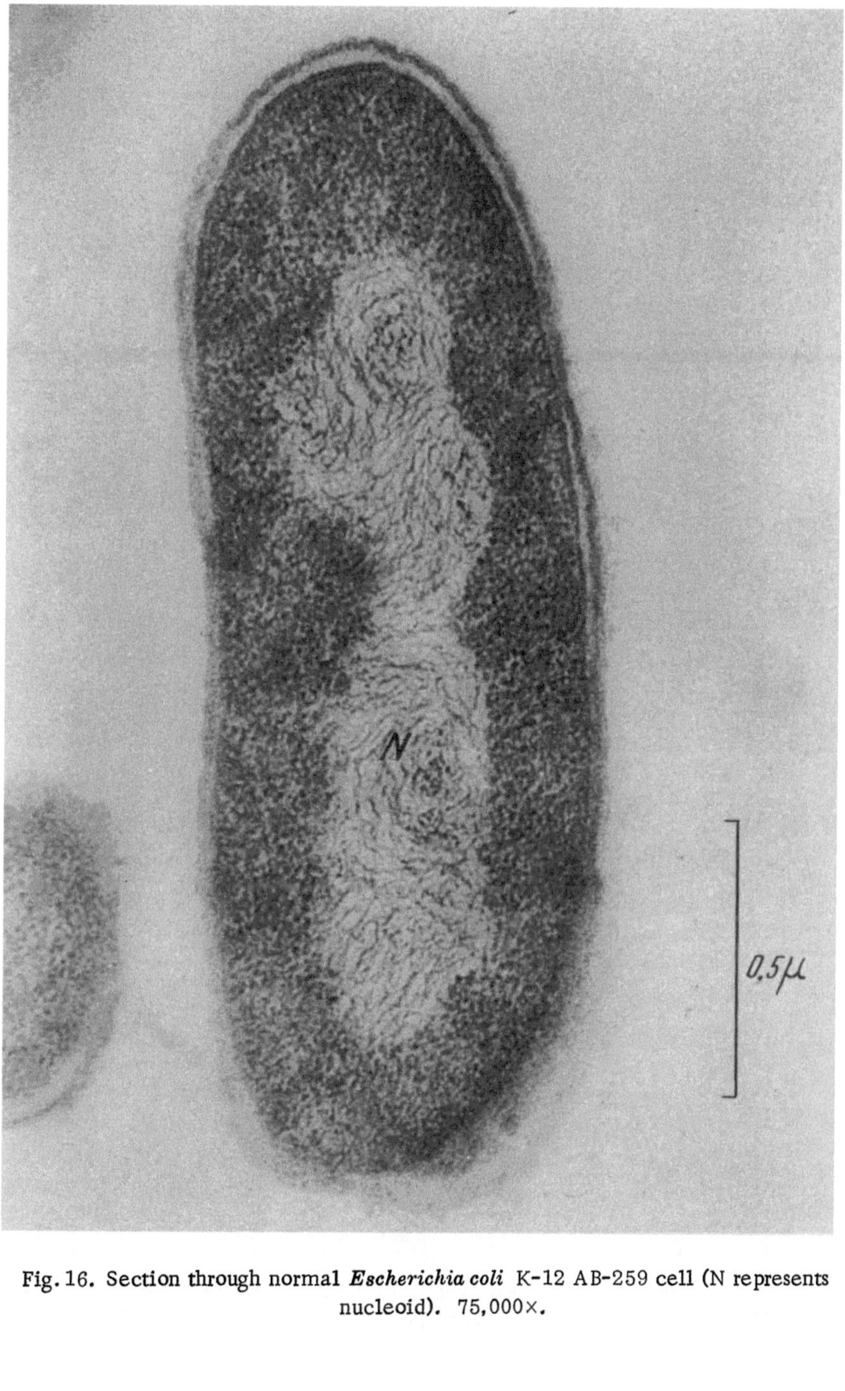

Fig. 16. Section through normal *Escherichia coli* K-12 AB-259 cell (N represents nucleoid). 75,000×.

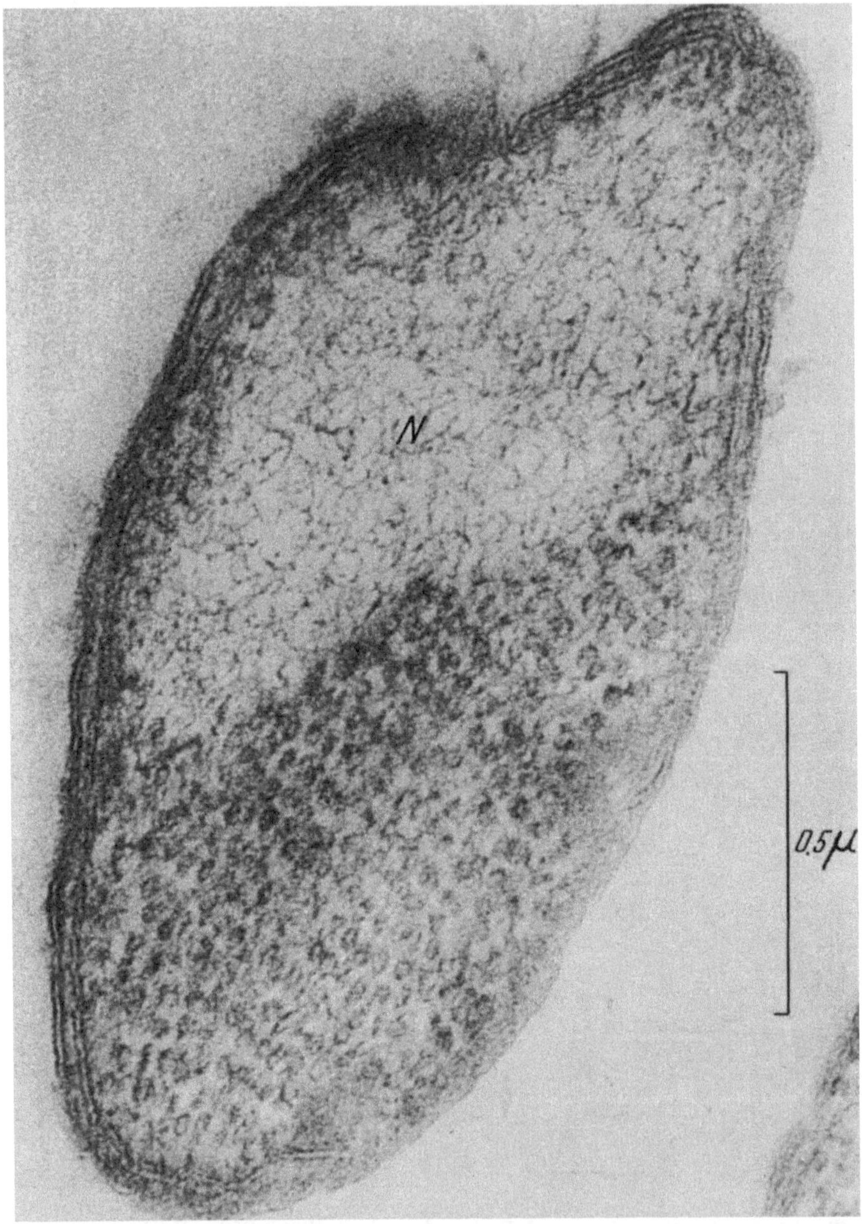

Fig. 17. Section through *Escherichia coli* K-12 AB-259 cell with intracellular phage (N represents nucleoid). 75,000×.

Franklin and Granboulan [179], who studied changes in the ultrastructure of *E. coli* cells infected with phage R17, found that with a one-stage cycle of reproduction, the cells show no morphological changes during the latent period. Clearly defined changes in the cell ultrastructure begin after intensive synthesis of virus and are observed in the polar zones of the cell. In the late stages of infection a paracrystalline arrangement of the virions becomes apparent. These workers noted that the synthesis of virus RNA takes place in the paranuclear region of the cell. Investigations by the same workers [186], using a combination of electron microscopy and autoradiography, showed that during infection of cells with the RNA-phage R17, synthesis of RNA takes place predominantly in the cytoplasm, but later (at the end of the latent period and during the stage of active virus reproduction) the label is localized in the polar zones of the cell. In the ultimate stages of development of these viruses, RNA is found only around the paracrystals formed by phage particles. The study of the synthesis of phage protein showed that it also is localized in the polar zones of the cell. On the addition of chloramphenicol during infection, synthesis of the protein of the virus envelope is inhibited, and RNA label is found in the paranuclear zone, indicating that RNA synthesis takes place there.

Morphological findings also indicate that synthesis of virus RNA and virus protein takes place mainly in the cell cytoplasm, and confirm the results of biochemical investigation. It can be postulated that the exceptionally high burst size of RNA-containing phages, coupled with the relatively short latent period of their intracellular reproduction (about 30 min in my own experiments), is due to the fact that these phages, unlike the DNA phages, develop independently of the genetic regulatory apparatus (the nucleus) of the host cell, and that no intermediaries are evidently required for the transmission of information during synthesis of daughter phage particles.

Other workers studying the intracellular development of RNA-containing viruses have obtained similar results [104, 301, 302, 303, 335].

Structure and Biological Properties of Phage of Type ϕX174

A typical representative of the spherical phages containing single-stranded DNA is phage ϕX174. It was first studied morphologically by Sinsheimer [342], Hall and co-workers [191], Tromans and Horne [366], and Daems and co-workers [140]. These investigators found that particles of phage ϕX 174 are icosahedral in shape and similar in their morphology to some small spherical viruses of animals and plants. Unlike the latter, in the particles of this phage each apex of the icosahedron ends in a projecting spine, the role of which has not yet been established for certain. Tromans and Horne [366] suggest that these outgrowths participate in the transmission of DNA to the bacterial cell. Kay [226] suggests that only one of these outgrowths in phage ϕR is responsible for adsorption, and that its function is analogous to that of the tail of other phages.

The negative contrasting method showed that the capsid of phage ϕX 174 consists of separate capsomeres about 70 Å in diameter. Some investigators [213, 366] consider that each capsomere, in turn, consists of five smaller structural units.

The unique structural features of these phages and the discovery that they contain single-stranded DNA [226, 342, 360] have attracted considerable attention. It has been shown [182, 318] that the single-stranded DNA of phage ϕX 174 is a closed ring.

Discoveries of new phages [99, 100, 207, 227, 273], indistinguishable from phage ϕX 174 in their structure and size (Table 2), have been reported. However, no detailed investigation of their biological properties and no attempts to identify them with other well-studied phages of this type have yet been made.

Il'yashenko and co-workers [18] have investigated the morphology and other biological properties of several, new, small intestinal bacteriophages containing DNA and isolated from natural sources. Phage ϕX 174 was used for comparison.

They centrifuged 10–20 ml of the water sample to be tested for 20–30 min at 7000–8000 rpm, and applied it in a volume of 2–5 ml by the agar layer method to a series of dishes containing an indicator culture of *E. coli* C. They found that in order to isolate small phages it is more convenient to investigate samples of water directly without preliminary incubation with the culture. Otherwise, mainly contaminating phages, also active against *E. coli* C, accumulate preferentially. Only the larger of the plaques thus formed were selected. A pure line of phage was isolated by 7-10 successive seedings on solid medium and by subsequent reproduction on *E. coli* C in nutrient broth. The titers of the phages were $2\text{-}5 \cdot 10^{10}$ particles/ml. Concentrated suspensions of the phages were prepared from lysates obtained on synthetic medium with aeration, followed by differential centrifugation [15]. The biological properties of the phages were investigated by Adams' method [1], and inactivation by formaldehyde by Thomas' method [67]. The DNA of these phages was extracted from concentrated suspension with hot phenol [189]. Infectivity of the phage DNA was determined and their treatment with nucleases was carried out by Il'yashenko's method [16].

For the electron-microscopic investigation, they used mainly unpurified lysates obtained by washing from solid medium the lysed growths of a culture with small volumes of 0.85% NaCl solution, followed by dialysis against distilled water.

From 46 samples of water investigated, 7 pure lines of new small bacteriophages were isolated and designated by the symbols 1ϕ1, 1ϕ3, 1ϕ7, 1ϕ9, dϕ3, dϕ4, and dϕ5.

Like phage ϕX 174, all the phages isolated are characterized by rapid formation of plaques. After incubation for 18 h at 37°C, the phage colonies attain a diameter of 8-10 mm. The colony morphology is of the virulent type: a transparent zone in the center, surrounded by a peripheral semitransparent zone with a clearly defined outer edge.

An electron-microscopic investigation of phage ϕX 174 showed that its particles have a highly specific morphology. Two-dimensionally, they appear as a six-pointed star with short prongs. The particle is an icosahedron, each apex of which ends in a short conical projection. In some cases this projection can be seen to be a hollow tube (Fig. 18). The diameter of the phage particle without the projections is 250 ± 10 Å. The projections measure $(50 \pm 10) \times (50 \pm 10)$ Å.

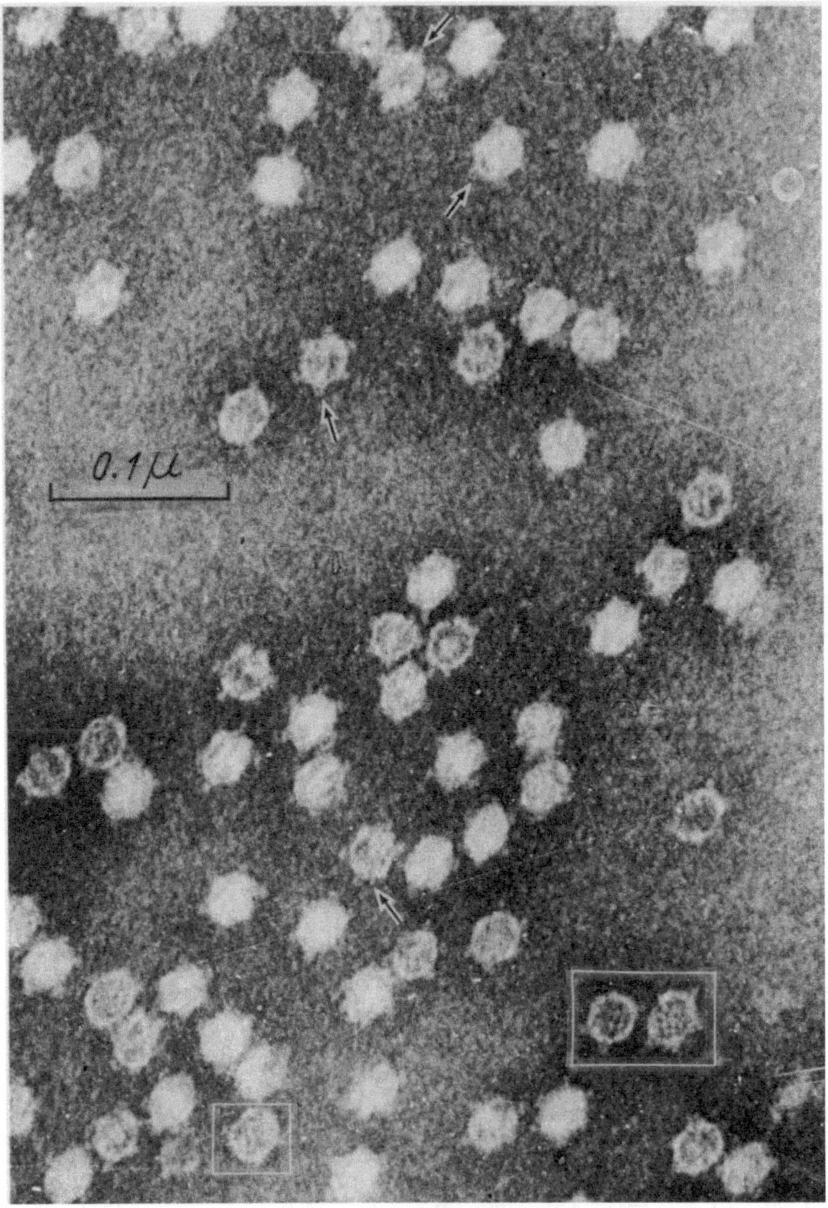

Fig. 18. Particles of phage ϕX174. Hollow projections of particles indicated by arrows. Particles with lower prongs are surrounded by squares. PTA. 260,000 ×.

Table 3. Differentiation of Phages of Type ϕX 174 by Their Spectrum of Lytic Activity

Strain of bacteria	Phages							
	ϕX174	1ϕ1	1ϕ3	1ϕ7	1ϕ9	dϕ3	dϕ4	dϕ5
E. coli 4	+	+	+	+	+	–	–	–
Shigella flexneri 45	+	+	+	+	+	–	–	–
S. flexneri 939	+	+	+	+	+	–	–	–
S. flexneri 3890	+	+	+	+	+	–	–	–
S. sonnei 776	+	+	+	+	+	–	–	–
S. sonnei 1413	+	+	+	+	+	–	–	–
Salmonella typhosa 58	+	+	+	+	+	–	–	–
S. typhosa B	+	+	+	+	+	–	–	–

Note. Plus denotes strain sensitive to phage; minus denotes resistant strain.

Particles of the new phages 1ϕ1, 1ϕ3, 1ϕ7, 1ϕ9, dϕ3, dϕ4, and dϕ5 are completely indistinguishable in size and morphology from phage ϕX 174 (Fig. 19). Like particles of phage ϕX 174, particles of the newly isolated phages also are hexagonal in shape on section and consist of an icosahedron with conical projections at each apex (12 projections). In a two-dimensional picture of the particles only six projections can be seen, one at each apex of the hexagon. On some particles, without their internal dense contents (DNA), the projection of the lower spines can be seen (Figs. 18 and 19). I consider that these projections are analogous to a tail and affect the specific interaction between phage and bacterial cell.

Despite the complete morphological identity of the phages thus isolated, differences have been found between them in certain biological properties (Table 3).

The lytic activity of the phages was tested on 51 strains, of which 17 belonged to *E. coli*, 26 to *Shigella flexneri*, 4 to *Shigella sonnei*, and 4 to *Salmonella typhosa*. Of all the strains tested only two (*S. sonnei* 714 and 1225, not included in the table) were sensitive to all phages. These two strains, together with the host strain *E. coli* C, mark the limit of the small number of strains showing sensitivity to phages of type dϕ. The remaining phages form another homogeneous group identical in their range of action with phage ϕX174 and characterized by a broader lytic spectrum.

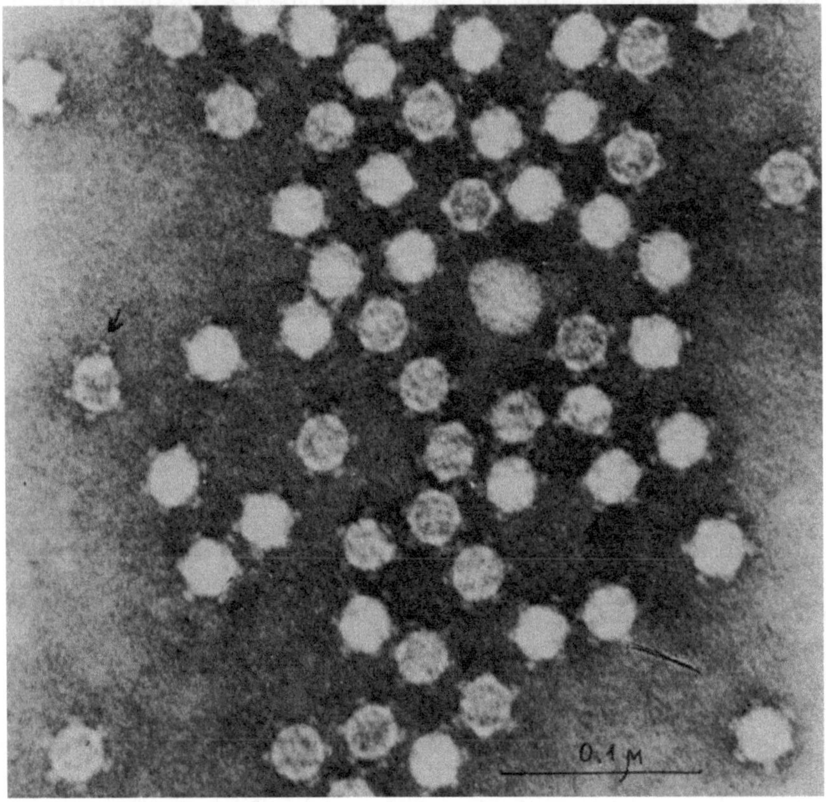

Fig. 19. Particles of phage 1φ7. Hollow projections of particles indicated by arrows. PTA. 260,000×.

Table 4. Serologic Differentiation of Phages of Type φX174

Serum	Neutralization velocity constants of phages (min^{-1})							
	φX174	1φ1	1φ3	1φ7	1φ9	dφ3	dφ4	dφ5
anti-φX174	92	56	46	51	48	0	0	0
anti-1φ1	78	78	75	78	72	0	0	0
anti-1φ7	90	92	88	92	80	0	0	0
anti-dφ3	0	0	0	0	0	90	46	0
anti-dφ4	0	0	0	0	0	60	92	4.6

No strains resistant to phages of type 1ϕ, but sensitive to type dϕ, were found. It was concluded from comparison of the number of strains of the different species tested and the number found to be sensitive that the activity of these phages is selective against *S. sonnei* and *S. typhosa*. Among the strains of *E. coli* and *S. flexneri* only one and three sensitive strains, respectively, were found, and these were sensitive only to phages of type 1ϕ. Evidently in relation to their spectrum of lytic activity, the newly isolated phages, like phage ϕX 174, would be more correctly included in the dysentery—typhoid group rather than directly in the enteric group.

I believe that these phages cannot be regarded as being highly specific and possessing a finely differentiated adsorption-receptor apparatus relative to the bacterial host, because mutation of sensitive bacteria to resistance for one of these phages is accompanied by the formation of resistance to other phages. All tested mutants, *E. coli* C ϕX 174, *S. sonnei* 1225/1ϕ7, 1225/dϕ3, 1225/dϕ4, and 1225/dϕ5, showed cross resistance to all phages as a result of loss of the power of adsorption. These results indicate a low degree of differentiation of the receptor apparatus, whose simplicity is evidently directly connected with the relative simplicity of the particle structure of these phages.

Division of the phages of this type into two subtypes, one resembling ϕX 174 and the other slightly different from it in biological properties, is confirmed by the results of the crossed neutralization reaction (Table 4). Despite their small size, these phages possess high antigenic activity. Antiphage sera with a neutralization constant of the order of 80-90 min^{-1} are formed after a few injections.

The results indicate that phages of type 1ϕ differ from phage ϕX 174 by the possession of an additional antigen, because anti-ϕX 174 serum neutralizes them less strongly than it does the homologous phage. No serologic differences are found between phages of type 1ϕ and they are probably identical. The antigenic structure of the three phages of type dϕ is quite different from them; two phages (dϕ3 and dϕ4) are closely related serologically, while one phage (dϕ5) is distinct.

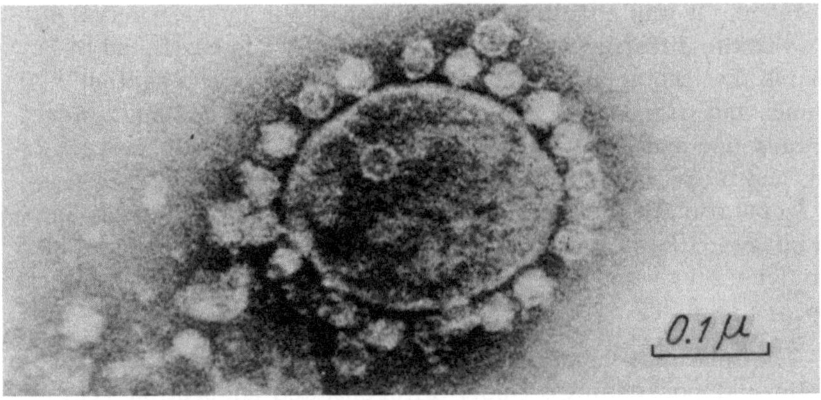

Fig. 20. Particles of phage 1ϕ1 adsorbed on the intracellular membrane of *E. coli* C. PTA. 160,000×.

Table 5. Interaction between Phages ϕX 174 and Host Cells

Phage	Maximal velocity of adsorption, ml/min/10^{-9}	Latent period, min	Duration of phage liberation, min	Burst size
ϕX174	4.6	18—19	15—20	200
1ϕ1	3.6	18—20	15—25	150
1ϕ3	3.7	18—20	15—20	130
1ϕ7	4.0	18—19	15—20	180
1ϕ9	3.9	18—20	15—25	170
dϕ3	4.8	18—20	15—20	150
dϕ4	3.8	18—20	15—25	200
dϕ5	4.2	18—19	15—20	200

Interaction between phages of type ϕX 174 and host cells is characterized by a number of special features in the adsorption phase. At 37°C adsorption of phage begins soon after mixing with the bacteria and for the first 60 sec it takes place at maximum velocity with fixation of 50-65% of the virions. Subsequently, the increase in the proportion of adsorbed phage becomes much slower, and the limiting value of 80-90% is not reached until 4-5 min. In the absence of Ca^{++} ions in the nutrient broth, adsorption of the phages does not exceed 40-50%. The optimal concentration of bacteria for adsorption of these phages is higher than for the T-phages, namely, 1-2 · 10^8 cells/ml. Details of the various phases of interaction between phages and host cells are given in Table 5.

Determination of the burst size by the method of one-stage growth of phages of type ϕX 174 evidently gives results which are too low. During electron-microscopic investigations of unpurified lysates, I have observed that many phage particles are present on the intracellular membranous structures liberated from the bacterial cell during lysis (Fig. 20). In all probability, these structures are mesosomes of the bacterial cell [94]. Bearing in mind the high degree of readsorption of phage on membranous structures of the disintegrated cells, it must be assumed that the burst size is much higher for small phages than for large phages.

Because of the similarity of the structure and biological behavior of the isolated phages, and considering the possibility of isolating the DNA of phage ϕX 174 in an infective state, tests of the biological activity of the isolated nucleic acids of these new phages were undertaken.

It had previously been shown [15, 189, 206, 337] that *E. coli* cells can be infected by purified native single-stranded phage DNA if the intact bacterial wall is first rendered permeable to DNA molecules isolated from phage particles.

As might be expected, preparations of nucleic acids of all the new phages were found to be infective toward lysozyme-treated spheroplasts of the *Enterobacteriaceae*. This fact was used to ascertain the type of nucleic acids of the phages by specific inactivation of infective preparations with deoxyribonuclease and ribonuclease. On the basis of the complete inactivation of the preparations by deoxyribonuclease and preservation of practically 100% of their activity after treatment with ribonuclease, it can be concluded that the genetic material of all the phages which I investigated is DNA. This conclusion was confirmed on purified DNA preparations from phage 1ϕ7 [17] by chromatographic identification of the nitrogenous bases and also by determination of deoxyribose by the reaction with diphenylamine. It was discovered that, among the inactivating agents used, formaldehyde is highly effective against these phages. A 0.19% solution of formaldehyde at 18-20°C for 15 min inactivates more than 99% of the phage. Inactiva-

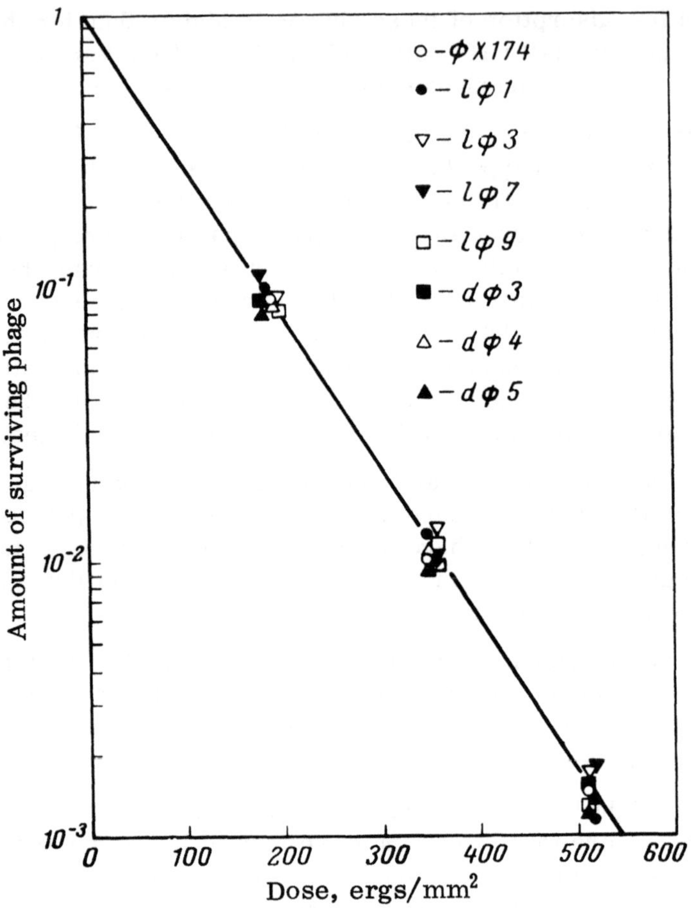

Fig. 21. Kinetics of inactivation of phages of φX174 type by ultraviolet light.

tion by formaldehyde under these conditions is most probably due to selective injury to the protein components of the phage particle. Isolated DNA of phages φX 174 and 1φ7, with single-stranded structure [17], under analogous experimental conditions, keeps its biological activity unchanged, and is inactivated only at 37°C.

Inactivation of phages by ultraviolet light behaves as an exponential function of the dose of irradiation. The curve of this function adheres strictly to the "one-hit" character (Fig. 21).

All phages of this type possess equal sensitivity to ultraviolet light, identical with that of phage ϕX174, and more sensitive to it than larger phages [340]. The velocity of inactivation of phages under experimental conditions is about 1.92 min^{-1} and coincides with the inactivation velocity of the isolated single-stranded DNA of phage 1ϕ7 [13]. This is indirect evidence to suggest that the DNA of the other small phages, likewise, is single-stranded in structure.

Phages of the ϕX 174 type are evidently widespread in nature, but despite their different habitats, exhibit considerable uniformity of size and shape. Moreover, different phages of this type possess identical characteristics of their relationship with the host cell, identical morphology of their plaques, and they are equally inactivated by formaldehyde and ultraviolet light. Their antigenic properties and spectrum of lytic activity can now be used as criteria for their differentiation.

Phages with equally specific morphology are known at the present time only for bacteria of the coli — typhoid — dysentery group.

Comparison of the phages investigated by the author, both with one another and with phages ϕX 174, S13, and ϕR, shows that all phages of this type, containing single-stranded DNA, are very similar in their fine structural details and morphologically they form a distinct group.

Chapter 4

Short-Tailed Phages (Group III)

The third group includes those phages which possess a small, yet clearly defined tail.

Phages with a short tail have been isolated from many genera and species of microorganisms (nonsporebearing and sporebearing bacteria and actinomycetes).

In this group, the overwhelming majority of phages which have been studied contain DNA of the usual type, i.e., double-stranded [21, 65, 76, 85, 88, 144, 145]. It must be considered that this type of DNA is characteristic of all the phages included in this morphological group.

The diameter of the head of all the phages in this group varies from 400 to 640 Å (Table 6).

The head of all these phages appears two-dimensionally as a hexagon, and most of them are isometric polyhedra. Only phages ϕ29 and GA-1 of *Bacillus mycoides* [85, 105] differ in having a head shaped like an elongated polyhedron.

Determination of the three-dimensional shape of the head from its two-dimensional projection can be very difficult because both icosahedra and octahedra can appear hexagonal in their two-dimensional projection. On theoretical grounds, Caspar and Klug [124] consider that the most logical structure for the capsid of viruses composed of individual subunits is a polyhedron of icosahedral type. On this basis they suggest that an octahedral form of viruses is improbable. However, Bradley [101] considers that

Table 6. Dimensions of the Virion of Short-Tailed Phages

Phage	Diameter of head, Å	Size of tail, Å: Length	Size of tail, Å: Width	Species of host	Literature citation
	Subgroup I (phages resembling T3, T7)				
T3	550×550(470)	150	80	*E. coli* B	[108]
T3	550	150	—	"	[101]
T7	590—650	—	—	"	[145]
14	400	130	—	*Pseudomonas syringae*	[102]
15	400	150	—	"	[102]
20	500	300	—	*Pseudomonas fluorescens*	[102]
21	600	200	—	"	[102]
Y, PTM, R	500	150	—	Pasteurella	[246]
EV	530±20	190±10	—	"	[49]
3, 6, 7, 10, 44 513, M, X *,	600±20	160±10	—	Brucella	[49]
F_1, F_2, F_3, F_4, F_5, F_6, F_7, F_8, F_9, F_{10}, F_{11}	590×660	230	100	"	[119]
10/I, 24/II, 45/III, 212/XV, 371/XXIX, 12, 3, 6, 7, P, T_B F25N, F44, F48, F2S, FP2, Fim, F, U, FO_1, F_1, F4S	600	200		"	[300]
Phage Brucella	550	150	—	"	[108]
317/XXIX and 22 others	500—600	200	—	"	[298, 299]
317/XXIX T_B	600	160	—	"	[112]
Phage Brucella	650	160	—	"	[280]
PS-1001, PS-192, PR-590a, PSR-1012	600	—	—	Agrobacterium	[317]
277	500	--	—	*Bacteroides varius* Anaerobe	[214]
114 †	560±20	170±10	—	*Thermoactinomyces viridis*	[49]
9248	611	185	—	Proteus	[307]
VI ‡	570±20	180±10	—	*Proteus mirabilis*	[49]

the head of phage T3 of *E. coli* B is octahedral in shape. Kiselev and co-workers [21] also concluded that the head of phage s_d is octahedral in shape.

From the example of phages ϕ29 and GA-1 of *B. subtilis* and from the description of phages contained in subsequent morphologi-

Table 6 (continued)

Phage	Diameter of head, Å	Size of tail, Å		Species of host	Literature citation
		Length	Width		
	Subgroup II (phages resembling s_d, P22) §				
s_d	570—615	—	—	*E. coli* SK	[21]
s_d	640	200	220	"	[43, 57]
P22	600	70	70	Salmonella	[81]
P22	530	70	70	"	[394]
27, 1(37), 1(40), 6(18), 14(6,7), PZt22, ε34, ε15	600	180	—	"	[375]
12B	700 and 500	—	—	*Pseudomonas syringae*	[102]
SM4	570	—	—	*Serratia marcescens*	[106]
PL26, PL37, PL25,	600	130	—	*Proteus morganii*	[129]
10041/2815	544	182	167	"	[307]
65	518	148	222	*Pr. hauseri*	[307]
34/13	630	167	204	"	[307]
12/57	589	185	204	"	[307]
9213/9211B	608	152	204	Proteus	[307]
9211/9295	533	148	196	"	[307]
∅29	415×315	130	60	*Bacillus subtilis*	[85]
GA-1	570×400	350	—	"	[105]
AA-1	650	185	130	Acetobacter	[105]
80	400	300	—	*Clostridium perfringens*	[376]
∅17	595±25	—	—	*Streptomyces chrisomallus*	[89]
Chlorellophage	410±10	240±10	100	*Chlorella pyrenoidosa*	[58]

* Obtained from M. Z. Papkhadze (Research Institute of Vaccines and Sera, Tbilisi).

† Isolated by A. Kosmachev (Institute of Microbiology, Academy of Sciences of the USSR).

‡ Obtained from U. Taubeneck (Institute of Microbiology and Experimental Therapy, Jena, East Germany).

§ All phages possess an end plate.

cal groups, it is clear that the head of some of these phages is not a regular polyhedron, but is elongated in shape as a prolate polyhedron. Therefore, it is obvious the experimental findings are contrary to the theoretical argument and they clearly illustrate the wide variety of shape assumed by viruses in nature.

For convenience of description of the morphologically distinguished phages constituting this group, I felt it advisable to divide it into two subgroups. This subdivision is based on the structural features of the short tail characterizing members of this group.

The first subgroup contains phages with a short, conical tail without an end plate. The second subgroup consists of phages in which the short tail terminates in an end plate.

SUBGROUP I: PHAGES OF TYPE T3 and T7

The phages included in the first subgroup are similar in their morphology to the well-studied phages T3 and T7, belonging to the T series of phages infecting *E. coli* B. The characteristic feature distinguishing the phages of this subgroup is the short conical tail without an end plate, arising from one apex of the polyhedral head. Phages with this type of tail structure have been described for many species of nonsporebearing bacteria, but none have yet been found among the phages infecting bacilli.

It must be assumed that the capsid of the head of these phages consists of separate capsomeres. However, these morphological units have not been described, most probably because they are too small and are beyond the limits of resolution of present-day electron microscopes. As Table 6 shows, a conical type of tail has been found, not only on phages T3 and T7 of *E. coli*, but also on phages infecting various species of *Proteus*, *Pseudomonas*, *Brucella*, *Agrobacterium*, etc. [49, 102, 108, 112, 119, 214, 298, 299, 300, 307, 317].

I have observed particles of this shape with a short conical tail on phage EV infecting bacteria of plague vaccine strain EV, on phage 114, active against a thermophilic actinomycete (*Thermoactinomyces viridis*), and also on certain dysentery phages.

It is interesting to note that a virus infecting blue-green algae, described by Smith and co-workers [346], is very similar in its morphology to phages of the T3 and T7 type.

The short tail of phage particles of this type is comparatively simple in structure. It consists of a hollow conical tube. Brad-

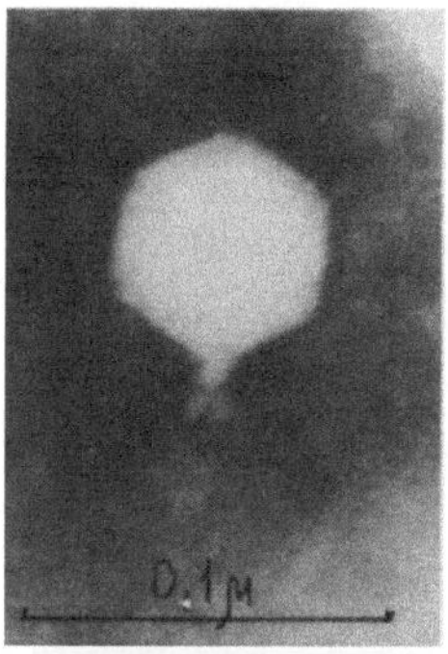

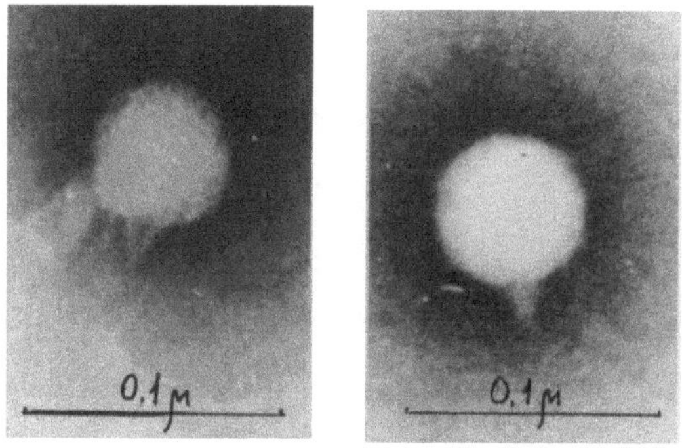

Fig. 22 Fig. 23

Fig. 22. Phage 114 of *Thermoactinomyces viridis*. PTA.

Fig. 23. Particles of phage EV of plague vaccine strain EV. PTA. 260,000 ×. a) Hollow in conical tail can be seen; b) hollow in conical tail cannot be distinguished.

ley [101] reports having found two thin filaments branching from the conical tail of phage T3 and possibly playing the same role in adsorption as the tail fibers of T-even phages.

I found no tail fibers on phages of this subgroup which I studied, including phage T3. However, the tail structure of phage 114 of *T. viridis* differs slightly from that of phages resembling T3. At the end of the tail of this phage there are two short fork-shaped projections (Fig. 22).

As an example of the structural organization of phages of this type, I offer illustrations of phage EV (Fig. 23a, b) and *Brucella* phage M (Fig. 24). It will be clear from Fig. 23a that the conical tail is a hollow tube. Incidentally, the group of *Brucella* phages is extremely uniform in its morphology.

I studied nine strains of *Brucella* phages isolated from different sources. Morphologically they all were found to be completely identical [49].

Other workers [108, 112, 119, 280, 298, 299, 300] who have studied *Brucella* phages isolated from different sources (milk, animal excreta, blood, etc.) and from different parts of the world (USSR, Poland, Africa, Australia) also report a striking morphological uniformity among these phages. It is now well

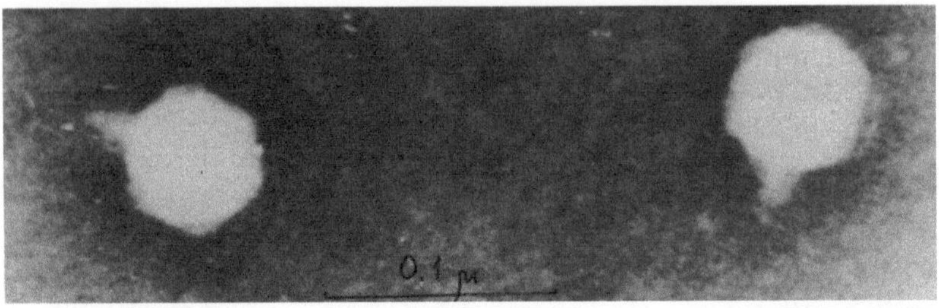

Fig. 24. Particles of phage M of *Brucella abortus*. PTA. 250,000 ×.

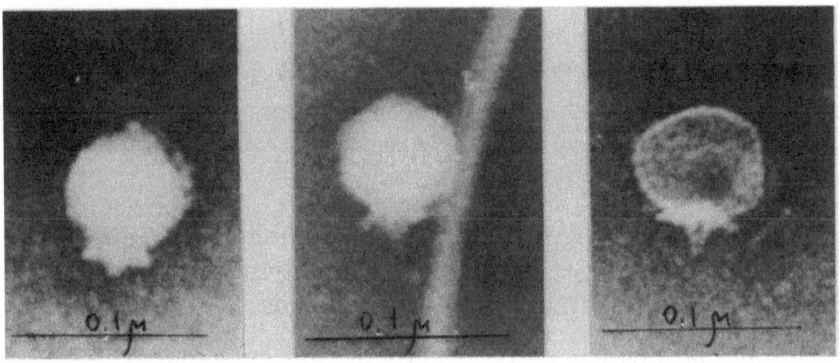

Fig. 25. Particles of phage VI of *Proteus mirabilis*. PTA. 250,000 ×. a,b) An additional disk is present on the tail; c) hollow inside the tail and condensation resembling a valve at the point of attachment of the tail to the head can be seen.

known that the same strain of bacteria can be infected by several phages differing from each other sharply in their morphology. Heterogeneity of this type has not yet been found among the phages infecting *Brucella*.

Before describing the structure of phages included in the second subgroup, I shall describe the morphology of phage VI of *Proteus mirabilis* which I have studied and which I consider to be intermediate in form between the phages of these two subgroups. Such a morphological type has not been described previously.

The particles of phage VI consist of a head, shaped like a regular polyhedron, and a short tail of peculiar structure. The dimensions of phage VI of *P. mirabilis* are given in Table 6. At the base of its head, phage VI has a plate about 300 Å in width and up to 20 Å in thickness, from the middle of which a conical tail about 60 Å in length arises. At the sides of the plate there are additional short spines (Fig. 25a, b, c). A further detail of this phage must be mentioned, which is most clearly distinguishable in particles which have lost their DNA. This structural detail consists of an electron-dense plate located inside the head at the plate of attachment of the tail (Fig. 25c). The importance of this structure is not yet known, although similar plates within the head have often been found in phages of more complex structure (phages of groups IV and V). Dawson and co-workers [147] have described a similar structural detail within the head of a phage of *Bacillus cereus* with a long tail and they postulated that it presumably plays some part in the transmission of phage DNA from the head to the host cell. I consider that grounds exist for the validity of this suggestion.

SUBGROUP II: PHAGES OF TYPE P22, s_d

The phages belonging to the second subgroup differ from phages of the T3 or T7 type in the structure of their tail. Despite its small size, their tail is more complex in structure.

The structural organization of phages of this type was first described by Anderson and Yamomoto [81, 394] on the example of temperate phage P22 isolated from *Salmonella typhimurium*. At the end of the short tail of phage P22 an easily distinguishable end plate was found, about 200 Å in width and 35 Å in thickness, having six hexagonally arranged projections about 35 Å in width and 75 Å in length. The end plate is attached to the head of the phage by a short cylinder measuring 70 × 70 Å.

Almost simultaneously with these investigations, particles of similar structure were described by the author [43] in the virulent phage s_d of *E. coli* SK (Fig. 26). The head of phage s_d, in the opinion of Kiselev and co-workers [21], is an octahedron.

During the study of a large number of preparations of phage s_d, I found that its tail, although small in size (200 × 200 Å), has a complex structure. The particles of this phage at first glance differ in their tail structure. However, after careful analysis of their structure, I concluded that this difference is only apparent. It is due to the fact that the phage particles may lie in different

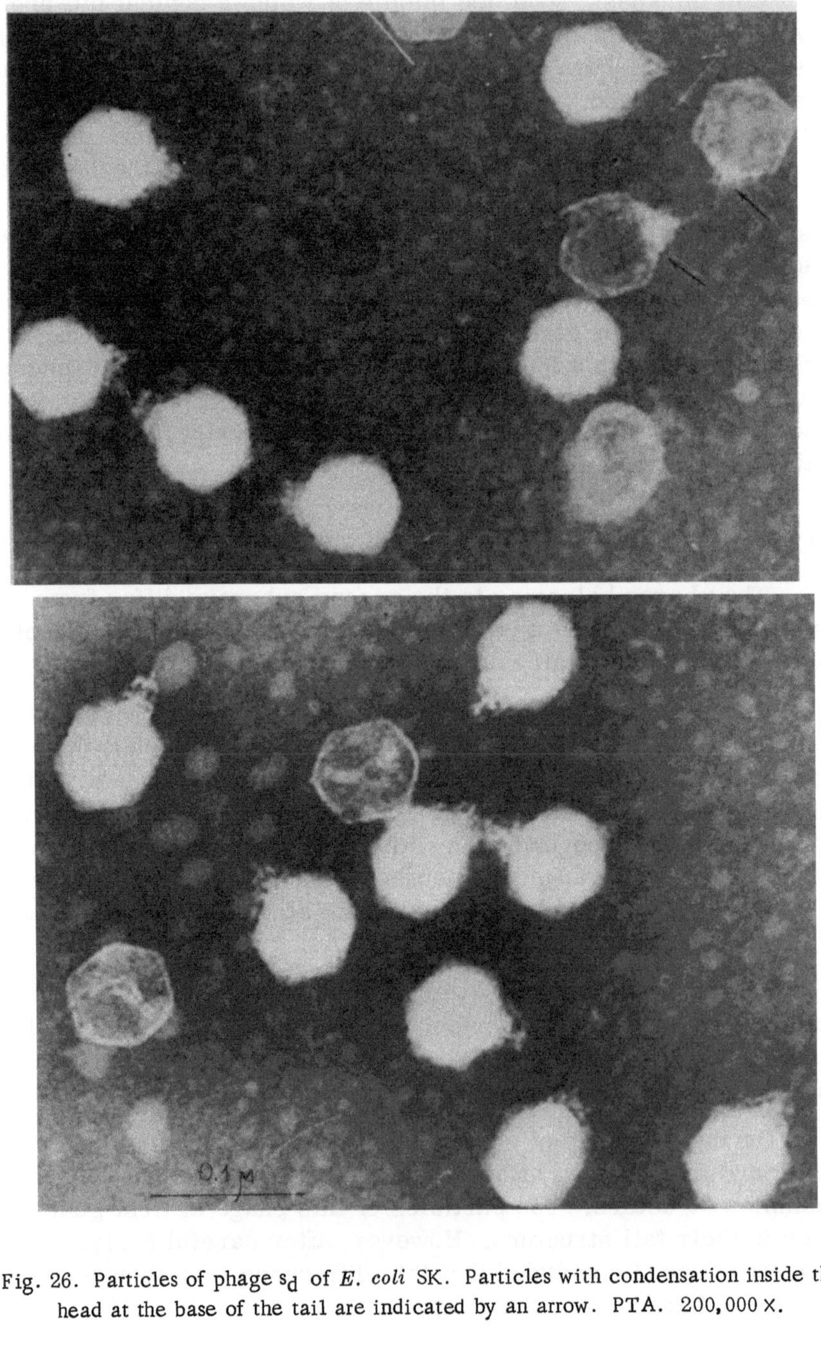

Fig. 26. Particles of phage s_d of *E. coli* SK. Particles with condensation inside the head at the base of the tail are indicated by an arrow. PTA. 200,000 ×.

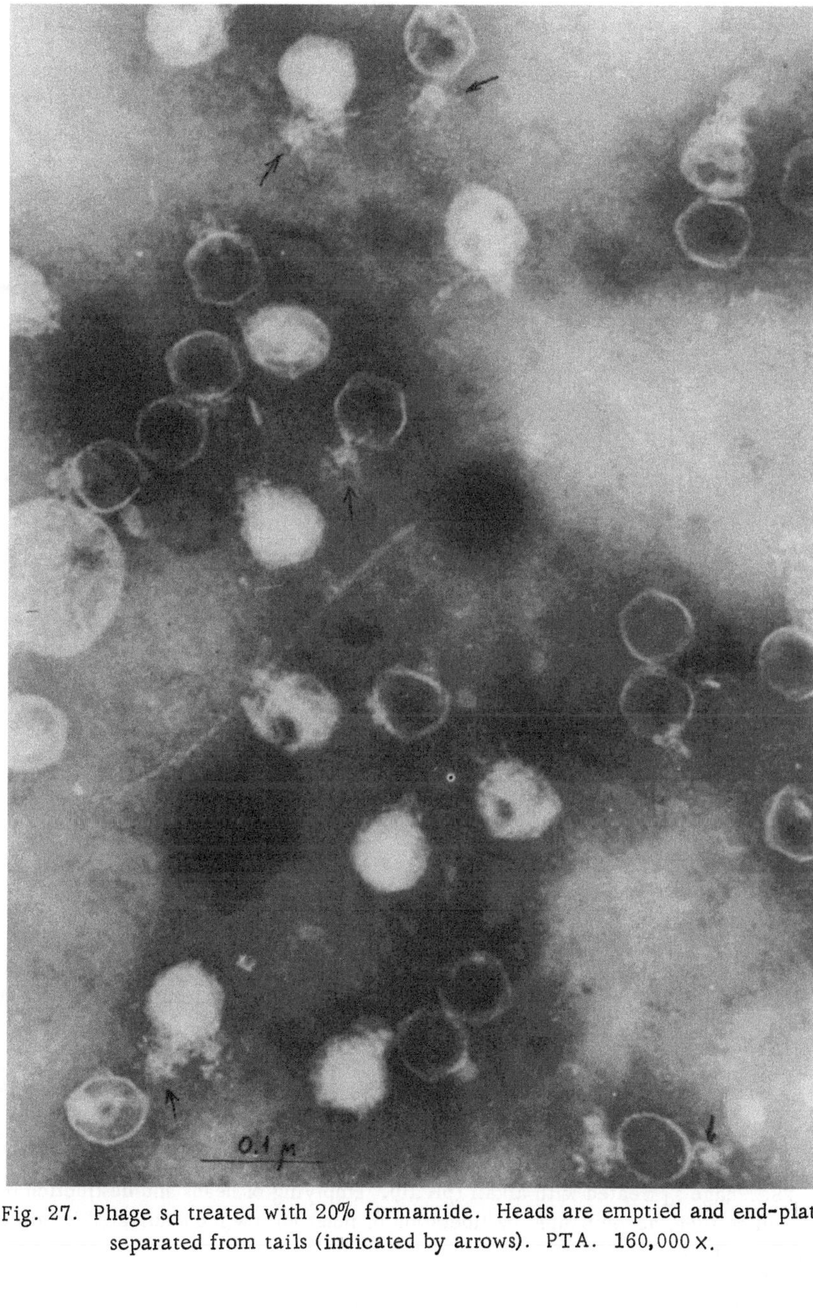

Fig. 27. Phage s_d treated with 20% formamide. Heads are emptied and end-plates separated from tails (indicated by arrows). PTA. 160,000 ×.

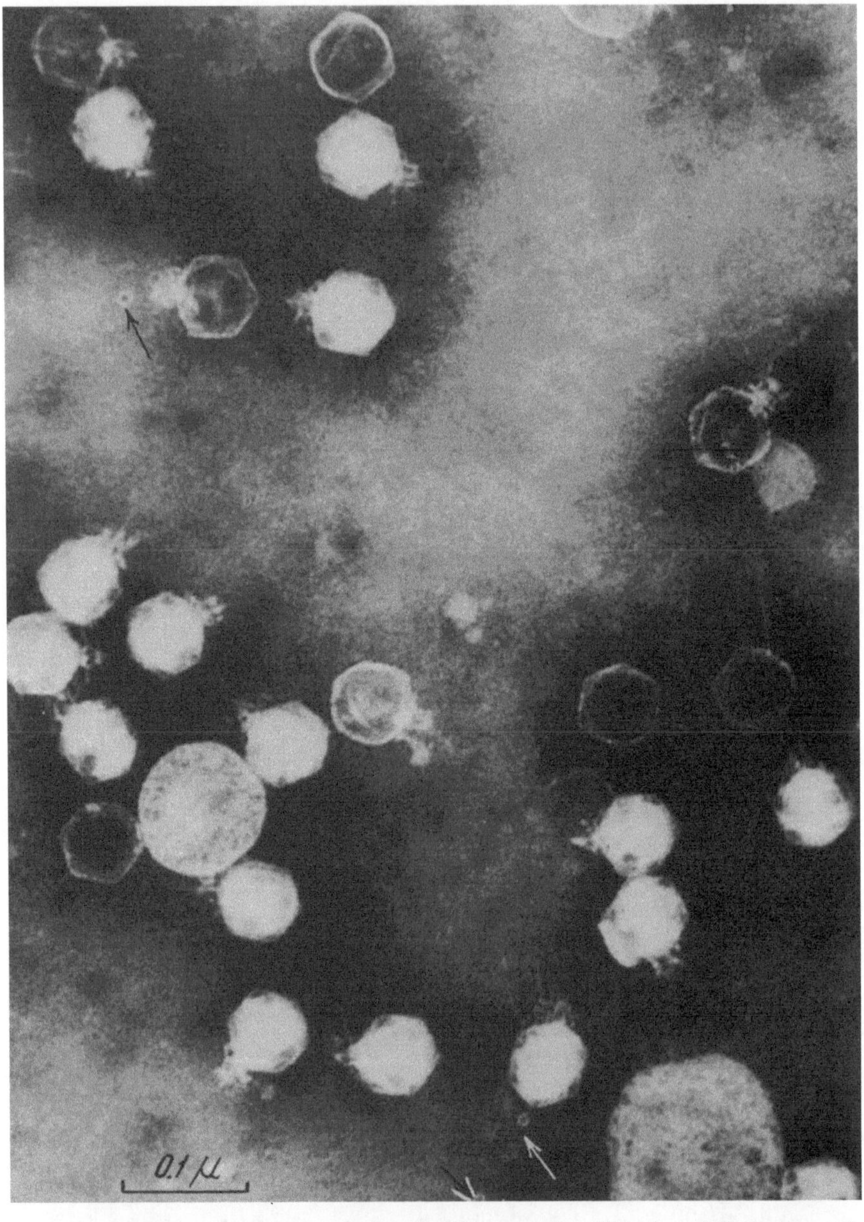

Fig. 28. Phage s_d treated with alkali (pH 10). Emptying of heads and destruction of tails can be seen, accompanied by liberation of inner hollow rod (indicated by arrows). PTA. 160,000×.

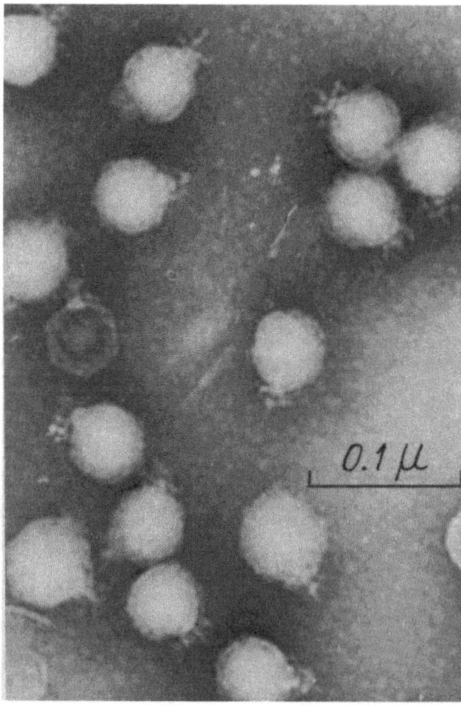

Fig. 29. Particles of phage s_d kept in PTA solution (pH 7.2) for 7 days. Partial destruction of the tail is observed, so that it has the appearance of tentacles. 150,000 ×.

planes on the support film, and for this reason the tail may differ in its appearance in different positions. From a comparison of the tail structure of phage s_d in several particles, I concluded that it consists of an outer sheath and an inner hollow structure resembling a rod, such as is clearly defined in phages possessing a tail with a contractile sheath (see Group V). On the short tail of some phage s_d particles, electron-dense transverse plates are clearly distinguishable (Fig. 26). This structure resembles the end plate of long-tailed phages. Seen from the end it appears as a plate with six projections diverging from it (Fig. 27).

Under the influence of certain factors, such as freezing and thawing, heating, treatment with alkalies or detergents, or after prolonged treatment with a neutral solution of potassium phospho-

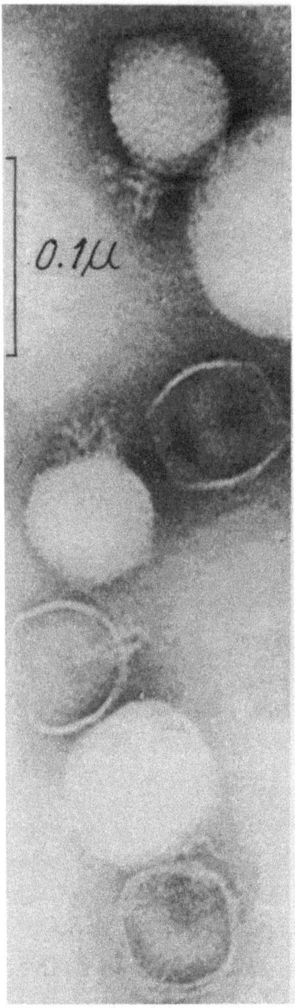

Fig. 30. Particles of phage s_d after freezing and thawing. Capsomeres of the capsid and partial destruction of the tail can be seen, leading to exposure of the inner hollow rod. PTA. 250,000×.

tungstate, partial destruction of the end plate takes place and the short tail of phage s_d then has the appearance of tentacles (Figs. 28, 29, 30).

The short tail of phage s_d thus consists mainly of an end plate which is joined almost immediately (through a very short neck) with the head. Inside the tail there is a thin, hollow rod. The free structure of the hollow rod in the tail of phage s_d can be observed after destruction of the phage particles by treatment with various chemical agents (Fig. 28) [57].

The capsid of the head of phage s_d consists of capsomeres approximately 30 Å in diameter (Fig. 30).

Kiselev and co-workers [21] found that the capsomeres of phage s_d are approximately 25 Å in diameter. Capsomeres of the same diameter were found in actinophage ϕ17 by Bacq and Horne [89].

Inside the hollow capsid of the head of phage s_d, just as in the case of phage VI, there is an electron-dense plate, situated at the point of attachment of the tail to the head (Figs. 26 and 27).

Phages with this type of tail structure were later described for many species of nonsporebearing and sporebearing bacteria, cocci, and actinomycetes, and in all probability they are a widespread structural type.

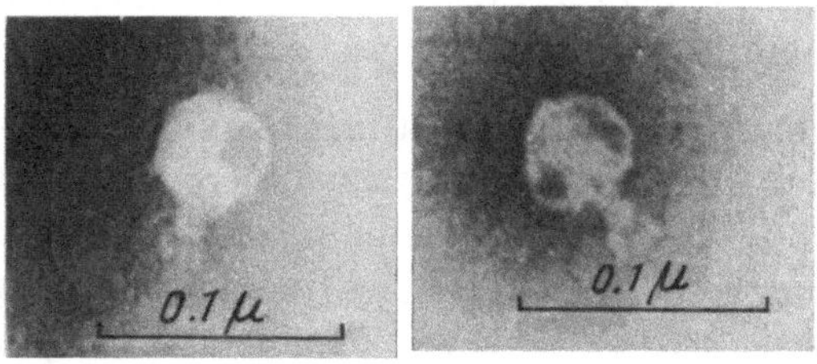

Fig. 31. Particles of virus infecting *Chlorella* PTA. 220,000 ×.

Phages with a short tail, but with a well-marked end plate, have been found for bacteria of the genera *Pseudomonas* [102], *Proteus* [129, 307], *Salmonella* [81, 375, 394], *Serratia marcescens* [106, *Acetobacter* [105], certain species of bacillus [85, 105, 312], and also for staphylococci [316] and actinomycetes [89].

Phages ϕ29 and GA-1 of this subgroup infecting *B. subtilis* are of particular interest. In contrast to the other phages of this type, phage GA-1 [105] has a polyhedral head of elongated shape (570 × 400 Å) to which an end plate with six spinous projections about 70 Å in length is directly attached. A tail, consisting of a hollow tube 350 Å in length and 60 Å in width, leaves the head through the end plate.

Phage ϕ29, described by Anderson and co-workers [85], has a unique shape. Like phage GA-1, it has a somewhat elongated head (415 × 315 Å). The distinguishing feature of this phage is that spinous projections 140 Å in length and 20 Å in width branch out radially from the capsid, the thickness of which is about 25 Å. The importance of the projections on the head of this phage is not yet known. The short tail of phage ϕ29 consists of two plates or collars, as these workers described them. The upper plate is directly joined to the head. The lower plate gives off 12 spindle-shaped projections which, surround it symmetrically. The thin axial tube, 130 Å in length and variable in thickness, passes through the plate. It is thicker in its distal part than its proximal part.

The volume of the head of phage ϕ29 (1.4×10^7 Å^3) is about 14% of the volume of the head of phage T2, which is 3.3×10^8 Å^3 [93]. However, the length of the DNA molecule of phage ϕ29 [85], measured on electron micrographs, is approximately 5-5.7 μ (molecular weight 10.9–11.3 · 10^6 Dalton), and this is fairly large, considering the small size of the head of this phage.

It is interesting to note that a tail possessing a structural organization similar to that of phage s_d was discovered by Tikhonenko and Zavarzina [58] on an agent producing lysis of the unicellular alga *Chlorella pyrenoidosa* (Fig. 31). Although this agent is a plant virus, we called it "chlorellophage" because its possession of a tail makes it resemble a bacteriophage (the dimensions of the chlorellophage particle are given in Table 6).

It is thus clear from the description of the morphology of the phages of group III that their particles possess the typical shape of bacterial viruses. They have two well-defined structural elements, a head and a tail, and the tail of phages of s_d type, despite its small size, is complex in structure.

The information needed for such a structural differentiation of the protein component of these phages is most probably satisfied by the higher DNA content than that found in the phages of the first two morphological groups. The molecular weight of the DNA of phage T7 is 19 · 10^6 [145], of phage T3, 23 · 10^6 [92], and of phage s_d, 66–88 · 10^6 [21].

Chapter 5

Phages with Noncontracting Tail (Group IV)

Phages with a long, noncontracting tail are the most widespread of all bacterial viruses. They have been found for nearly all known microorganisms and they infect both nonsporebearing and sporebearing bacteria, cocci, mycobacteria, actinomycetes, stalked bacteria of the genus *Caulobacter*, *Asticcacaulis*, and even the multicellular bacteria of the genus *Caryophanon*. Dimensions of several phages of this group are given in Table 7.

When giving a general description of this group, it is important to note that it includes phages with heads of different shapes and sizes. The members of this group have a head which is shaped like an isometric or a prolate polyhedron. Its size varies within wide limits, from 540 to 1000 Å among the different phages of this group. A general feature characteristic of the group as a whole is that all these phages have a comparatively long and thin, noncontracting tail. This tail may be slightly or considerably curved. Periodic striations can be seen on it and these give the tail the appearance of a crinkled tube, a highly characteristic feature of the structural organization of the tails of all the phages in this group.

In cases where this periodicity in the tail structure has not been found in particular members of the group, the reason has been an inadequate resolving power of the electron microscope rather than the absence of these structures.

This view is confirmed by analysis of the work of Bradley, published in 1960 [108] and in 1963 [102]. In 1960, when electron-

Table 7. Dimensions of Vibrion of Phages with a Long, Non-contracting Tail

Phage	Size of head, Å	Size of tail, Å		Species of host	Literature citation
		Length	Width		
T1	600×600	1400—1600	70	*E. coli* B	[49]
T1	620×620 (500)	1300(1500)	100	"	[108]
T5	750×750 (650)	1800	120	"	[108]
ZG/3A	750×600	1900	—	*E. coli*	[103]
C1	900	Long tail	—	"	[101]
F1	Similar to	»	—	"	[101]
β4	600	1500	—	"	[101]
γ2	600	1500	—		[101]
3000	550	1400	—	*E. coli* (male and female strains)	[103]
λ	540	1400	70	*E. coli* K12	[228]
λ	—	1530	170	"	[157]
q	Similar to	—	—	*E. coli* (male and female strains)	[103]
ω	Similar to	1300	70	"	[103]
SiBL	500×500	1300	100	Typhoid	[108]
1	750×750	1800	90	"	[108]
DDUP	600×615	1400—1500	100	Coli-dysentery	[49]
∅χ	670×675	2200—2230	120	Salmonella	[282]
P221	530	1800	100	*Salmonella Typhimurium*	[394]
886*	470	1300	70	*Aerobacter aerogenes*	[49]
2600/D52 †	655—675	1800	100	*Proteus mirabilis*	[49]
9	826	1837	89	*Proteus hauseri*	[307]
12	593	2165	115	"	[307]
14	660	2045	115	*Proteus hauseri*	[307]
$\frac{24}{25}$/14	715×604	1715	108	"	[307]
47	556	1481	85	*Proteus morganii*	[307]
9213/9211a	626	1696	137	*Proteus*	[307]
9000/9402	682	2304	148	"	[307]
7480	634	2185	126	*Proteus rettgeri*	[307]
7480	367	330	68	"	[307]

* Obtained from the State Research Institute for Veterinary Preparations, Moscow.

† Obtained from U. Taubeneck, Institute of Microbiology and Experimental Therapy, Jena, East Germany

Table 7 (continued)

Phage	Size of head, Å	Size of tail, Å		Species of host	Literature citation
		Length	Width		
7479	737	1852	85	*Proteus rettgeri*	[307]
7478/325	604	1741	115	"	[307]
7476/322	533	1600	77	"	[307]
Kappa (temperate)	600	1100	100	*Serratia marcescens*	[341]
SMB1	650	1350	—	"	[106]
SMPA	650	2250		*Serratia marcescens* *E. coli* C 3000 (F^+)	[106]
PS4	550	1700	120	*Pseudomonas syringae*	[277]
B3	520—600	1630	80	*Pseudomonas aeruginosa*	[345]
Pc	650×650	1600	110	"	[108]
Pz	650×650	1600	100	"	[108]
24	750	1500	—	*Pseudomonas marinalis*	[102]
A64/A62	750	2500	100	*Alcaligenes faecalis*	[272]
A5/A6	750	2400	90	"	[272]
8764	600	1700	110	"	[272]
Marine phage	600	860—1000		Cytophaga	[368]
Arthrobacter phage	750×630	2200	—	*Arthrobacter polychromogenes*	[138]
76*	885×600	2750—2800	100—110	*Caulobacter vibrioides*	[49]
φCb3, φCb6, φCb13	1700×500	2000—2500	100	Caulobacter	[331]
φAc20	650×700	1500	—	Asticcacaulis	[331]
St_{kaz}	780±10	4250—4350	120±10	*Caryophanon tenue*	[28]
β, B, Bh	450—500	2500	—	*Corynebacterium diphtheriae*	[278]
Rs 29†	640×650	3500—3700	110±10	"	[49]
Temperate‡	1100×500	2200	150	*Mycobacterium tuberculosis*	[49]
Polonus II	700×700	2500	105	"	[49]
HP(polonus)	850×450	1700	100	Mycobacterium	[354]
B-1	550	1400—1500	90	"	[354]
$MyF_3P/59a$	520±40	1230±110	—	"	[283]
HC	950×500	1800—1900	—	"	[365]

* Isolated by É. S. Shavina and Ya. I. Rautenshtein [70].

† Obtained from R. N. Rebrova (Ryazan'), isolated by Professor Ciuca (Rumania).

‡ Obtained from Warsaw through T. G. Chanishvili.

Table 7 (continued)

Phage	Size of head, Å	Size of tail, Å		Species of host	Literature citation
		Length	Width		
βa Temperate	580	1300—1600	80—90	*Actinomyces erithreus*	[36]
3	580	1300—1600	80—90	"	[36]
121	580	1400—1600	80—90	"	[36]
1527	580	1300—1400	80—90	"	[36]
119 *	600	1800—1850	100	*Thermoactinomyces viridis*	[49]
4 type	700×450	1500—1550	110±±10	*Actinomyces streptomycini*	[49]
MSP8	700×550	1500	100	*Streptomyces venezuelae*	[248]
MSP2	580	1610	70	"	[293]
Actinophage	810—820×620—630	1800—1950	110±±10	Actinomyces	[268]
28 ‡	550	1800—1900	100	*Streptococcus lactis*	[49]
3M	550×400	1000	90	"	[108]
187	600×600	1700—1800	120	Staphylococcus	[102, 108]
187	580	1700	—	"	[259]
77	600×600	2500	100	"	[108]
77	550	2200	—	"	[102]
77	550	2200	—	"	[259]
71	630×630	1700	100	"	[108]
71	550	1500	—	"	[259]
71	500	1500	—	"	[102]
52	550×550	1500	110	"	[108]
52	550	1600		Staphylococcus	[259]
52A	500	1500		"	[259]
P42D	550	2300		"	[102]
581	550	2400		"	[102]
b581	550	2400		"	[102]
72	550	1500		"	[102]
P52A	500	1500		"	[102]
P71	600	1500		"	[102]
3B	800×600	3000	100	"	[108]
3B	920×420	3000	75	"	[259]
6	920×400	3000	100	"	[102, 108]
6	850×550	3000	75	"	[259]
594n	960×550	3000	—	"	[102]

* Isolated by A. Kosmachev (Institute of Microbiology, Academy of Sciences of the USSR).

† Obtained from Ya. I. Rautenshtein (Institute of Microbiology, Academy of Sciences of the USSR).

‡ Obtained from L. Yu. Medvinskaya (Institute of Microbiology, Academy of Sciences of the Ukrainian SSR).

Table 7 (continued)

Phage	Size of head, Å	Size of tail, Å		Species of host	Literature citation
		Length	Width		
b^{594n}	960×550	3000	—	*Staphylococcus*	[102]
70 PTA	980×530	3000	95	"	[102]
Uranyl acetate	750×300	2800	85	"	[102]
29	580	2250	—	"	[259]
42D	560	2300	—	"	[259]
55	570	2250	—	"	[259]
75	500	2400	—	"	[259]
52A	500	1500	—	"	[259]
53	560	1700	—	"	[259]
80	580	1750	—	"	[259]
3A	900×400	3000	75	"	[259]
3C	830×400	3000	75	"	[259]
42E	780×490	3000	75	"	[259]
7	850×550	3000	75	"	[259]
47	920×500	3000	75	"	[259]
54	920×450	3000	75	"	[259]
STJ	550±10	1900—2000	70—90	*Bacillus anthracis*	[49]
VA-9 *	730—735	4000	90—95	"	[49]
D†	520—525	1700—1720	80	*Bacillus cereus*	[49]
Temperate					
A	640±50×640±40	2000±20	95±10	"	[147]
	630±30×680±30	2000±50	80±10	"	[147]
	620±30×590±40	2000±50	75±5	"	[147]
D	620±40×580±30	2155±90	75±5	"	[147]
N6P	560±20	2150±50	100±10	*Bacillus mycoides*	[49, 50]
Temperate					
N5	940—960	5300—5350	120±10	"	[49, 50]
№ 2	780±10	4250±50	120±10	"	[49, 50]
t	600—620	1700±30	70±7	*Bacillus megaterium*	[74]
α	580—600	1215±25	89±2	"	[128]
I	730	1925	75	*Bacillus thuringiensis*	[127]
II	990	5450	135	"	[127]
IV	710	1940	85	"	[127]

* Obtained from the Moldavian Institute of Epidemiology and Hygiene through E. N. Levin (Gamaleya Institute of Microbiology and Epidemiology, Academy of Medical Sciences of the USSR).

† Obtained from L. S. Khachatryan and Ya. I. Rautenshtein [71].

microscopic methods of preparation used to detect the fine structural details of biological objects were only just beginning to be developed and learned, periodicity in the tail structure of phages was not found in every case. In investigations published in 1963, after more experience with these methods, Bradley was able to demonstrate that a periodic structure also exists in the tails of those phages in which hitherto it had not been found.

This periodic structure of the tail is determined by the fact that it is formed by a helically coiled strand, which in turn consists of serially connected morphological subunits. Clear confirmation of this can be found in half disintegrated tails of N5 phage particles of *Bacillus mycoides* which I found broken up into separate fragments.

These fragments consist of turns of the helix which form the tail. It is apparent from tail fragments lying endways that they are hollow. This demonstrates that the tail is a hollow tube. Each separate turn of the helix forming the tail of this phage consists of six morphological subunits (Figs. 32a, b).

The length of the tail varies in different members of this group from 1300 to 5350 Å and its width from 70 to 120 Å.

The most characteristic feature distinguishing the phages of this group is that their tail cannot contract. Morphologically, the tails of these phages resemble some of the rod-shaped plant viruses, such as tobacco mosaic virus or beet yellows virus [211].

The tails of the different phages of this group vary in their flexibility. In all probability this is determined by the strength of the bonds between the separate morphological subunits forming the turns of the helix.

This extensive morphological group of phages with a noncontracting tail, it must be admitted, is extremely difficult to describe systematically. On the one hand, its individual members show great similarity, even though they infect different species and genera of bacteria, but, on the other hand, the shape of the head and the length of the tail and some of its structural details account for many individual structural details among the members of this group.

Phages with a long, noncontracting tail may have a prolate polyhedral head or an isometric polyhedral head. Some species of phages with a prolate head have been found among those infecting staphylococci and streptococci [102, 108, 259].

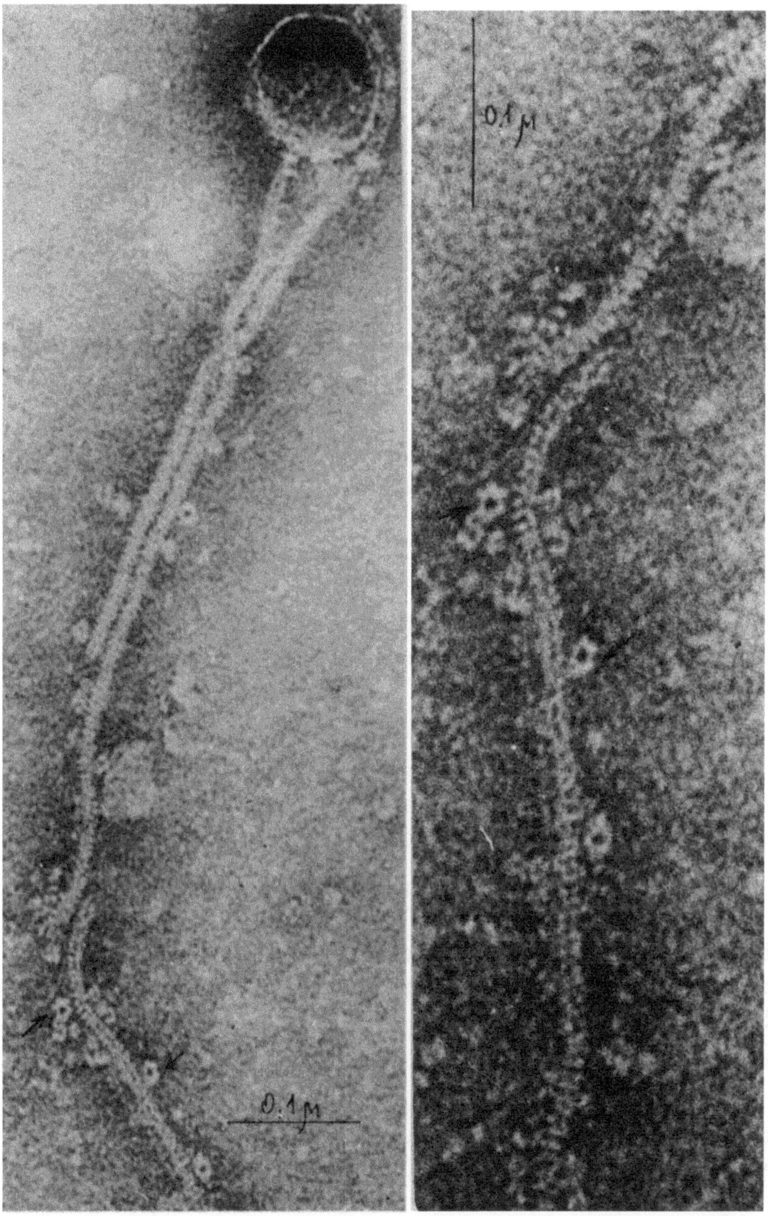

Fig. 32. Particles of phage N5 of *Bacillus mycoides*. PTA. a) Readily distinguishable helical structure of the tail. 170,000 ×; b) magnified fragment showing separate turns of the helix forming the tail, consisting of 6 morphological subunits (indicated by arrows). 250,000 ×.

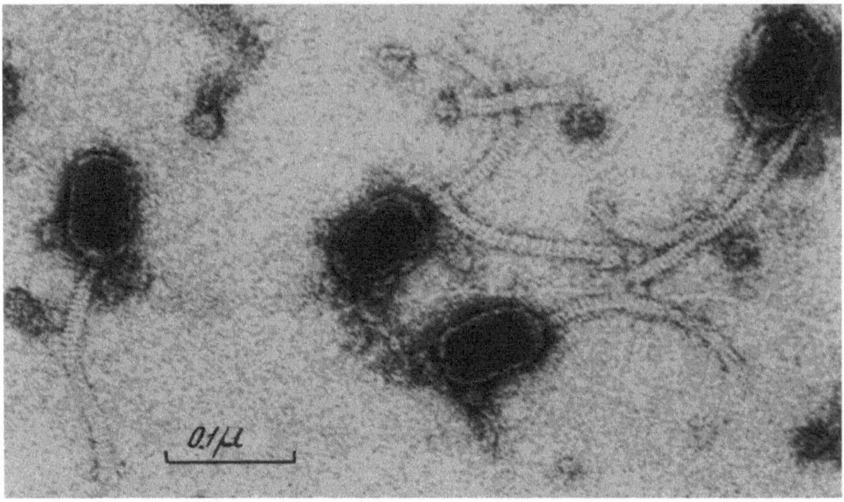

Fig. 33. Particles of phage 4 of *Actinomyces streptomycini.* Uranyl acetate. 170,000 ×.

Takeya and Amako [354] described phage HP which is active against many species of mycobacteria, and also has an elongated head.

I have studied the following phages with elongated head [49]: actinophage 4 (Rautenshtein's type II; Fig. 33), phage 76, producing lysis of *Caulobacter* (Fig. 34a, b), and phage Polonus I, active against *Mycobacterium tuberculosis* (Fig. 35a, b, c).

However, the overwhelming majority of phages of this group have an isometric polyhedral head consisting of an icosahedron or octahedron. For example, phage Polonus II, producing lysis of the same strain of *M. tuberculosis* as phage Polonus I, has an isometric polyhedral head (Fig. 36).

Among the phages of group IV, considerable variation is also seen in the structure of their end plate. However, it is sometimes difficult to determine the structure, and even the general shape of the end plate, because it is comparatively small in size and its details are easily masked. The structure at the end of the tail is evidently very delicate and its integrity can easily be disturbed during preparation of the specimens. In addition, difficulties arise in assessing the spatial configuration of the end plate because most frequently this structure is seen by the investigator in one plane.

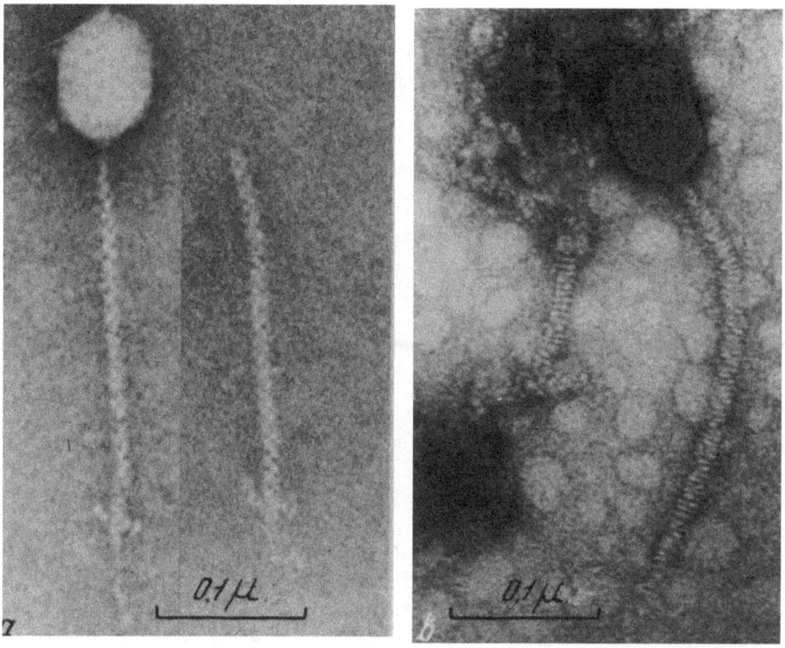

Fig. 34. Phage 76 of *Caulobacter vibrioides* 200,000×. a) PTA; b) uranyl acetate.

Takeya and Amako [354] illustrate this state of affairs using mycophage B-1 as an example and point out that the expansion at the end of the tail appears two-dimensionally as a trilobate corona. In cases when the whole surface of the end plate is visible, in this phage it is pentagonal in shape, with short projections attached to the five corners, and a central hole between them. In all probability, the central hole is the end of the tail tube.

All phages whose tail terminates in an end plate which appears two-dimensionally as a number of lobes evidently possess a structure which in cross section is either pentagonal or hexagonal in shape. This structure is formed by short or long projections joined together into an end plate. Different phages may have 5, 6, or more of these projections.

However, an end plate with lobate projections cannot be distinguished in all phages. Some phages of this group possess a tail with a tapering, conical end or a tail with no additional structures on its end. In some cases a very thin filament or several

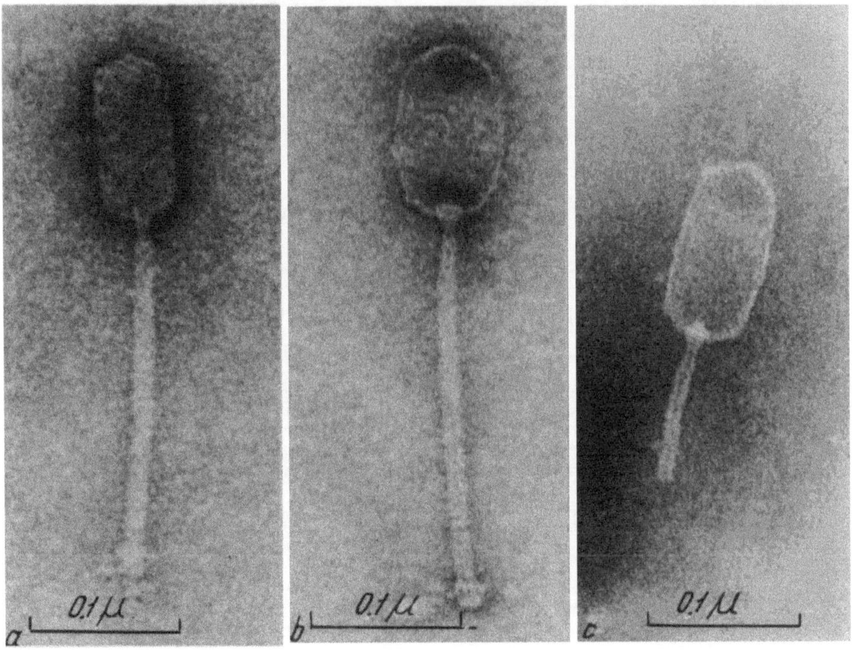

Fig. 35. Phage Polonus X of *Mycobacterium tuberculosis*. 200,000 ×. a,b) The segment of the tail near the head is narrower and consists of the inner rod. A valve-like structure can be seen inside the head. Uranyl acetate. c) Phage particle with fragment of the tail without its outer sheath. The inner valve is clearly visible at the point of attachment of the rod to the head. PTA.

such filaments analogous to those first discovered on the T-even phages, belonging to the next morphological group (group V), are attached to the end of the tail.

On the basis of structural variation observed at the end of the tail among phages of this group, I recognize three distinct types illustrated schematically in Fig. 37.

This subdivision is, of course, purely arbitrary, because in all probability it does not reflect the whole range of variations in end-plate structure existing in nature among these phages. In addition, the probability must not be forgotten that types I and II

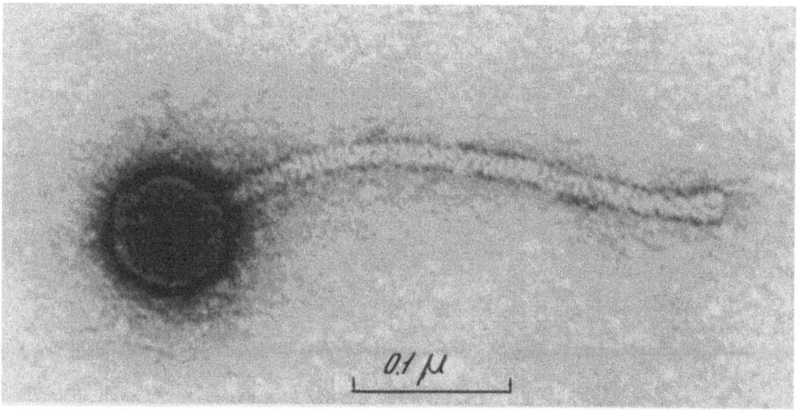

Fig. 36. Phage Polonus II of *Mycobacterium tuberculosis*. Uranyl acetate. 210,000 ×.

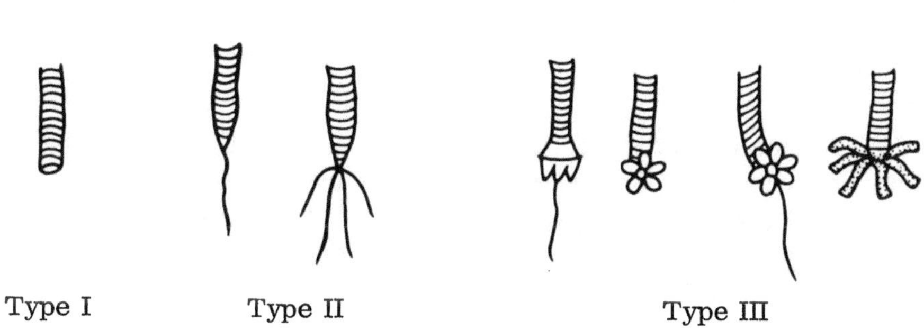

Fig. 37. Types of terminal structures of the tail of group IV phages.

(more especially type I) may arise as a results of the destruction of part or all of a type III end plate. This can be illustrated by the example of actinophage 4 of *Actinomyces streptomycini* (Fig. 33), where phage particles whose tails end in structures of types I and III can be observed simultaneously. It is assumed that the tail of actinophage 4 ends in an end plate of type III. Particles without additional structures on the end of their tail most probably appear as the result of destruction of the end plate, which is an extremely labile structure easily damaged during preparation of specimens.

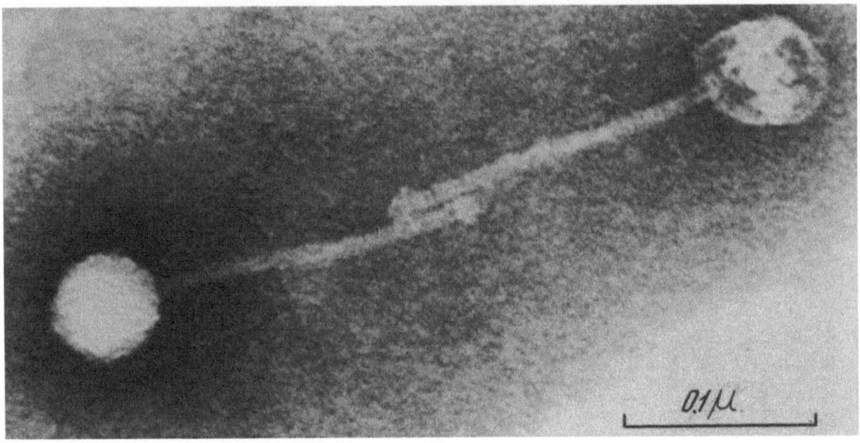

Fig. 38. Phage 28 of *Streptococcus lactis*. PTA. 260,000 ×.

STRUCTURAL VARIATION AMONG PHAGES WITH A NONCONTRACTING TAIL

Among the many phages included in this group, even though they produce lysis of different species or even genera of microorganisms, there is often a very considerable resemblance in the size of the head and in certain structural details.

Of the phages I have studied, the following were found to be identical in morphology: phage 28 of *Streptococcus lactis* (Fig. 38), temperate phage N6II of *Bacillus mycoides*, phage STI of a vaccine strain of *Bacillus anthracis* (Fig. 39), phage 2600/D52 of *Proteus mirabilis* (Fig. 40), and phage 119 of the thermophilic actinomycete *Thermoactinomyces viridis* (Fig. 41).

All these phages have an isometric polyhedral head, whose size varies within narrow limits from 520 to 650 Å. The tails of these phages are about equal in length, namely 1700–2000 Å. The capsomeres of the capsid are clearly distinguishable in some of these phages. Phages 2500/D52 have quite large capsomeres. Cross striation of the tail of these phages also is well defined, as a rule. The tail of these phages terminates in an end plate with short lobate projections (type III).

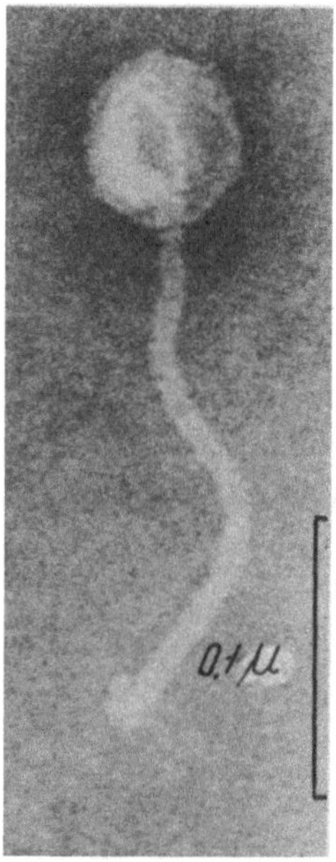

Fig. 39

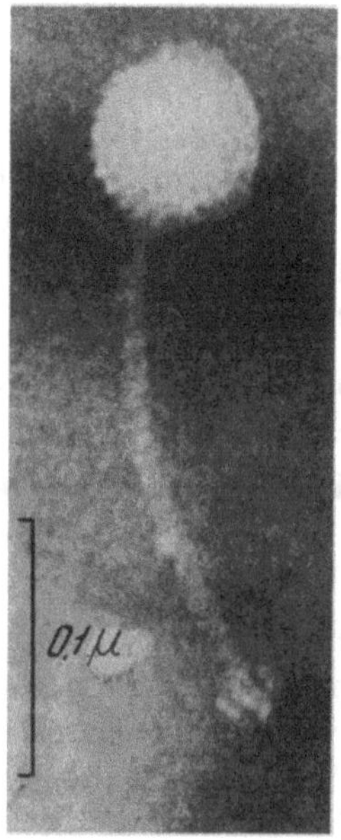

Fig. 40

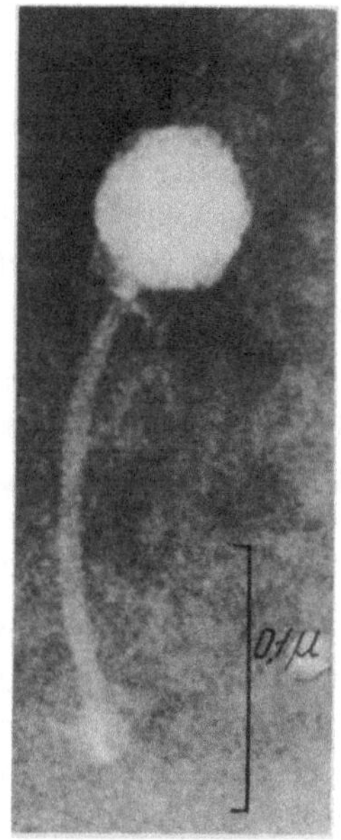

Fig. 41

Fig. 39. Phage STI of vaccine strain of *Bacillus anthracis*. PTA. 260,000×.

Fig. 40. Phage 2600/D52 of *Proteus mirabilis*. PTA. 240,000×.

Fig. 41. Phage 119 of *Thermoactinomyces viridis*. PTA. 250,000×.

Phages with this morphology have also been described by other investigators. They include the four phages A, B, C, and D of *Bacillus cereus* [147], phages 187, 77, P71, and 52 of *Staphylococcus* [102], mycophage B-1 [354], phages Pc and Pz of *Pseudomonas* [108], phage Kappa of *Serratia marcescens* [341], phage P221 of *Salmonella typhimurium* [394], temperate phages of *Bacillus stearothermophilus* [387], temperate phage 535/222a of *Lactobacillus fermenti* [243], and many others.

Some phages with an elongated head also possess an end plate of type III with short processes. These include actinophage 4 of *Actinomyces streptomycini* (Fig. 33) and phage Polonus I (Fig. 35a, b) causing lysis of *M. tuberculosis*. Another phage, Polonus II, with a head consisting of an isometric polyhedron, has the same tail structure (Fig. 36). Other actinophages infecting various species of actinomycetes are very similar to actinophage 4 in size and morphology [248, 268, 293].

Phage HP and other phages active against certain species of saprophytic mycobacteria are similar in their morphology to phage Polonus I [354, 224]. In addition, phages with a prolate head and comparatively short tail have been described by other workers for *Bacillus subtilis* [378, 379] and *Pseudomonas aeruginosa* [356].

Phage 76 of *Caulobacter vibrioides* also has a prolate head. However, the tail of this phage terminates in an end plate with long projections. If the end plate is projected on a flat surface, only two prongs can be seen. A clearly distinguishable thin filament emerges from the center of the end plate (Fig. 34a).

The same structure of the end plate was described by Slayter and co-workers [345] for phage B3 of *Pseudomonas aeruginosa*, and by Matthews and Bradley [277] for phage PS4 of *Pseudomonas syringae*, the head of which is an isometric polyhedron. These last workers consider that the tail of this phage terminates unusually. In my opinion, this structure is one variant of the shapes assumed by type III end plates.

I found a type III end plate with long hairy projections in phage BA-9 of *Bacillus anthracis* (Fig. 42) and phage Ct_{kaz} of *Caryophanon tenue* [28] (Fig. 43a, b). These phages have a large head consisting of an isometric polyhedron and an extremely long tail.

The capsid of phages Ct_{kaz} and BA-9 consists of separate capsomeres about 50-55 Å in diameter. In the capsid of phage BA-9 of *B. anthracis* (Fig. 42) the structure of the capsomeres could be distinguished more clearly. They are short hollow tubes.

The long tail of these phages is formed by a spirally coiled strand, as shown by the well-marked periodic striation. One turn of the tail helix of phage Ct_{kax} is about 30 Å in thickness and the intervals between adjoining turns of the helix are about 25 Å. The total number of turns in the tail is 100-105. At the end of the tail of phage Ct_{kaz} (Fig. 43a) an end plate with six long projections resembling tentacles can be clearly distinguished.

As mentioned previously, the structure of the end plate is very delicate and it can easily be destroyed during preparation of specimens. In phage BA-9 the number of projections attached to

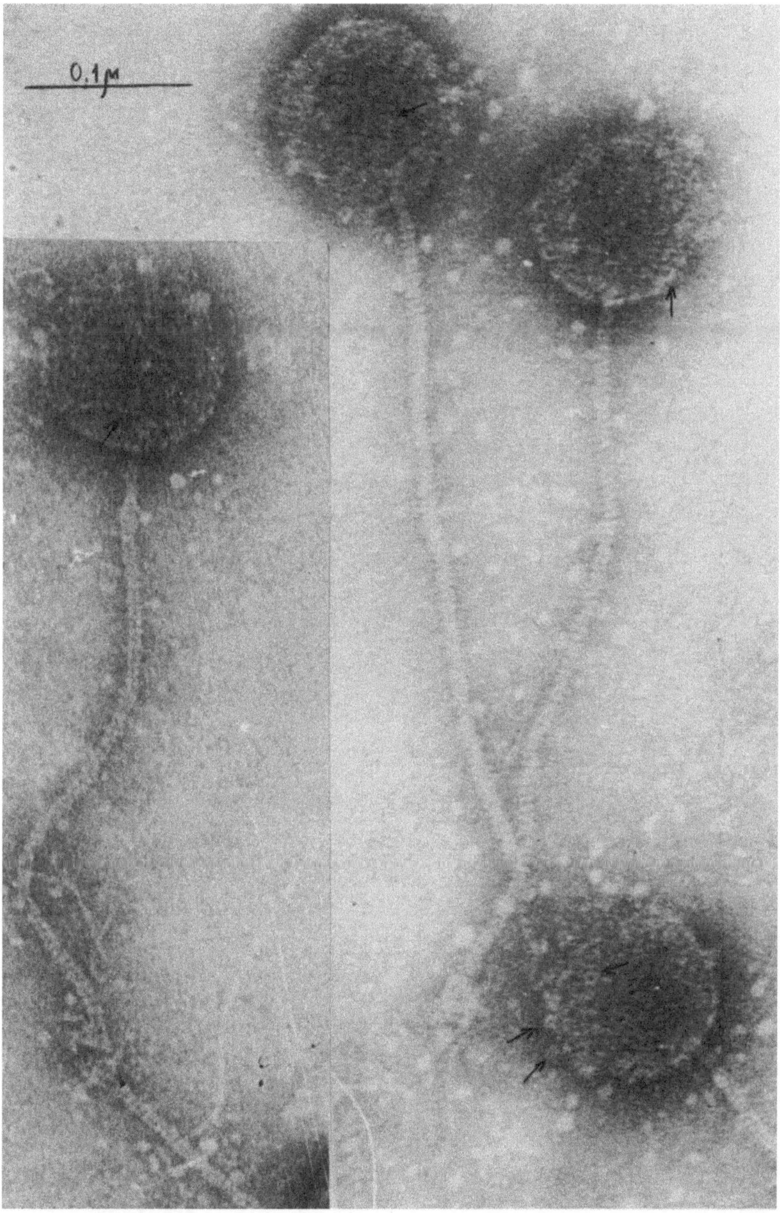

Fig. 42. Phage VA-9 of *Bacillus anthracis*. Capsomeres of the capsid are indicated by arrows. 200,000 ×.

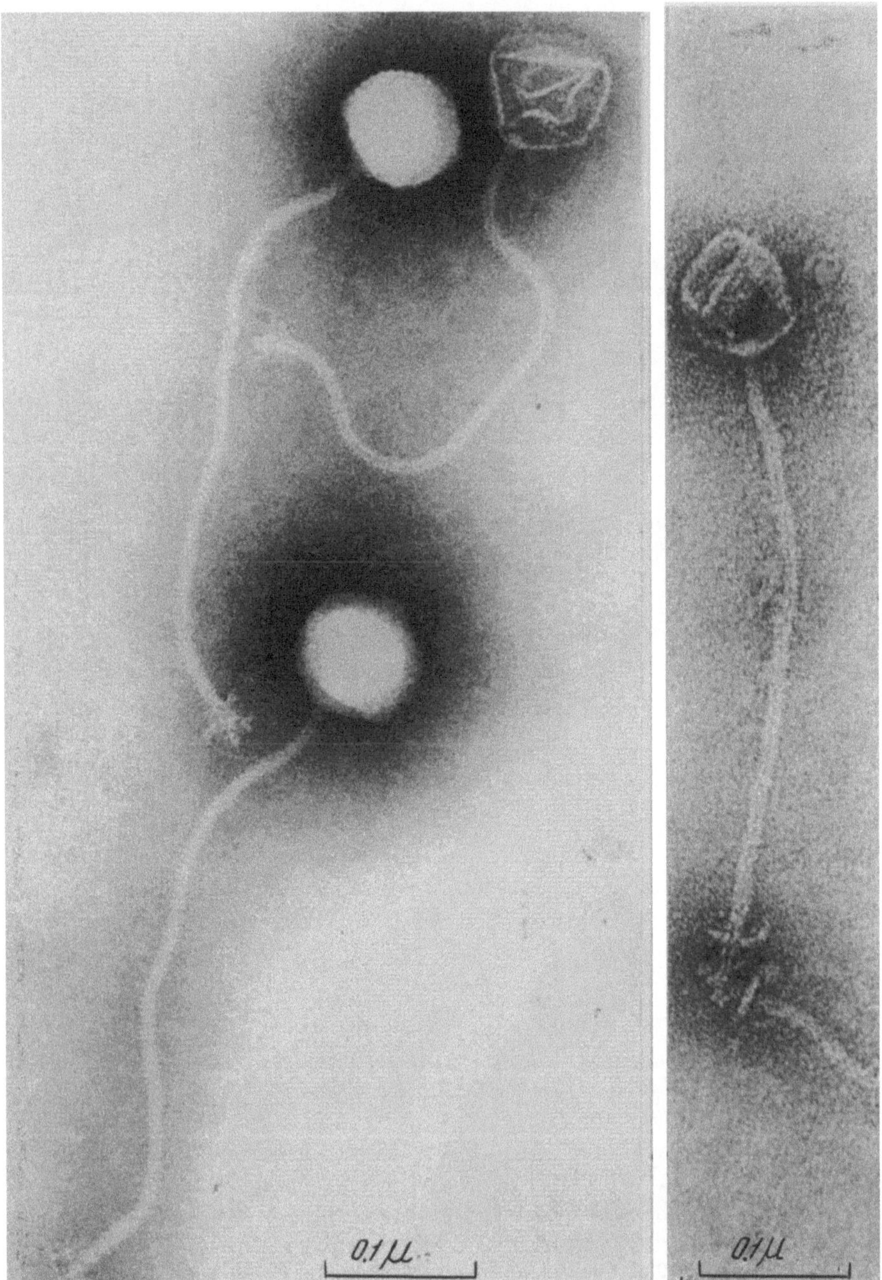

Fig. 43. Phage Ct_{kaz} of *Caryophanon tenue*. 200,000 ×. a) PTA; b) uranyl acetate.

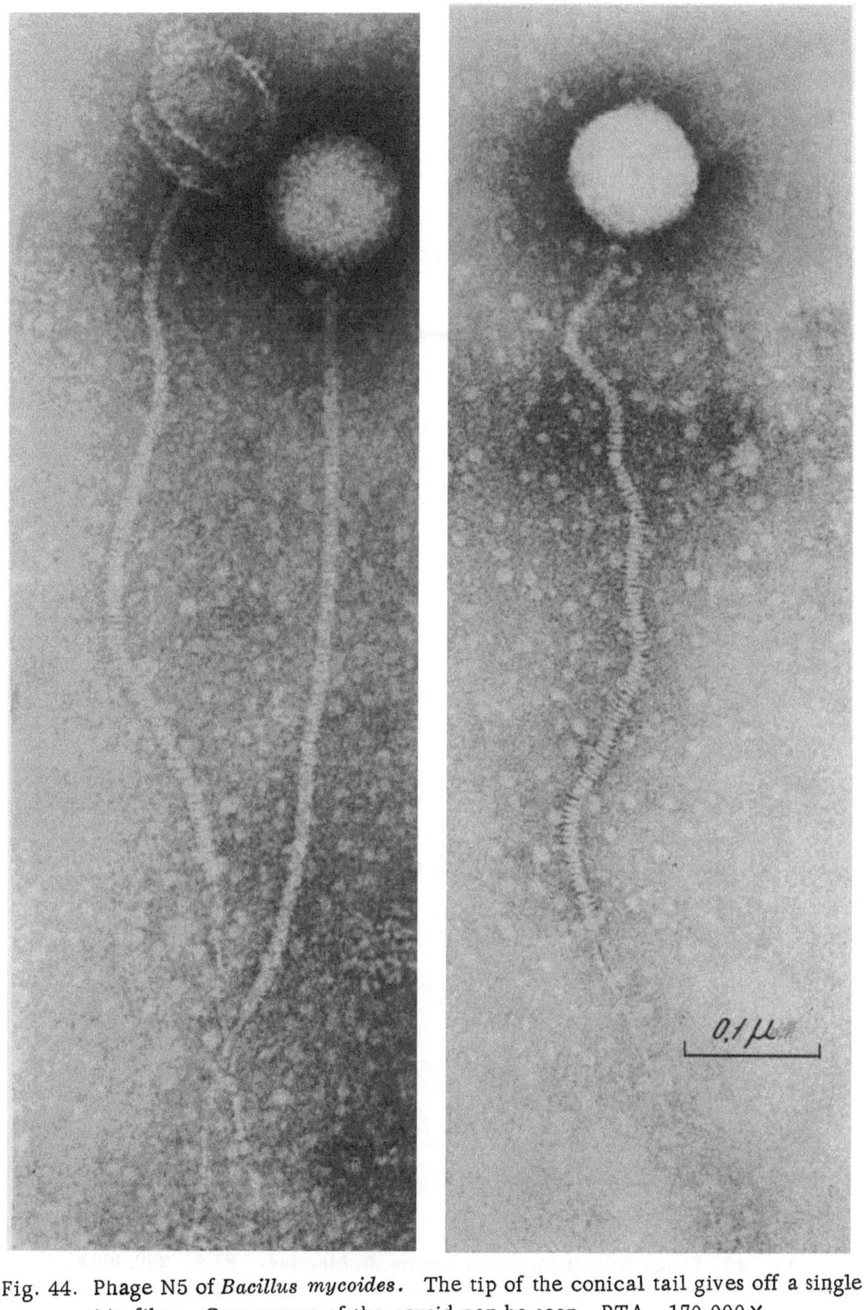

Fig. 44. Phage N5 of *Bacillus mycoides*. The tip of the conical tail gives off a single thin fiber. Capsomeres of the capsid can be seen. PTA. 170,000×.

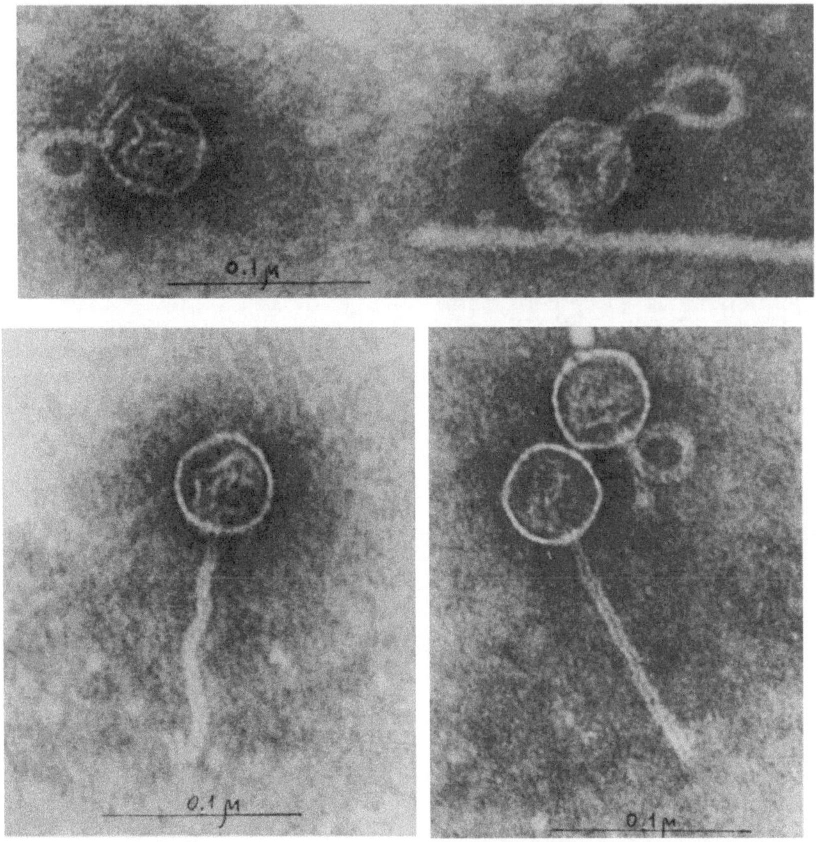

Fig. 45. Phage 886 of *Aerobacter aerogenes*. A condensation can be seen at the point of attachment of the tail to the head. PTA. 270,000×.

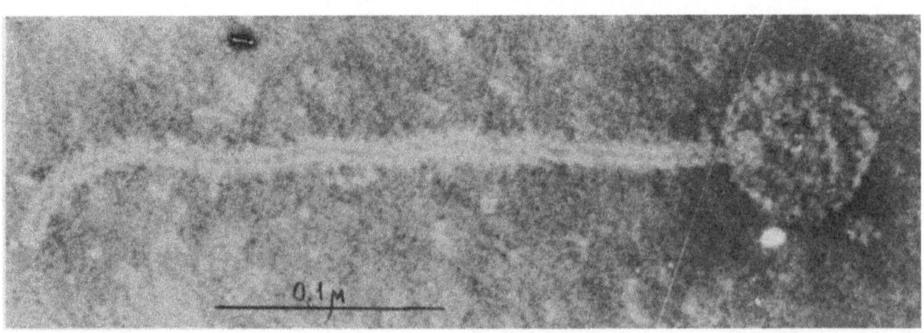

Fig. 46. Phage R_S29 of *Corynebacterium diphtheriae*. PTA. 260,000×.

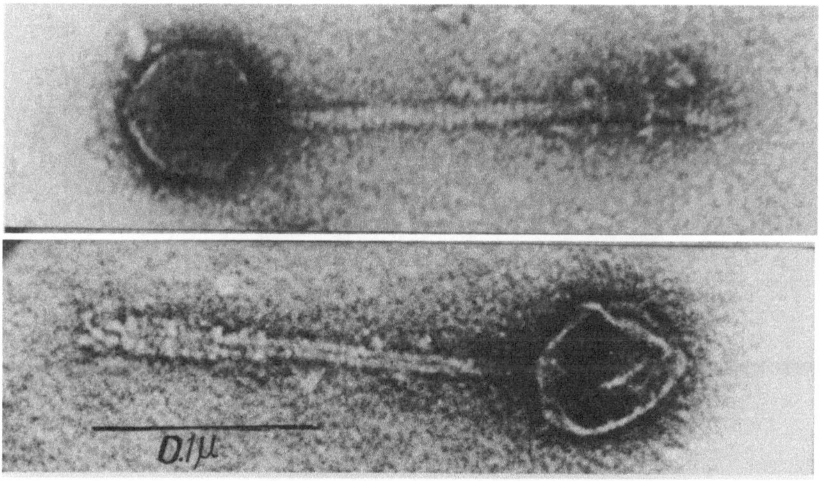

Fig. 47. Phage D of *Bacillus cereus* with ring-like structures on the distal end of the tail. Uranyl acetate. 300,000 ×.

the end plate is more difficult to determine than in phage Ct_{kaz}. The degree of lability of the end plate obviously differs from one phage to another, and the degree of its preservation also depends on the substance used for contrasting.

For example, if phage Ct_{kaz} is stained with uranyl acetate, two projections can be seen on the end plate (Fig. 43b), while if PTA is used, six can be seen (Fig. 43a). It is also possible that the end plate of phage 76 of *Caulobacter* has more than the two projections visible after contrasting with PTA (Fig. 34a). However, if this phage is stained with uranyl acetate, the end plate is completely destroyed (Fig. 34b).

An end plate of hexagonal shape when seen endways, with six fairly long projections, has been found on several different types of phages producing lysis of staphylococci and streptococci [108]. Bradley calls end plates of this structure "anchor-shaped."

Tails tapering to a cone at the end (type II), to which one thin filament is attached, were found in my examination of phages No. 2 and N5 of *B. mycoides* (Fig. 44). In the size and fine structure of the head and tail these phages are similar to phage Ct_{kaz}, but they differ from it in the terminal structure of the tail.

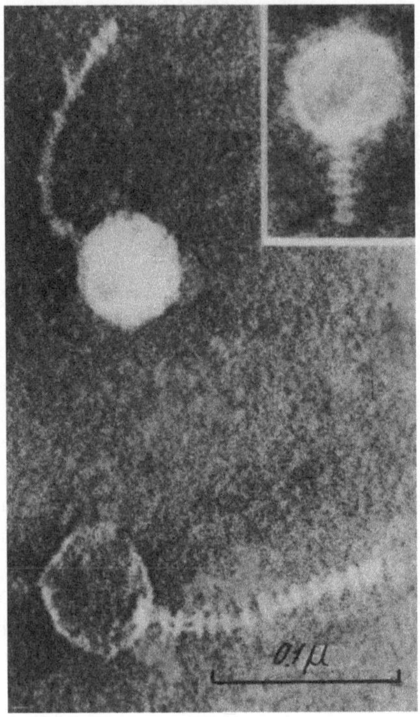

Fig. 48. Temperate phage Za of *Actinomyces erythreus* with ring-like structure of its tail. PTA. 240,000 ×.

A terminal structure of the tail like that of phages No. 2 and N5 of *B. mycoides* have been found for coli phages T5, C1, F1 type SBL (β 4, γ 2, 3000), ZG/3A, and λ for phage 24 of *Pseudomonas* [101, 102, 103], and for several phages of *Proteus* [307]. One or more thin filaments are attached to the end of the conical tail of these phages.

Phages whose tail has no additional structures on its end (type I) are identified as follows: VII, producing lysis of the coli–dysentery group of bacteria, phage T1 of *E. coli* B, and phage 886 of *Aerobacter aerogenes* similar to it in size and morphology (Fig. 45), diphtheria phage Pc 29 (Fig. 46), phage D of *B. cereus* (Fig. 47), and one temperate phage, 3a (Fig. 48), and three virulent phages, 3, 121, and 1527 (Fig. 49), producing lysis of *Actinomyces erythreus* [36].

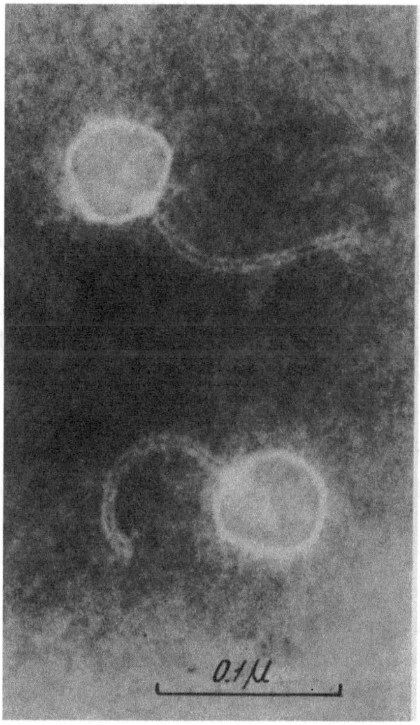

Fig. 49. Virulent phage 1527 of *Actinomyces erythreus* with a smooth tail. PTA. 240,000×.

Many phages described by different workers have a tail of the same structure.

To complete the morphological description of the characteristics of this group of phages, so complicated for systematic classification, the unusual structural details which I found on the tails of some phages must be mentioned. Rautenshtein, myself and Retinskaya [36] discovered that the tail of temperate phage 3a of *A. erythreus* and phage D of *B. cereus* possesses accessory structures in the form of wider transverse rings, projecting considerably beyond the margin of the tail.

The shape and size of the head and tail of temperate phage 3a (Fig. 48) are identical with those of virulent phages 3, 121, and 1527 of *Actinomyces erythreus* (Fig. 49). However, in its fine structure, the tail of temperature phage 3a differs from that of the virulent phages. The tail of the temperate phage throughout its length possesses transverse rings dividing it into segments (Fig. 48). The diameter of these rings is 130 Å, much greater than the diameter of the main tube of the tail which is 80-90 Å. The number of transverse rings on the tail differs for different phage particles. On the particles with the longest tails there are 13-15. The segments of the tail formed by the transverse rings are easily broken, and phage particles can be seen in the specimens with a very short tail (Fig. 48). The rings are evidently connected to the outer layer of the tail tube, but when they are destroyed the tube remains intact (Fig. 48). The tail of these particles resembles that of the virulent phages (Fig. 49).

Phage D of *B. cereus* (Fig. 47) also has wide transverse rings, 3-4 in number, on its tail. They are situated nearer its distal end and their diameter is greater than that of the main tube of the tail. The role and importance of these rings are not yet known. Possibly the discovery of even finer details in the structure of the phage particle in the future will help to elucidate the relationship between the shape of a phage and the character of its specific interaction with the host cell.

Despite some individual differences in structure between the phages described above, it can thus be seen that their noncontracting tail is a hollow tube of constant diameter throughout its length, formed by a spirally coiled strand consisting of morphological subunits.

I found a tail of slightly different structure on phage Polonus I of *Mycobacterium tuberculosis*, which can also be included among the group of phages with a noncontracting tail. However, the short segment of the tail of this phage directly connected to the head is narrower (75 Å) than the rest of the tail (150 Å) (Fig. 35a, b). The narrower part resembles the inner rod and the wider part the outer sheath of the tail of the phages of group V, the structure of which will be described in the next chapter. The impression is thus formed that the tail of phage Polonus I consists of an outer and an inner structure. After destruction of the outer sheath, it can be seen that the narrower part is in fact the inner hollow rod, passing along the whole length of the tail (Fig. 35c).

These observations suggest the existence of transitional forms of tail between noncontracting and contracting. The tail of phage Polonus I is evidently one of these transitional forms, because in the structure of its tail it resembles the phages of morphological group V with an outer sheath capable of contracting and an inner rod, while because of the inability of its sheath to contract it must be classed with the phages with a noncontracting tail.

Inside the head of nearly all phages of morphological group IV is an electron-dense plate with the appearance of a valve, located at the point of attachment of the tail. It is clearly visible in phages which have lost their DNA (Figs. 33, 35b, c, 38, 43a, 44b, 45, 46, 47, 48, 49).

The phages of this group thus show considerable structural variation, manifested mainly in the fine details of their tail structure. It must be assumed that these individual structural features determine the specificity of different phages relative to a particular type of bacteria. Incidentally, many phages of this group are temperate.

Chapter 6

Phages with a Tail Possessing a Contractile Sheath (Group V)

The most characteristic feature of the phages of group V is the structural organization of their tails which is quite different from that of other phages.

The phages belonging to this group consist of a head which may be of different sizes and shapes, and a powerful tail, terminating as a rule in a well-defined end plate of complex structure. The end plate of nearly all these phages gives off long, thin fibers.

The dimensions of the phages of group V are given in Table 8. The tail consists of an outer sheath and an inner hollow rod. The tail sheath may exist in two different states: stretched, characteristic of the intact particle, and contracted. During contraction the tail sheath becomes shorter and wider, thereby exposing the inner rod. A change in the state of the tail sheath is accompanied by a change in its size, ultrastructure, and, sometimes, its shape, although the volume of the sheath remains constant irrespective of its state [44, 111].

The contractility of the tail sheath is evidence of the existence of an elementary contractile organ even in the simplest representatives of the biological kingdom.

More detailed information on the properties of the contractile proteins of phages will be examined in Chapter 9.

Table 8. Dimensions of the Virion of Phages with a Contractile Tail Sheath (in A)

Phage	Dimensions of head	Normal tail			Contracted sheath		Width of end plate	Species of host	Literature citation
		length	width	width of end plate	length	width			
T	1000×700 (950×650)	1100 (1000)	250	—	—	—	70	*E. coli* B	[110, 111]
T2	1100±50×800±50	1150—1250	190±10	230±20	400±50	250±30	70	"	[49]
T2	950×650	1150	200	200×360	—	—	80	"	[228]
T4	—	—	160—170	—	380—400	260—270	—	"	[234]
T4	850×1150	950	180	220	380	260	80	"	[233]
T-even	950—1050×600—800	1100—1150	160—175	200—250×300—350	330—350	200—300	75—80	"	[213]
DD VI *	1100—1200×850—860	1250—1350	180±10	230±20	—	—	80	Coli-dysentery typhoid	[49]
108/106 †	840×1100	1400	170	—	—	—	—	*Thermoactinomyces viridis*	[49]
3T	900×650	950	150	—	—	—	60	Coli-typhoid	[108]
C4	1100×750	1000	200	—	—	—	70	"	[108]
11F	900×650	920	150	—	—	—	60	"	[108]
66F	900×700	950	150	—	—	—	—	"	[103]
α1	Similar to T4	—	—	—	—	—	—	"	[101]
66t	Similar to T4	—	—	—	—	—	—	"	[101]
PST	950×1260	1150	250	—	—	—	—	Pasteurella	[246]
2	720×660	1100	220	—	—	—	100	Coli-typhoid	[108]

Vi1	950×900	1100	180	—	—	—	—	"	[108]
E1	800	1100	—	—	—	—	—	*E. coli, S. typhi*	[101]
ϕ2	800	1100	—	—	—	—	—	"	[101]
PK, PK_{vir}	480×520	1040—1100	150 170	—	380—420	160—180	60—70	*Shigella sonnei*	[222]
P1 large	900	2200	200	+	950	300	100	*S. typhimurium*	[81]
P1 small	650	2200	200	+	950	300	100	"	[81]
P2	680	1400	180	—	550	250	100	*Salmonella typhimurium*	[81]
9/0 ‡	1100—1200×800—820	1300—1400	180±10	230±20	560±30	250±20	70—80	*Proteus vulgaris*	[49]
13_{vir}	600	1019	167	—	—	—	60	*Proteus hauseri*	[307]
78	611	889	163	—	—	—	60	"	[307]
67b	589	981	174	—	—	—	74	"	[307]
57	619	882	178	—	—	—	56	"	[307]
50	970×670	1252	159	—	—	—	52	*Proteus morganii*	[307]
5845	1022×763	1252	156	—	—	—	74	"	[307]
9266	1193×822	2152	248	—	—	—	96	*Proteus*	[307]
8893	926×741	1296	178	—	—	—	74	*Proteus rettgeri*	[307]
12s	800	1000	—	—	—	—	—	*P. syringae*	[102]

* Obtained from T. G. Chanishvili (Research Institute of Vaccines and Sera, Tbilisi).

† Obtained from A. Kosmachev (Institute of Microbiology, Academy of Sciences of the USSR).

‡ Obtained from the Mechnikov Research Institute of Vaccines and Sera, Moscow.

Table 8 (continued)

Phage	Dimensions of head	Normal tail			Contracted sheath		Width of end plate	Species of host	Literature citation
		length	width	width of end plate	length	width			
E79	660	1500	170	—	620	250	75	*P. aeruginoza*	[345]
F116	580—700	790	80	—	—	—	—	"	[345]
6C	650	1250	140	+	410	190	60—70	*P. syringae*	[90]
SM2	1350	1700	—	—	—	—	—	*Serratia marcescens*	[277]
SM2	1100	1900	—	—	—	—	—	"	[106]
SMP	1350	2350	275	—	—	—	100	"	[106]
SMP5	570	1250	—	—	—	—	—	"	[106]
SMB3	570	1250	—	—	—	—	—	"	[106]
Phage Saprospira	1100—1200	1150—1450	220	100—400	—	—	—	*Saprospira grandis*	[261]
Twort	1040—1060	2000	170	600×230	975	300	74	Staphylococcus (Twort)	(373, 374)
Twort, 3K, 119, 130, 131, 200	750	1900	100	—	1000	180	—	Staphylococcus	[259]
1623*	900±50	2250—2350	180±20	290	900±50	290±20	90±10	*Staphilicoccus aureus*	[49]
P2, P3, P4, P8, P9, P10†	910±30	2400±50	190±20	270±20	1050—1100	310±20	90±10	"	[49]
RZL‡	900±50	2000—2100	200±10	240	900±50	310±20	80—90	*Streptococcus lactis*	[49]
№ 1	810	2000	140—170	180	900	200	75	*Bacillus mycoides*	[44]

№1M	330	2000	140—170	—	--	200	—	"	[53]
H17 N17 large	810—850	2000	180—200	250	1000	210	70—80	"	[50]
H17 N17 small	340	2000	180—200	250	1000	210	70—80	"	[50]
H19	950	2600	150	250	1650	210	70—80	"	[50]
μ	400	2200	200	—	—	—	75	*Bacillus subtilis*	[219]
GA-2	350	2100	—	—	—	—	90	"	[105]
phi	450	2000	180—200	—	1100	250	75	"	[3]
AR1	850	1300	150—180	—	700	200	80	"	[3]
AR2	950	1800	150—200	—	1100	200	80	"	[3]
AR3	900	1800	150—200	—	1100	250	80	"	[3]
AR9	1500	2700	370	370	1200	510	140	"	[5,6]
GF-2	1150	2800	—	—	—	—	—	"	[105]
SP3	1150×1100	2890	220	290×360	1500	240	100	"	[158]
SP8	1000	1650	200	850	700	260—300	80	"	[143]
SP50	920	2100	—	—	—	—	—	"	[157]
PBS1	1200	2000	220	400	910	—	90	"	[156]
SP50	1000	2300	—	—	—	—	—	"	[304]
III	905	2320	165	—	1210	245	80	*Bacillus thuringiensis*	[127]
A6	900	1100	160	—	—	—	—	*Alcaligenes faecalis*	[272]
A11/A79	650	1300	190	—	—	—	—	"	[272]
MX-1	750	1100	—	—	—	—	50	*Myxococcus xanthus*	[114]

* Obtained from the Tarasevich State Scienticic Control Institute, Moscow.

† Obtained from V. A. Soboleva (Research Institute of Vaccines and Sera, Tbilisi).

‡ Obtained from L. Yu. Medvinskaya (Institute of Microbiology, Academy of Sciences of the Ukrainian SSR).

The tail sheath of all phages of this morphological group does not cover the whole rod, but leaves part of it at the head end exposed. The sheath is thus not joined directly to the head, but is fixed above to the rod. The other end of the sheath terminates in the end plate.

The inner rod of the tail is a hollow tube of rigid structure. When the sheath contracts, as a rule the end plate is drawn upward along with it. In some cases it remains attached to the end of the inner rod.

In my opinion, the end plate of the tail is chiefly connected to the sheath. However, it also has a connection with the rod maintaining the sheath in a stretched state. If the end plate remains attached to the end of the rod when the sheath contracts, evidently an artificial rupture of the connection between the end plate and the sheath must take place as a result of the action of certain chemical or physical agents on the phages. Winkler and co-workers [392], for example, showed that after irradiation of phage T4 with ultraviolet light at 235 mμ, the end plate of many particles with a contracted sheath remains attached to the rod. Anderson and Stephens [84] observed a similar arrangement of the end plate after treating phage T6 with a dilute alkaline solution. These workers also noted that under the action of alkali the contracted tail sheath splits up into separate fragments. These observations are clear evidence of rupture of the connections not only between the sheath and the end plate, but also within the structure of the sheath itself.

The components listed above do not exhaust the structural complexity of the phages of this group. Additional structures have been found on some members, in the form of a collar or sleeve at the point of attachment of the rod to the head [44, 49, 81] and also an outer tail sheath formed of very thin filaments radiating from the end plate and attached to the collar on the rod [139]. However, a collar-like structure has also been discovered on phages with a noncontracting tail [103].

Most phages of group V contain double-stranded DNA, accounting for about 50% of the entire virion. All phages with this type of structural organization can be assumed to have double-stranded DNA.

Typical members of this morphological group are the T-even

phages of *E. coli* B, which are widely known and have received the most study.

A distinguishing feature of the DNA of the T-even phages is that instead of cytosine it contains hydroxymethylcytosine. The DNA of the T-even phages consists of a single giant molecule with a molecular weight of $130 \cdot 10^6$ Dalton [115, 118, 146, 319]. The DNA of phage Sp 50 of *Bacillus subtilis* also has a high molecular weight ($1 \cdot 10^8$) [172]. The molecular weight of the DNA of these phages is much greater than that of the DNA of phages with a simpler tail organization. For example, the molecular weight of DNA of phage T5, one of the T series of *E. coli* belonging to the group of phages with a noncontracting tail, is $66 \cdot 10^6$, and the length of its molecule is $34 \pm 1.7\mu$ [177]. According to measurements obtained by different workers, the length of the DNA molecule of the temperate phage λ, which also has a noncontracting tail, is 16.5 μ; 17.2 ± 0.9 μ; 16.3 μ [120, 269, 313], or approximately half the length of the DNA molecule of phage T5. This may perhaps be explained by the incomplete structure of phage λ, which is temperate in character. The length of the DNA molecule of phage T3, which has a short tail, is 14 ± 0.6 μ [92], whereas the length of the DNA molecule of phage s_d, also with a short tail, but with a well-defined end plate and inner rod, is 36μ, according to Kiselev and co-workers [21]. The length of the DNA molecule of phage T2 is 50μ, measured on electron micrographs [242].

The high molecular weight of the DNA of the group V phages can be thought of as necessary for transmitting the large volume of information required for replication of the more complex structure of these phages.

Depending on the shape of their head, phages with a contractile tail sheath can be divided into two groups: those with a regular, isometric polyhedral head and those with an elongated head consisting of a prolate polyhedron, such as is characteristic of the T-even phages of *E. coli* B.

The T-even phages of *E. coli* B and other phages active against nonsporebearing bacteria and actinomycetes have a head shaped like a prolate polyhedron. Among them may be mentioned the coli — dysentery phage DDVI, phage 9/0 of *Proteus vulgaris* and phage 108/106 of the thermophilic actinomycete *Thermo-*

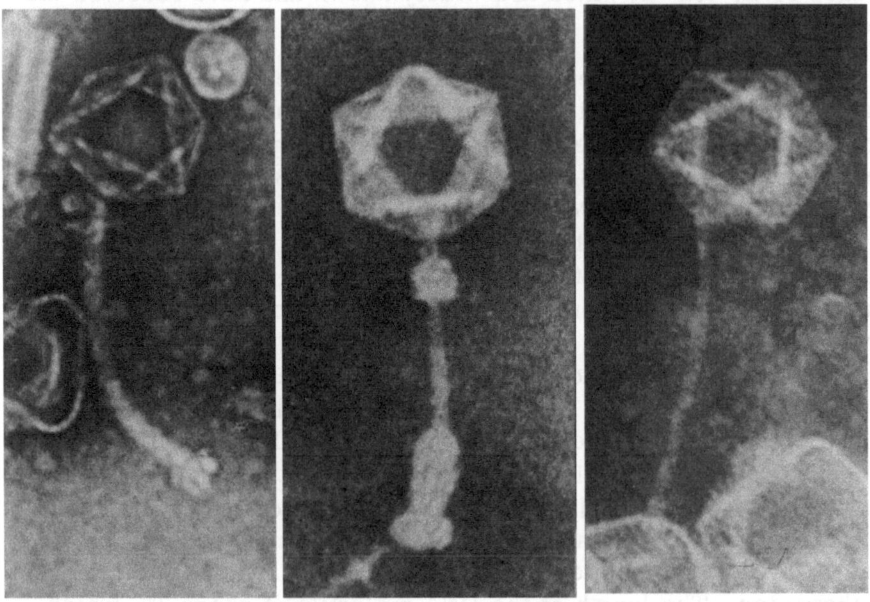

Fig. 50. Empty capsids of phage No. 1 of *Bacillus mycoides* with clearly distinguishable sides of an octahedron.

actinomyces viridis which I have studied, phages of the coli — typhoid group (II, C4, I, 66t) described by Bradley [102, 108], and phage PST of *Pasteurella pseudotuberculosis* [246]. All these phages show great similarity to the T-even phages not only in the shape of their head, but also in the structure and shape of their tail, which is shorter than the tails of the other phages of this group and is completely straight. Phage PST of *Pasteurella* resembles the T-even phages not only in its morphology, but also in its ability to produce lysis of several strains of the coli — dysentery group.

Many phages of this group have a head shaped like an isometric polyhedron. As mentioned above, establishment of the precise geometric shape of the phage head is a difficult task, because two-dimensionally phage heads of both icosahedral and octahedral shape can give a hexagonal outline. To solve this problem it is necessary to compare many phage particles whose heads lie in the same plane but in different positions. The most valuable information for this purpose can be obtained by studying the head outline of phages which have lost their internal contents.

It will be clear from the example of phage No. 1 of *B. mycoides* that its empty heads clearly reveal the sides of an octahedron (Fig. 50). Although Caspar and Klug [124] in their theoretical derivation of the geometric shape of spherical viruses consider that the icosahedron is the most rational shape and, therefore, the most realistic one, experimental data obtained by studying the shape of phage heads have conclusively shown that some are octahedral in shape with a 4:3:2 symmetry. These include phage No. 1 of *B. mycoides* [44, 49], coli phages ϕ2, E1, and C1 [101], phage 12S of *Pseudomonas syringae* [102], phages E79 and F116 of *Pseudomonas aeruginosa* phage SM2 of *Serratia marcescens* [345], and many others.

Many of the phages of this group, for example SP3 [158], SP8 [143], and SP50 [157] of *B. subtilis*, have an icosahedral head with 5:3:2 symmetry.

Phages with an isometric polyhedral head have been found for different species of cocci and sporebearing and nonsporebearing bacteria. They include phages No. 1, N17, and N19 of *B. mycoides* studied by myself, staphylococcal phages P2, P3, P4, P8, P9, P10, and 1623 phage RZh of *Streptococcus lactis*, phages AR1, AR2, AR3 of *B. subtilis* [3, 44, 49, 50, 51, 53, 55, 363], phages SP3, SP8, and SP50 of *B. subtilis* [143, 157, 158], phage Twort of staphylococcus (Twort) [259, 374], and many phages active against nonsporebearing bacteria [90, 101, 102, 222, 261, 345].

The tail of intact particles of these phages can be either slightly curved or straight. The tail sheath of some phages is uneven in width, and somewhat narrower when closer to the head than toward its end, giving it the shape of a truncated cone. The sheath of other phages is straight throughout its length and cylindrical in shape. The tail of these phages terminates in a well-marked end plate with projections. Sometimes the end plate projects considerably beyond the diameter of the tail.

Elongated heads have not yet been found among phages infecting cocci and sporebearing bacteria.

The possibility has not been ruled out that the slight structural variation of the tail among phages of group V is determined by the structural and chemical organization of receptor sites of the host cell.

A description of the ultrastructure of individual phages of this group is given below.

Phage T2

A typical representative of phages with a contractile tail sheath and an elongated head is phage T2 of *E. coli* B.

The study of the structure of this phage goes back for many years, and it is still being continued intensively. The ability of the phage tail to contract was first demonstrated in fact on phage T2.

The earliest electron-microscopic investigations showed that the head of phage T2 is a bipyramidal hexagonal prism [379]. It was subsequently shown [230] that the head of the T-even phages is shaped like a prolate polyhedron with symmetry 5 : 3 : 2.

It was shown by treatment with hydrogen peroxide, zinc cyanide, or by the action of gentle heat or freezing and thawing, that the outer cover of the tail can shorten and can move nearer to the head, thereby exposing the thin inner rod [231, 390, 251, 252]. Similar changes in the tail were observed by Kellenberger and Arber [231] after interaction between phage particles and isolated bacterial cell membranes.

By the negative contrasting method, the structure of phage T2 could be studied in greater detail [20, 110, 111, 167].

In addition to work carried out by other investigators, I established the shape of the capsomeres in the capsid of phage T2 [49], which can be distinguished in empty heads. The capsomeres are hollow structures, hexagonal in shape and about 60 Å in diameter, and, in turn they consist of six smaller structural units (Fig. 51).

Cummings [135] considers that the capsomeres in the head of phage T2 are ellipsoidal in shape and measure 270 × 19 Å. However, capsomeres of this shape have never been found.

The tail of phage T2 is a complex structure consisting of an outer sheath inside which runs a thin hollow tube, the rod. The sheath is cylindrical in shape and is formed from a spirally coiled strand, which consists of separate morphological subunits. The turns of the helix forming the sheath can be seen as transverse bands on photomicrographs. On the stretched sheath of phage T2, about 24 of these transverse bands (turns) can be counted (Fig. 52).

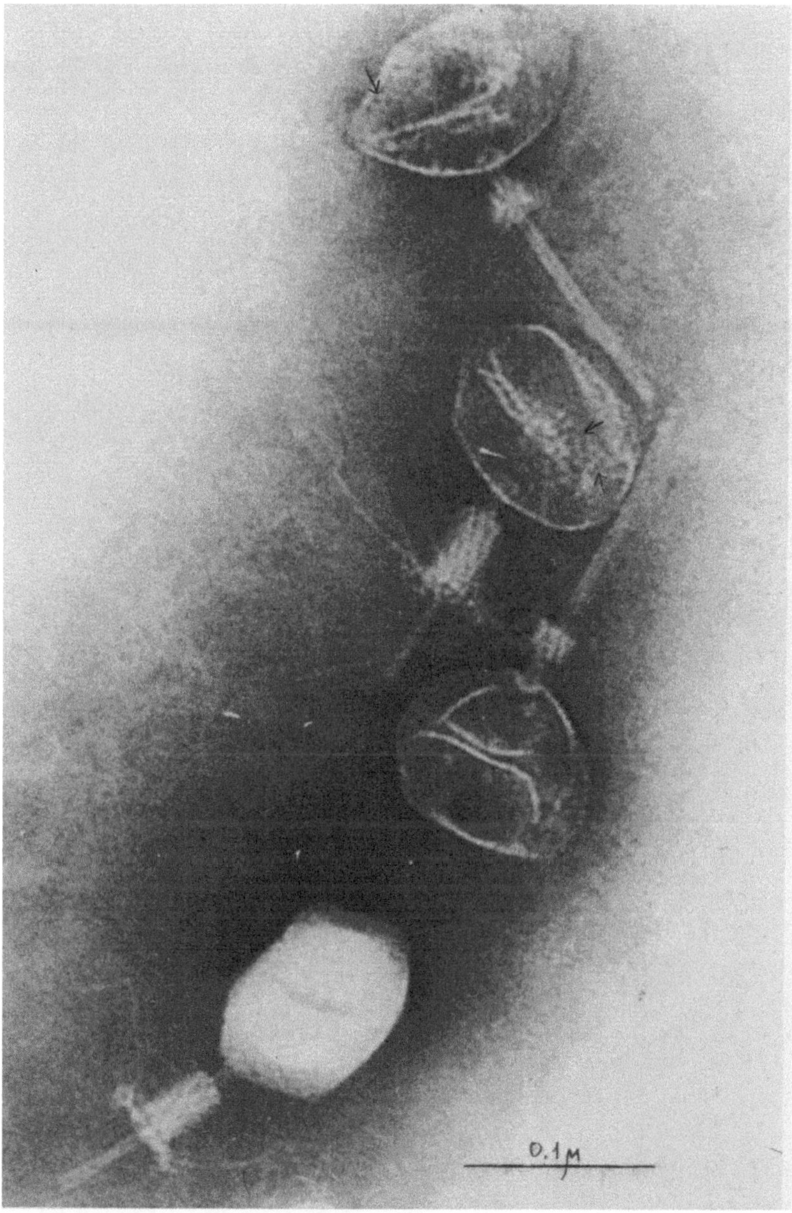

Fig. 51. Phage T2, treated with urea, with a contracted tail sheath. Capsomeres of the capsid, with the appearance of hollow short hexagonal tubes, indicated by arrows. PTA. 260,000×.

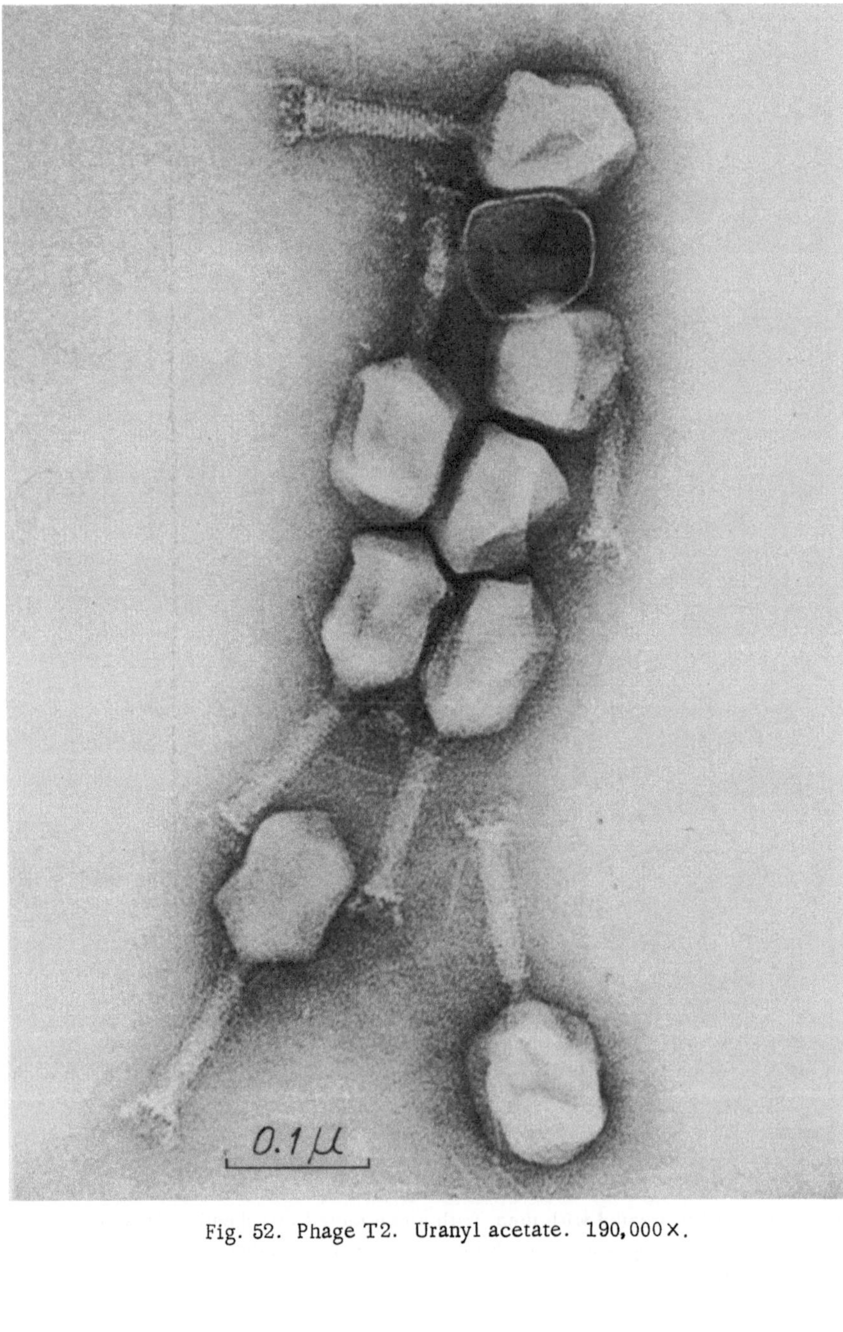

Fig. 52. Phage T2. Uranyl acetate. 190,000×.

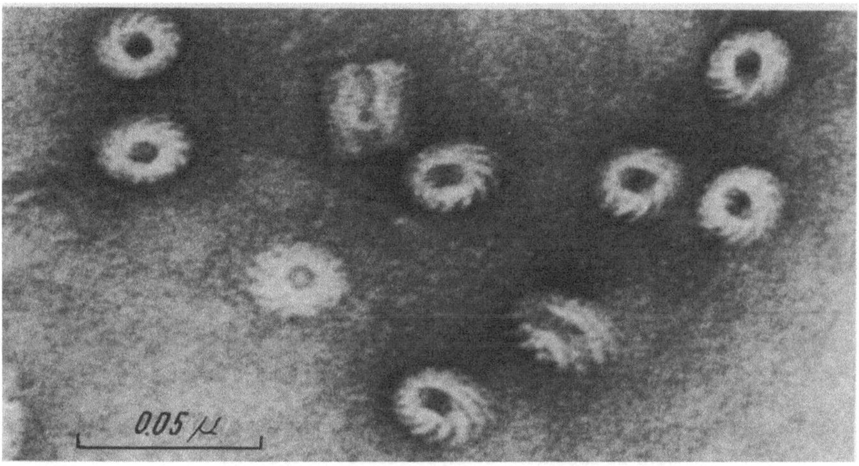

Fig. 53. Isolated contracted tail sheath of phage T2 with clearly distinguishable elongated subunits. PTA. 430,000 ×.

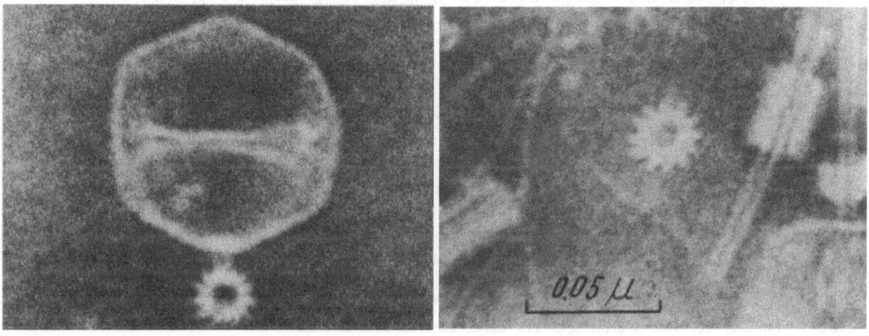

Fig. 54. Contracted tail sheaths of phage T2 lying on its end, with 12 subunits. PTA. 310,000 ×.

The same number of transverse bands was found by Kiselev and Poglazov [20]. As it contracts, the tail sheath widens and shortens by about half, but still retains its periodic cross striation. In this case only half as many transverse bands can be counted (10-12, Fig. 51). The morphological subunits are also clearly distinguishable in the contracted tail sheath. As the sheath changes from the stretched to the contracted state, the diameter of each turn of the helix is increased. Whereas one turn of the stretched sheath, ac-

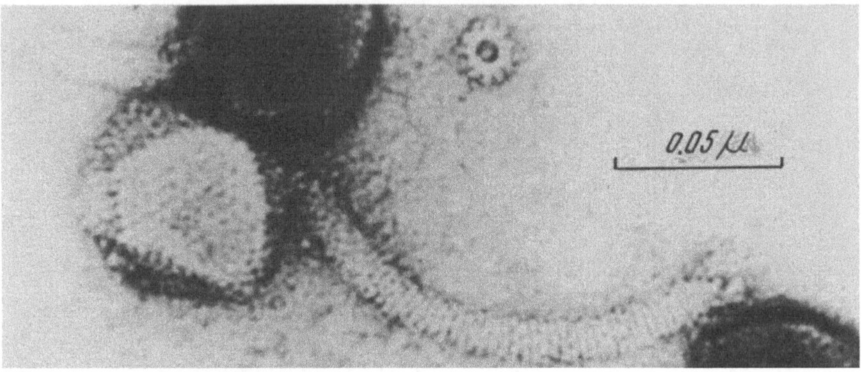

Fig. 55. Contracted tail sheath of phage No. 1 of *Bacillus mycoides*, lying on its end, with 12 subunits. Uranyl acetate. 400,000×.

cording to optical diffraction measurements, is composed of six morphological subunits [82], there are 12 such units in each turn of the contracted sheath. The 12 subunits composing one turn of the contracted sheath of phage T2 are clearly visible when the sheath lies endways (Figs. 53 and 54).

One turn of the helix in the tail sheath of phage No. 1 of *B. mycoides* when contracted also contains 12 subunits (Fig. 55).

Kiselev and Poglazov [20] also consider that in each turn of the contracted sheath of phage T2 there are 12 elongated morphological subunits. According to Brenner and co-workers [111], their number is 12-15. It thus follows that during contraction of the sheath there is no change in the total number of morphological subunits. The total volume of the sheath likewise remains unchanged in the transition from a stretched to a contracted state [111].

Several investigators consider that when the sheath changes from a stretched to a contracted state, changes take place in the conformation of the subunits [32, 61, 82, 234]. Morphologically, the subunits of the contracted sheath appear narrower and longer (Fig. 53).

The helical nature of the phage tail sheath is clearly illustrated by the structures found by Poglazov and the author [32] during partial degradation of normal phage particles. The structures which they found represent the uncoiled strand of the tail sheath (Fig. 56a, b, c). The last turn of the helix, consisting of 12 morphological units, can be seen in these figures.

The stretched helices of the tail sheath of phages T2 and T4 have been described by Brenner and co-workers [111] and by Kellenberger and Boy de la Tour [234].

The tail of phage T2 terminates in an end plate which gives off thin filaments (Fig. 57). In side view, the end plate has the appearance of a trident (Fig. 52). The work of Fernandez-Moran [167] and my own investigations [49] showed that seen from the end, the end plate looks like a round nut with a hole in the center. Six spinous projections, ending in long, thin, filaments, radiate symmetrically from it (Fig. 58).

In all probability the end plate is connected to the last turn of the tail helix and to the end of the rod. Partial destruction of the end plate, which can be produced in different ways, both physiologically and artificially, free it from its connection with the rod, and, if the sheath is in a stretched state, it begins to contract drawing the end plate after it. According to some investigators [20, 29], this action is stepwise in character, like cocking a gun. Nobody has yet returned a contracted sheath into the stretched state.

I consider that the process of contraction of the tail sheath must take place in stages, but that the time occupied by the sheath in contracting is very short. For this reason, the probability of finding intermediate stages of contraction of the sheath is very slight, so that the tail as a rule is observed in either the stretched or the contracted state. The suggestion that the tail sheath of T-even phages may change successively from the stretched to the contracted state was put forward by Anderson and Krimm [82] on the basis of their study of optical diffraction.

I have recorded an intermediate state of contraction of the tail sheath in other phages [51], 364]. This question will be examined more closely below.

The tail rod of phage T2 is a hollow rigid tube joining the head directly with the tail. The rod is built of separate, but tightly packed small subunits, which can sometimes be distinguished (Fig. 51).

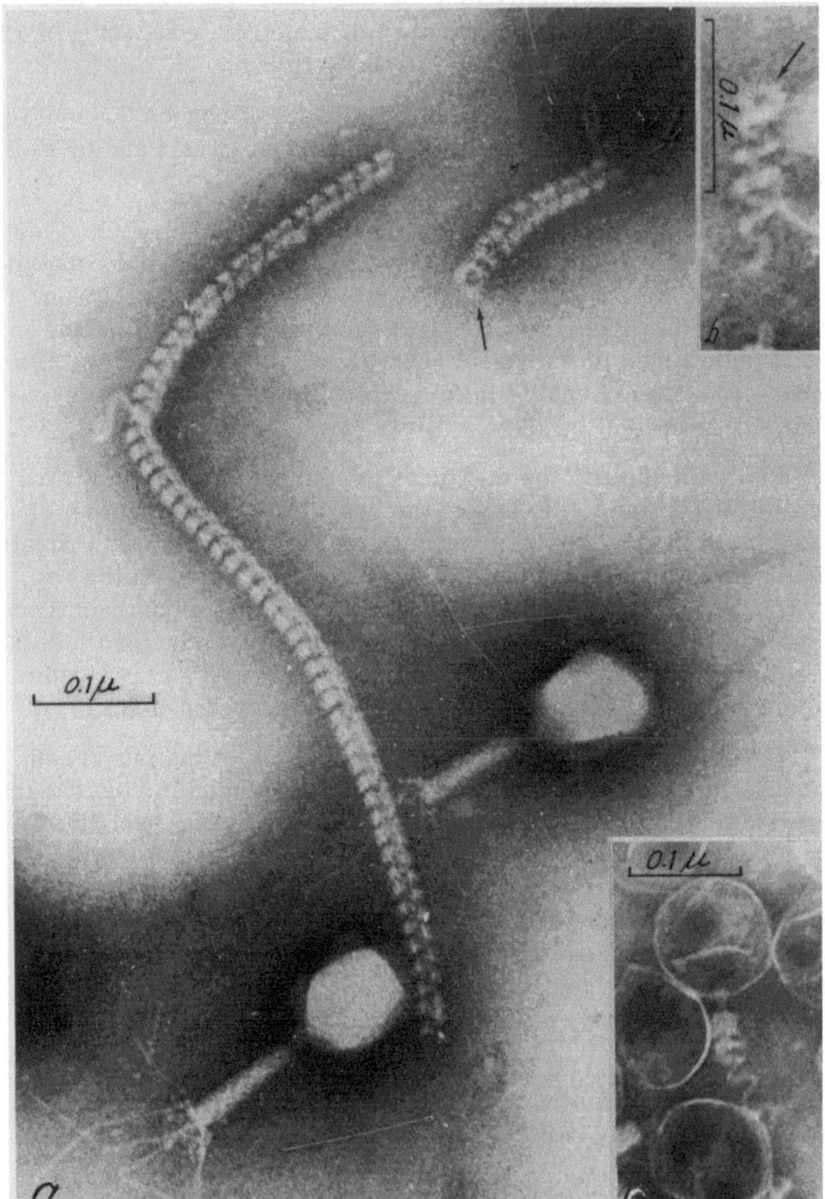

Fig. 56. Phage T2 with stretched strand forming the tail sheath. The turns of the helix consist of morphological subunits (indicated by arrows). PTA. a) 160,000×; b) 240,000×; c) 160,000×.

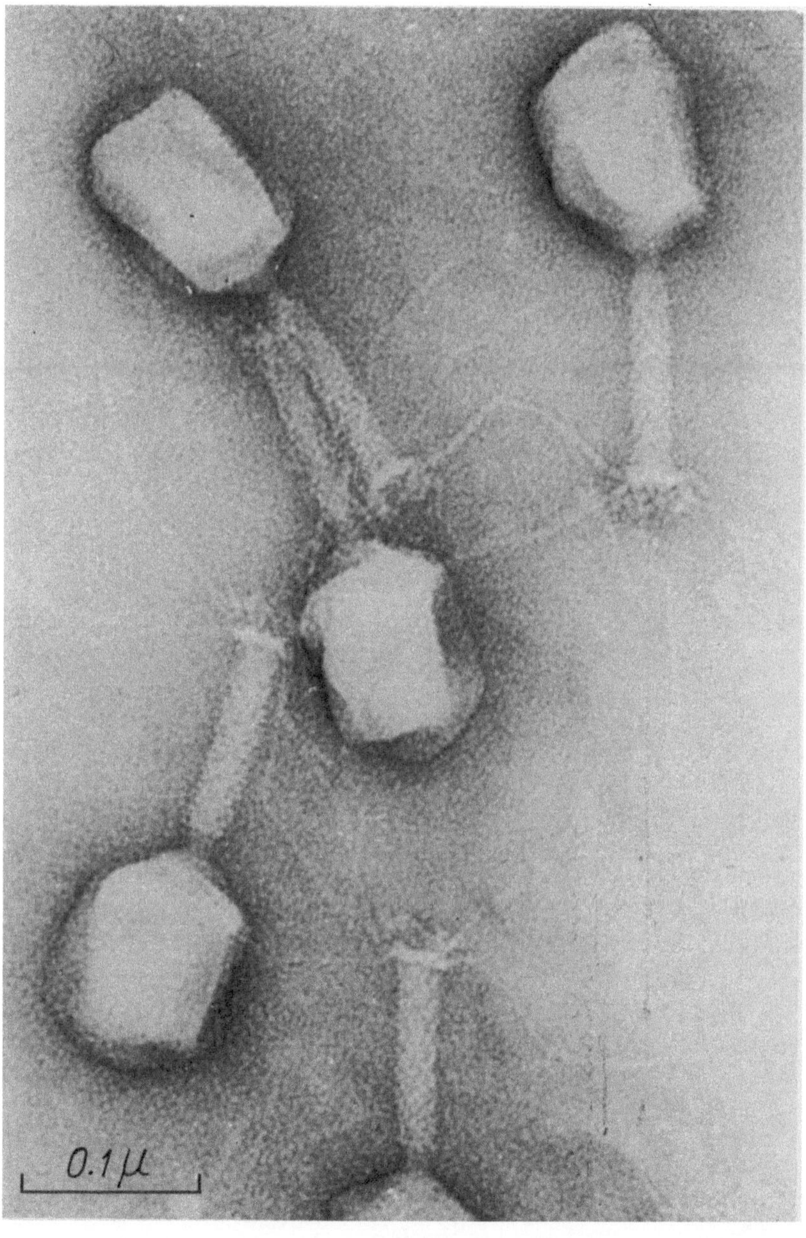

Fig. 57. Particles of phage T2 with clearly distinguishable tail fibers. Uranyl acetate. 250,000×.

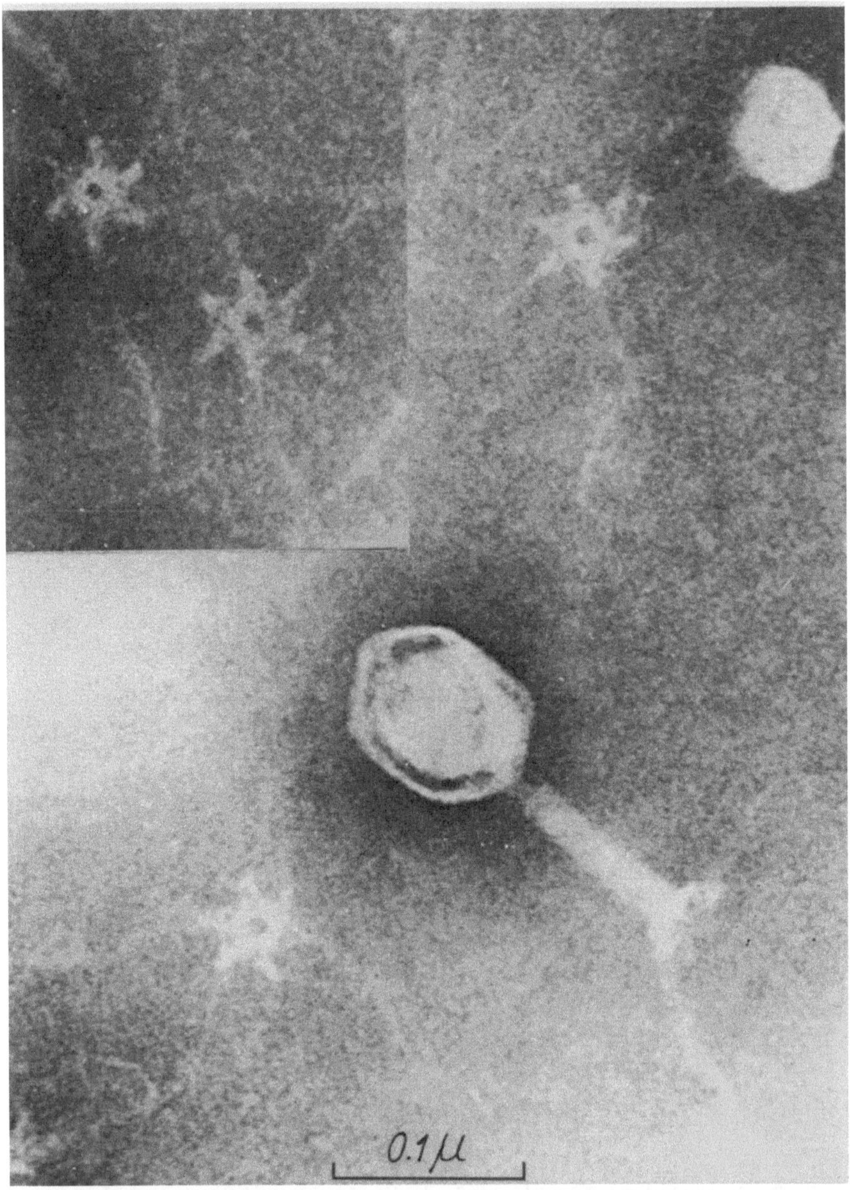

Fig. 58. End plate of phage T2. Negative staining of the phage particle with PTA at pH 10. 240,000×.

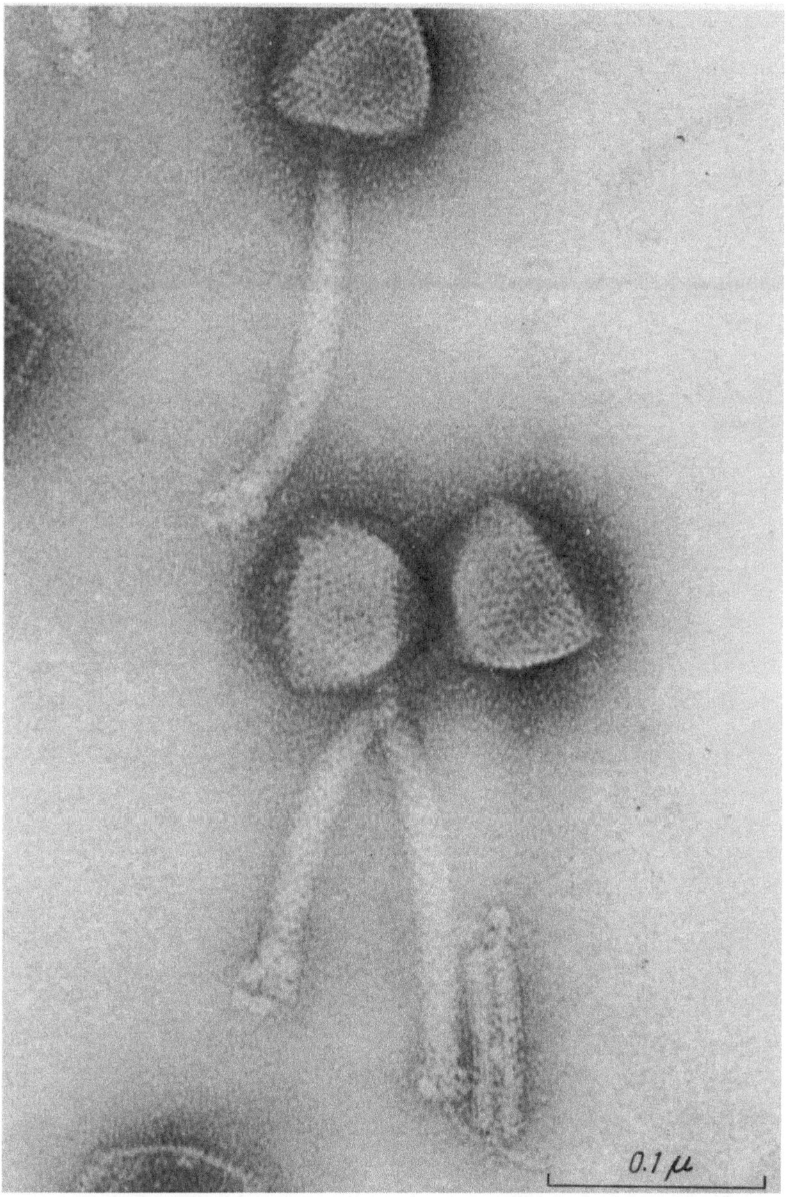

Fig. 59. Particles of phage No. 1 of *Bacillus mycoides* with clearly distinguishable capsomeres in the capsid. Uranyl acetate. 280,000 ×.

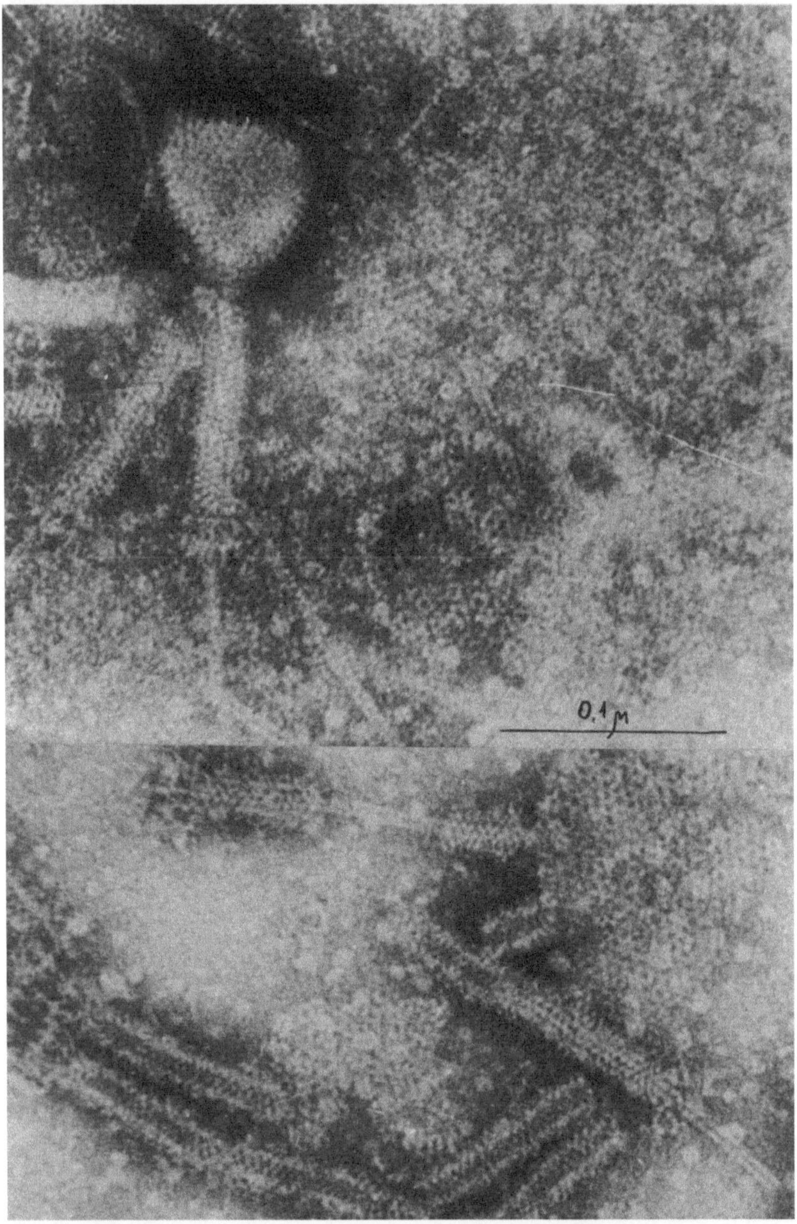

Fig. 60. Phage No. 1 of *Bacillus mycoides*, disintegrated by freezing and thawing three times. Capsomeres of the destroyed capsid, and tail sheaths and rods in various stages of fragmentation can be seen. PTA. 300,000×.

Coli — dysentery phage DDVI, phage 9/0 of *Proteus vulgaris* and phage 108/106 of *Thermoactinomyces viridis*, which I have studied, have the same shape and particle structure as phage T2.

Phage No. 1 of *Bacillus mycoides*

Phages causing lysis of bacilli and cocci are rather different in their morphology. A current feature of these phages is that thus far only particles having a head shaped like an isometric polyhedron have been described among them. A typical member of the phages of this morphological group is phage No. 1 of *B. mycoides*, the fine structural details of which have been studied by the author [44, 49].

The head of phage No. 1 is an octahedron. As a rule, on a flat surface, it lies on one side of the octahedron, so that in projection the head is usually hexagonal in shape. In some cases all sides of the octahedron are visible (Fig. 50).

The head capsid is formed from readily distinguishable capsomeres. On each side of the octahedron, the capsomeres are arranged in accordance with the rule of the greatest packing density of spheres on a flat surface. They form a characteristic hexagonal pattern, i.e., one capsomere is surrounded by six neighbors (Fig. 59). Similar results were obtained by Vainshtein and Kiselev [9] when they studied the structure of phage No. 1.

In a closer study of the capsid, I established the shape and structure of the individual capsomeres. They are short hollow tubes, hexagonal in shape, consisting of structural units. These structural units are easily distinguishable in individual capsomeres when the head capsid is ruptured. Examination of isolated capsomeres shows that most of them are composed of 6 structural units. More rarely capsomeres are found which are formed of four structural units (Fig. 60). The impression is sometimes obtained that the capsomeres are pentagonal in shape. However, because the capsid of phage No. 1 is octahedral in shape, it is to be expected that the capsomeres forming the sides of the octahedron will be built of six structural units, whereas the apex of the octahedron is formed by tetrahedral capsomeres. The presence of pentagonal capsomeres can, in all probability, be explained either by damage to the capsomere structure during preparation of the specimen or by inadequate resolution of the fine details of their structure.

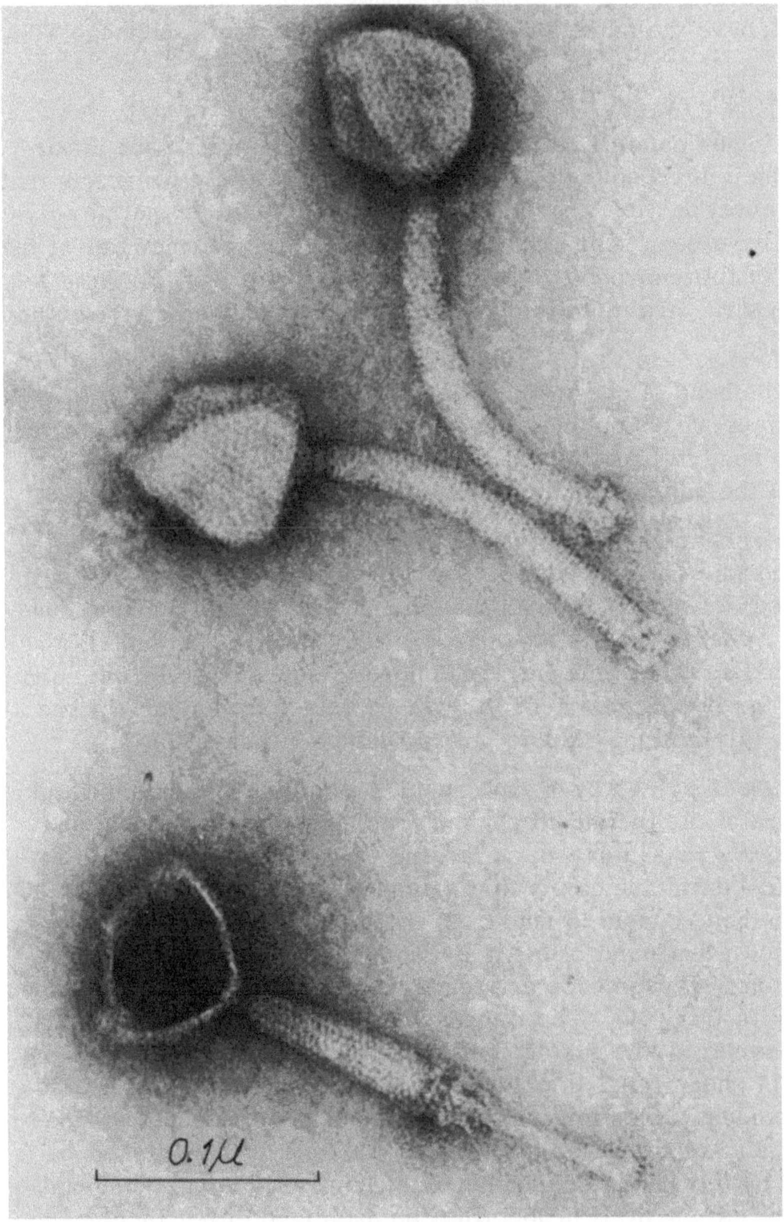

Fig. 61. Particles of phage No. 1 with stretched and contracted tail sheath. Uranyl acetate. 300,000 ×.

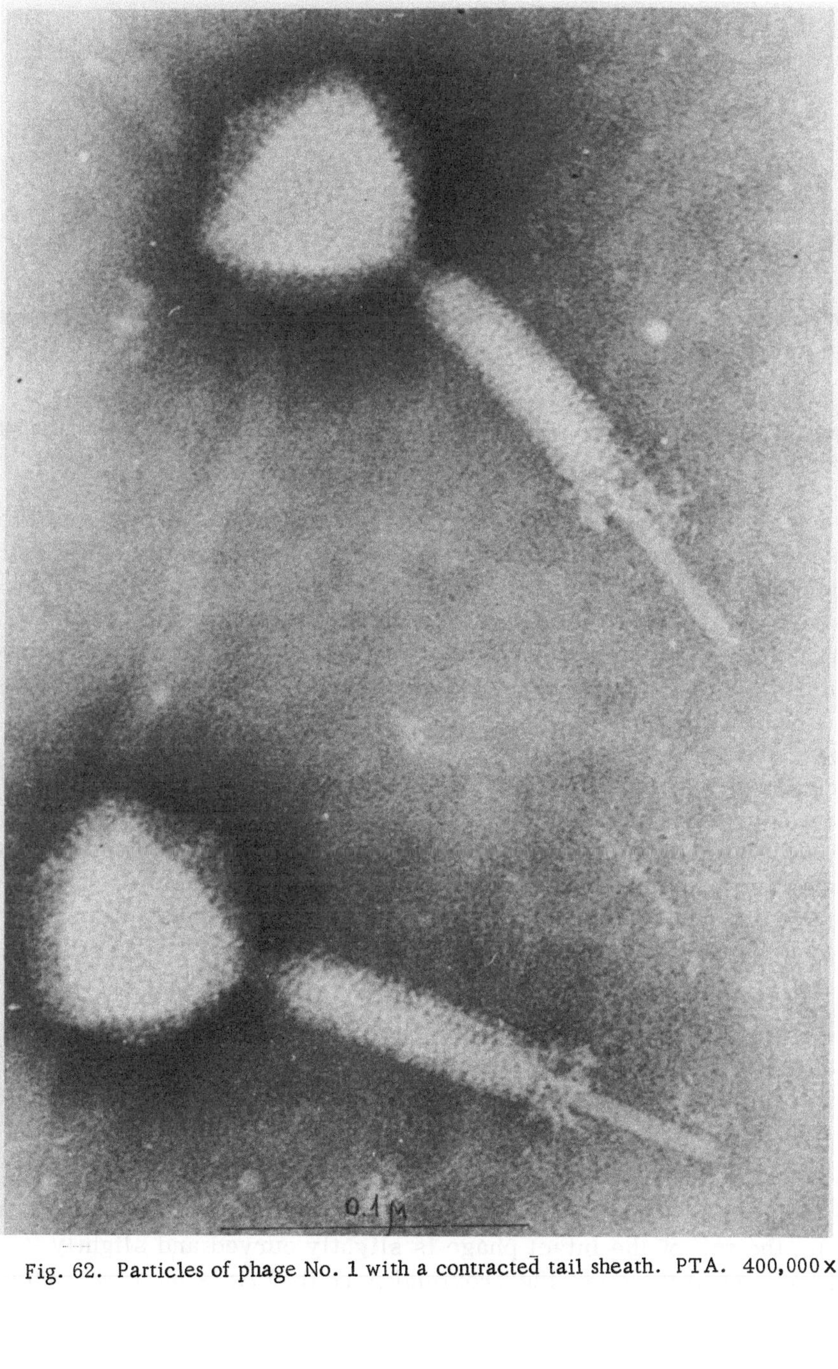

Fig. 62. Particles of phage No. 1 with a contracted tail sheath. PTA. 400,000×.

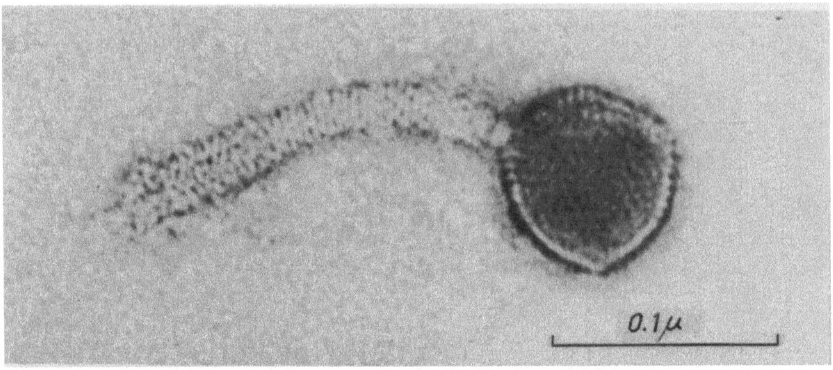

Fig. 63. Particle of phage No. 1 of *Bacillus mycoides* with semicontracted tail sheath (the distal part of the sheath is contracted, the proximal part stretched). Uranyl acetate. 260,000 ×.

Direct counting of the capsomeres on one half-surface of the head of phage No. 1 (four sides) gave a mean value of 446, i.e. 892 subunits for the complete surface. To verify the results of these counts, the number of capsomeres on the surface of the head was calculated in another way. Having determined the number of capsomeres on one edge of the octahedral head, it is possible to calculate the number of capsomeres over the complete surface of the head. On one edge of phage No. 1, 16 capsomeres can be distinguished. By calculation the figure of 904 is obtained for the total number of capsomeres. This figure, it will be understood, must be slightly reduced because a hole is certainly present at the apex to which the tail rod is attached. Hence, the number of capsomeres on the surface of the head, obtained by calculation in different ways, is consistent and is about 900 [44].

The edge of the octahedron is 810–840 Å in length. If these measurements are divided by 16 (the number of capsomeres), it follows that the approximate diameter of the capsomere is 50–55 Å. Direct measurement of individual capsomeres gives a figure of 60–70 Å.

As with the T-even phages, the tail of phage No. 1 is complex in structure. It consists of an outer sheath and an inner rod. As a rule, the tail of the intact phage is slightly curved and slightly wider toward the end: the proximal part (140 Å) is narrower than

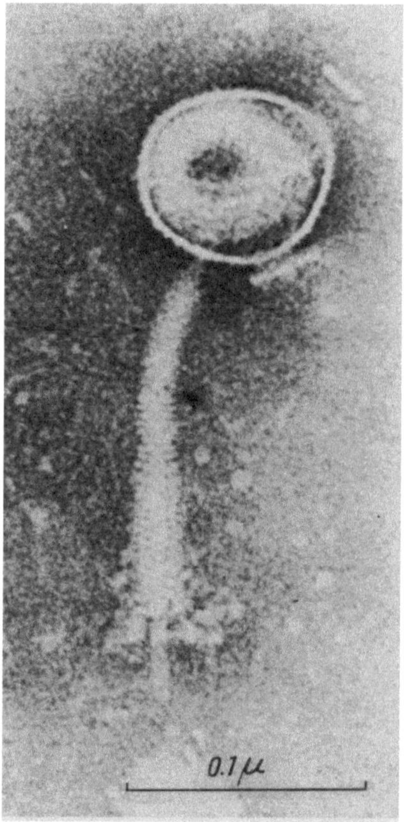

Fig. 64. Particle of phage 1623 of *Staphylococcus aureus* with semicontracted tail sheath. PTA. 260,000 ×.

the distal part (170 Å). The outer sheath of the tail is a helix composed of separate morphological subunits. The separate turns of the helix form a well-defined cross striation of the sheath (Fig. 61). Results obtained by Vainshtein and Kiselev [9] and my own calculations [49] show that the stretched tail sheath of phage No. 1 contains about 50 transverse bands.

In the contracted state, the turns of the helix forming the sheath become wider and the sheath is shortened by about half (Figs. 61 and 62). The helical structure of the contracted sheath is particularly clearly distinguishable when no rod is present (Fig. 60). Each turn of the helix of the contracted sheath of phage No. 1

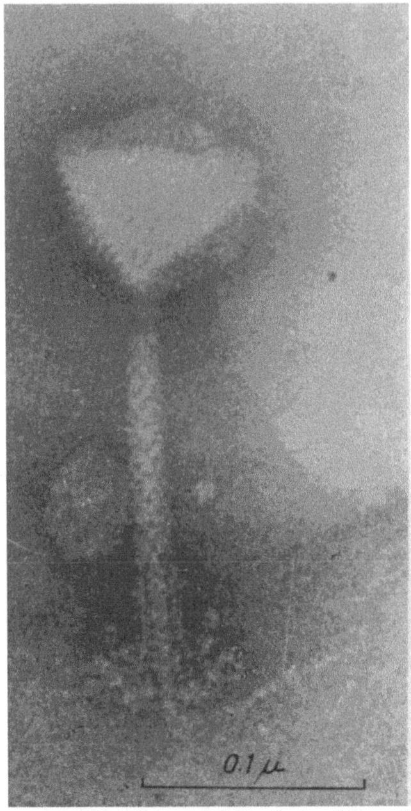

Fig. 65. Particle of phage AR3 of *Bacillus subtilis* with semicontracted tail sheath. PTA. 260,000×.

consists of 12 morphological subunits, which are clearly seen if the sheath tube lies endways (Fig. 55). Knowing the dimensions of the individual structural elements of the phage particle, the volume of the sheath in its stretched and contracted states can be calculated. The volume of the contracted sheath without end plate, calculated from the formula for a hollow cylinder, is 2.37×10^7 Å^3. The volume of the stretched sheath, also without its end plate, calculated from the formula for a truncated cone, with deduction of the volume occupied by the rod, is 2.4×10^7 Å^3 [44]. It is clear from these calculations that the volume of the sheath is the same whether it is stretched or contracted. This indicates that, as it shortens, the tail sheath is not broken, but contracts. (The dimensions of the principal structural elements of phage No. 1 are given in Table 8.)

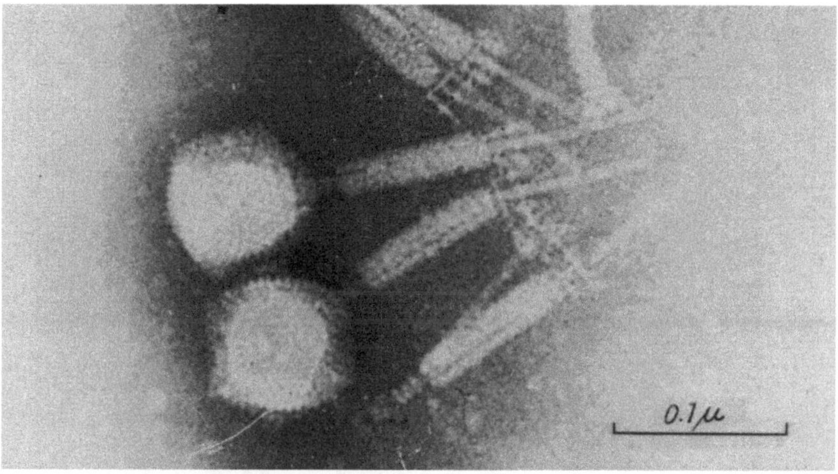

Fig. 66. Particles of phage No. 1 of *Bacillus mycoides* with contracted tail sheath and pointed projections from the end plate. A collar can be seen on the rod. PTA. 210,000×.

Contraction of the sheath is accompanied by regrouping of the subunits and by their more dense packing, so that the external appearance of the tail when contracted differs from that when stretched. In all probability, contraction of the sheath is accompanied by a change in the conformation of the subunits.

As was mentioned above, it is generally considered that contraction of the sheath takes place suddenly, because intermediate stages of contraction have not been observed. Tikhonenko and Belyaeva [49, 51, 364] have recorded intermediate stages of contraction of a tail sheath. A particle of phage No. 1 is illustrated in Fig. 63, where it can be seen that the distal part of the sheath is contracted, with the characteristic structural organization of the contracted sheath, whereas the proximal part still retains the structure of a stretched sheath. I have also seen intermediate stages of contraction of the sheath in phages 1623 of *Staphylococcus aureus* and AR3 of *B. subtilis* (Figs. 64 and 65). In the process of contraction, the sheath gradually begins to expose the inner rod of the tail. The exposed part of the rod, as can be seen in Figs. 64 and 65, in the intermediate stage of sheath contraction is much shorter than in particles with a completely contracted sheath. These observations

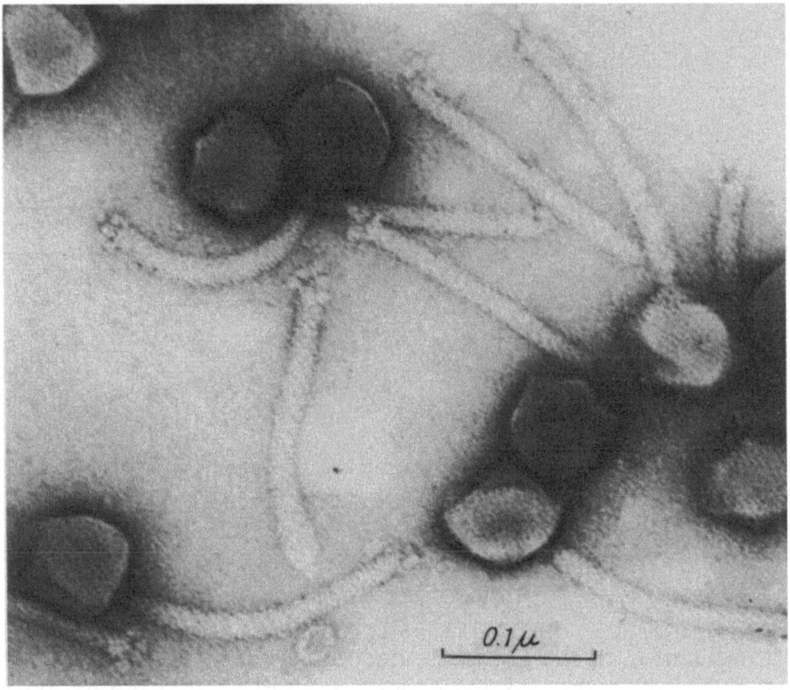

Fig. 67. Particles of phage No. 1 of *Bacillus mycoides* on which 6 rounded projections from the tail end plate can be seen. Uranyl acetate. 180,000×.

indicate, first, that contraction of the sheath does not take place suddenly but successively, and second, that the process of contractions of the sheath travels from the distal part toward the proximal part. In addition, this process is accompanied by regrouping of the morphological subunits, leading to structural changes in the sheath.

The tail sheath of phage No. 1, like that of phage T2, is formed of a spirally coiled strand, but stretched helices of the sheath of phage No. 1, such as are observed in phage T2 (Fig. 56a, b, c), have not been found. The most likely explanation is that subunits composing the helix of the sheath of phage No. 1 are less firmly joined together than the subunits forming the helix of the sheath of phage T2. On rupture of the bonds holding the turns of the helix in phage No. 1 in a compact state, it seems that at the same time the bonds are broken between individual morphological subunits forming the sheath helix, and because of this the sheath breaks up

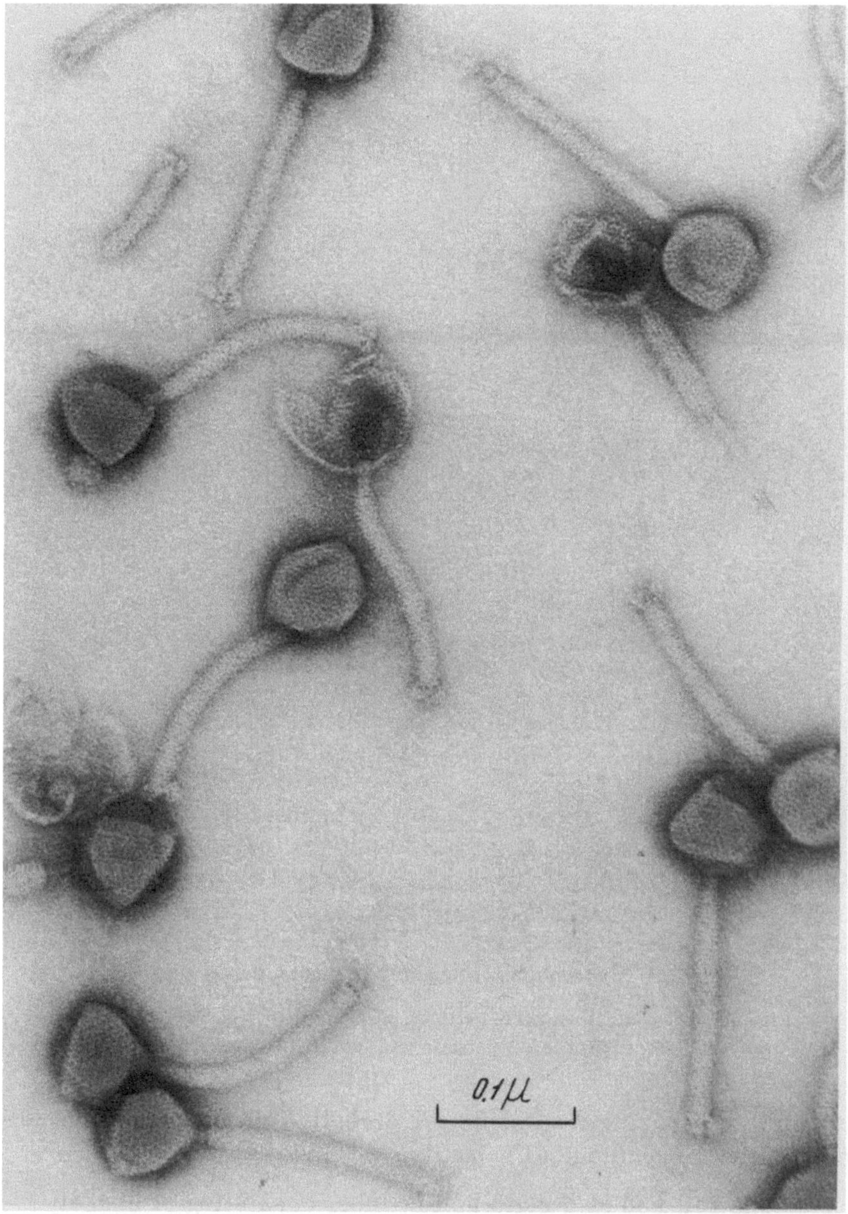

Fig. 68. Particles of phage No. 1 of *Bacillus mycoides* with stretched and contracted tail sheaths. Condensations at the point of attachment of the tail to the head can be seen inside the empty capsids. Uranyl acetate. 180,000×.

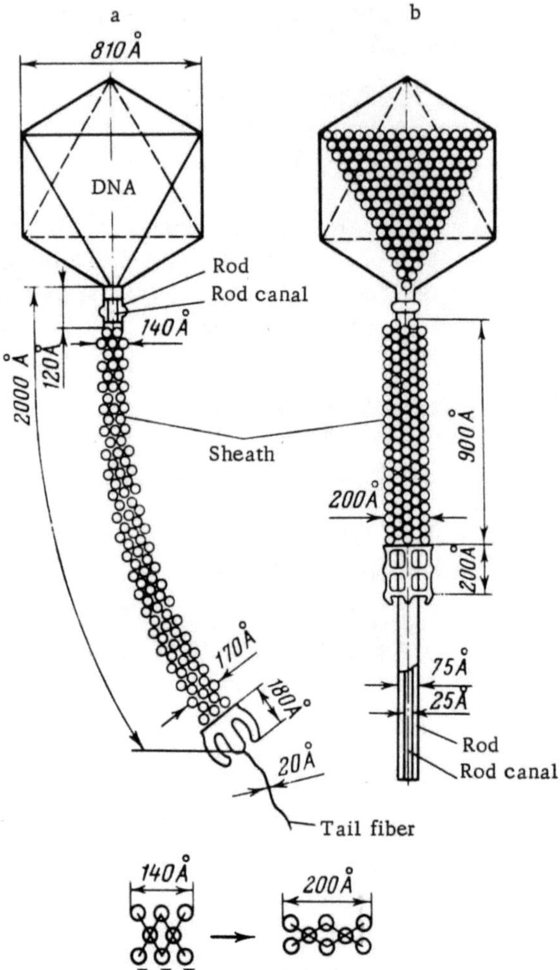

Hypothetical mechanism of contraction of sheath

Fig. 69. Diagram illustrating particles of phage No. 1 of *Bacillus mycoides* a) Intact particle; b) particle with contracted tail sheath.

either into separate fragments, or directly into its component elements, the morphological subunits.

The tail rod is a rigid hollow tube, consisting of densely packed morphological subunits (Fig. 60). The rod is responsible for joining the head to the tail, because the outer sheath arises from the rod at a distance of about 120 Å from the head. Near the head and on the rod is a thickening with the appearance of a collar or sleeve (Figs. 61 and 66).

Inside the head, at the point of attachment of the rod, an electron-dense structure can be distinguished, in the form of a membrane most probably directly connected with the rod (Fig. 68). This structural detail is possibly a special type of valve, playing an important role in the mechanism of transmission of nucleic acids from the head to the bacterial cell. Such a membrane is found inside the head of nearly all phage particles, whatever the length and structural organization of their tail (see Chapters 4 and 5).

The tail terminates in an end plate with six rounded prongs or projections (Fig. 67). In side view, three can be distinguished (Figs. 67 and 68). The structure of the end plate and, in particular, of its projections, is very labile, and in some cases it is apparently partly destroyed. The end plate is slightly wider than the tail. It has a single thin fiber (Figs. 61 and 68).

During contraction of the sheath the end plate is drawn up with it, and when this happens the projections become thinner and sharper. They are connected with each other by two transverse discs (Fig. 66). In my opinion, the tail sheath is kept in a stretched state by certain labile structures located on the end plate and fixing it to the end of the rod. If these structures are broken after contact with the bacterial cell or as a result of the action of external factors, the end plate is freed from its connection with the rod and the sheath begins to contract, in the course of which the projections which are attached to the end plate change their shape.

The conventional scheme for the structure of phage No. 1 of *B. mycoides* is illustrated in Fig. 69. On the same figure a hypothetical mechanism of contraction of the sheath is given, based on regrouping of its component morphological subunits. Evidently, a similar regrouping of subunits during the transition from the stretched to the contracted state of the sheath is characteristic of all phages possessing a contractile sheath.

Phage N19 of *Bacillus mycoides*

Phage N19 [49, 50, 51], which is active against the same strain of *B. mycoides* as phage No. 1, has a tail with a contractile

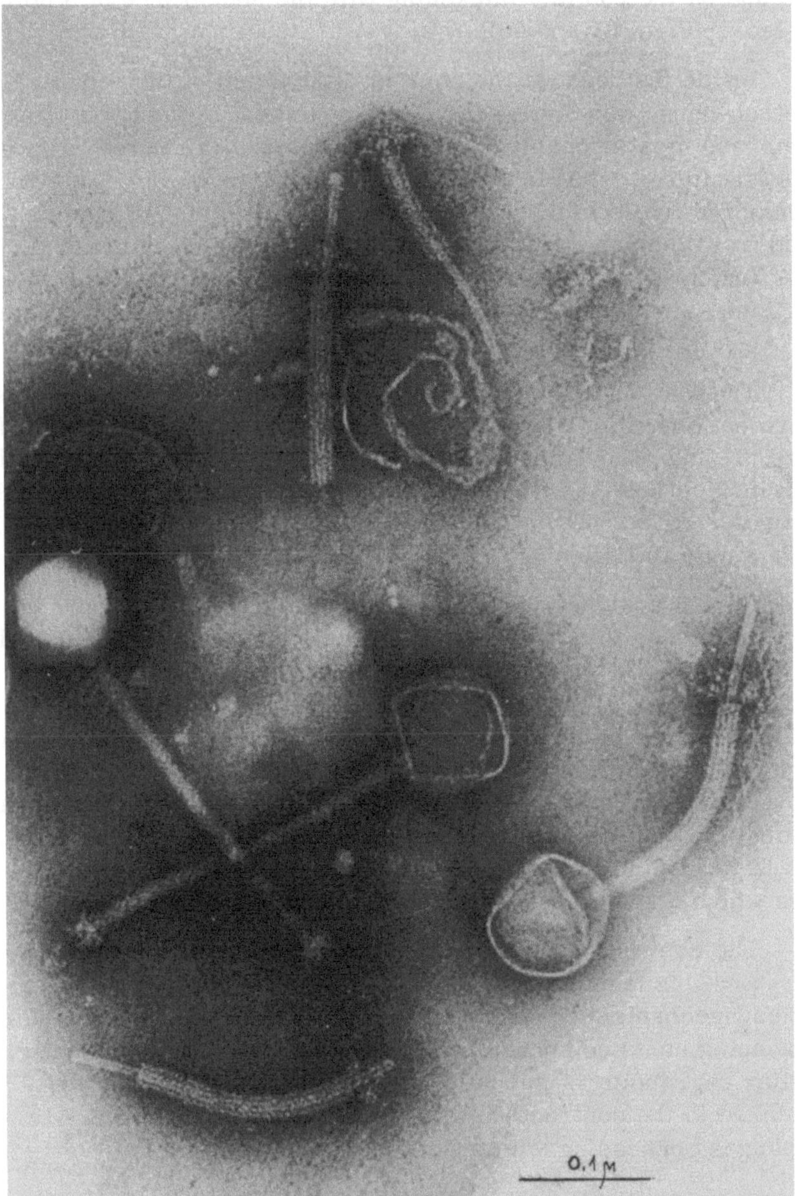

Fig. 70. Particles of phage N19 of *Bacillus mycoides* with stretched and contracted tail sheaths. PTA. 170,000×.

sheath. However, this phage differs from phage No. 1 in its size and in some structural details (Table 8). It has a larger head, consisting of an isometric polyhedron, the geometric shape of which has not yet been accurately established. Most probably, the head of this phage is icosahedral. The head capsid is made up of separate capsomeres which are smaller than those in phage No. 1.

A tail, or more accurately the tail rod, is attached to one apex of the polyhedron.

The tail of phage N19 consists of an outer sheath and inner rod. The proximal end of the tail sheath is attached to the rod a short distance away from the head. The distal end is attached to the end plate (Fig. 70). The end plate of phage N19 is complex in structure and differs in its configuration from the end plate of phage No. 1. Its diameter is a little larger than the diameter of the tail sheath, and, as a rule, the projections attached to the end plate are compactly arranged on the uncontracted tail, in the form of a cup. a single thin fiber is attached to the center of the end plate.

Just as in the case of phage No. 1, the uncontracted tail of phage N19 is slightly curved and its sheath varies in thickness along its length; the proximal part is narrower than the distal. The tail sheath is built from readily distinguishable subunits, coiled to form a helix around the rod. Contraction of the tail sheath is accompanied by regrouping of the morphological subunits composing it. During contraction the subunits are so arranged that the sheath appears like a tube formed from several longitudinal strands (Fig. 70).

The tail sheath of phage N19 does not contract to the same degree as that of phage No. 1, which shortens by about half its length. The sheath of phage N19 contracts by only one-third of its length. During contraction the end plate is drawn up along with the sheath. The projections of the end plate lose their compact shape when the sheath contracts and they open out to appear like a fully opened flower. In all probability, the change in shape of the end plate during contraction of the sheath of phage N19 is due to the same causes as those which operate in phage No. 1.

The tail rod of phage N19 is a hollow rigid tube built from separate morphological subunits (Fig. 70).

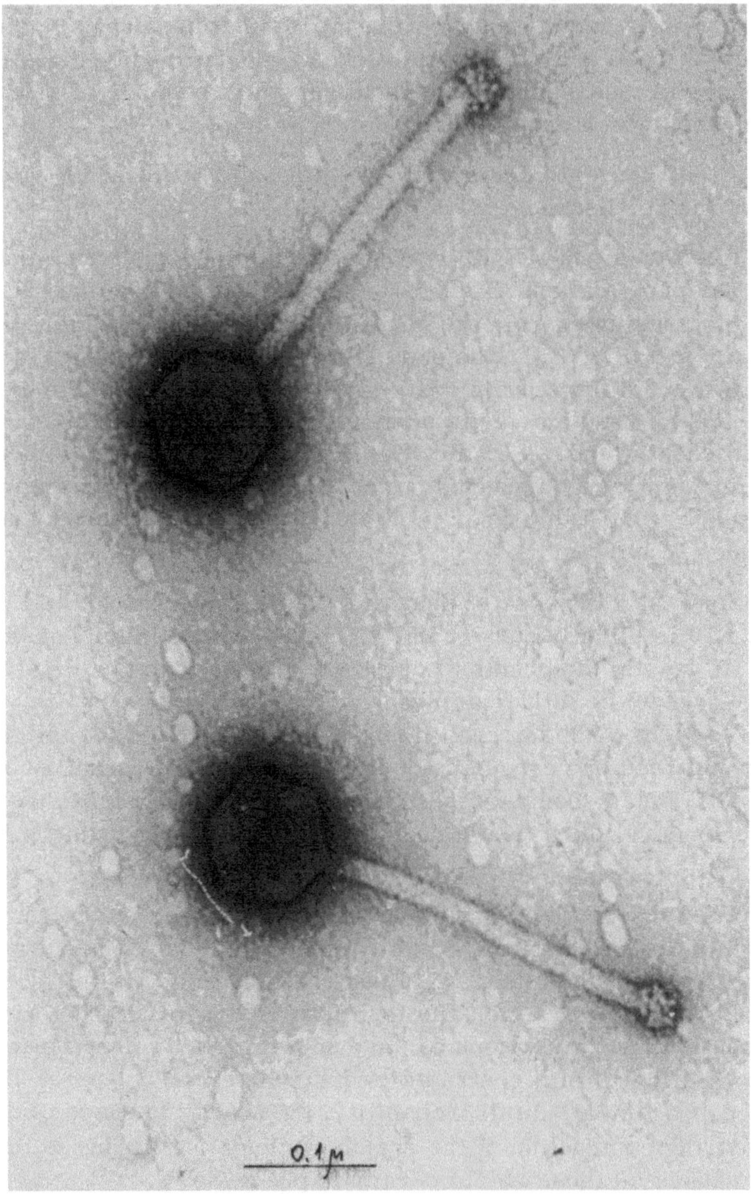

Fig. 71. Particles of phage N19 of *Bacillus mycoides*. Uranyl acetate. 170,000×.

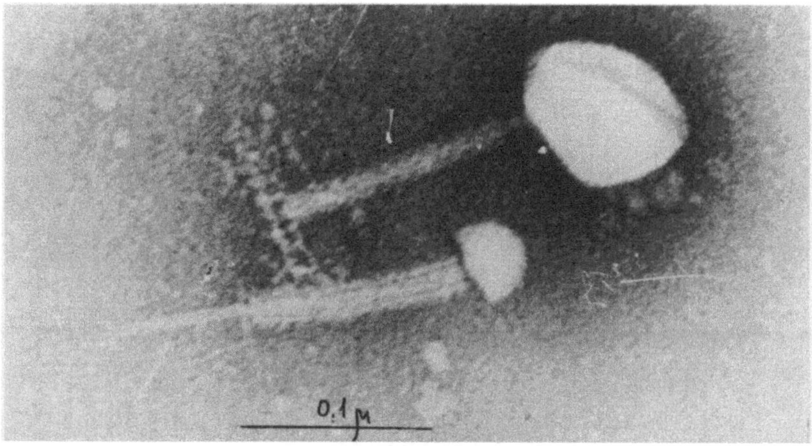

Fig. 72. Phage AR1 with a large head and phage φ with a small head of *Bacillus subtilis*. PTA. 220,000×.

After negative staining of phage N19 with phosphotungstic acid, particles with an empty head and contracted tail are more frequently observed in the specimens (Fig. 70). When uranyl acetate is used for negative staining, the specimens contain mainly particles with a stretched tail and full head. Phage particles with a contracted tail are rare in such specimens (Fig. 71). This observation applies not only to phage N19, but also to phage No. 1 of *B. mycoides*. When investigating intact particles of these phages, it is therefore advisable to use uranyl acetate for negative staining.

Phages of *Bacillus subtilis*

A number of virulent and temperate phages have been isolated by Azizbekyan and Kriviskii [2] from soil samples obtained in Moscow on various indicator cultures of *B. subtilis* strain Marburg. The study of material from plaques of these phages in the electron microscope revealed in every case two sharply different co-existing types of phages with a contractile sheath [3]. One type had a large head, the other a small head (Fig. 72). Whereas the phages with a large head differed slightly among each other in the size of head and tail, depending on the soil samples from which they were isolated, the phages with a small head were always identical in size and morphology and could be found accompanying any of the

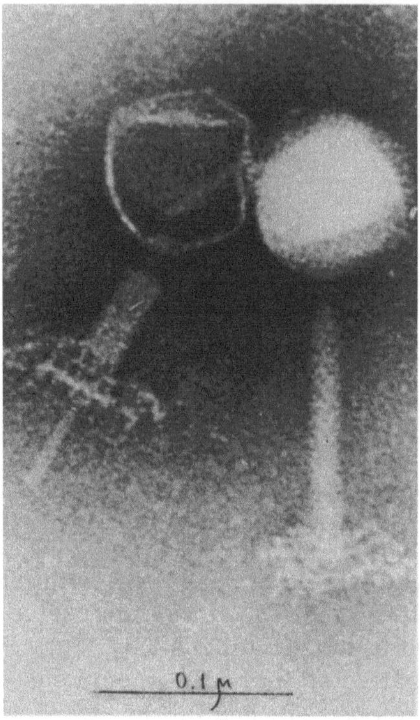

Fig. 73. Particles of phage AR1 of *Bacillus subtilis* with stretched and contracted tail sheaths. PTA. 220,000×.

phages with a large head. The large-headed phages were designated AR1, AR2, and AR3, and the phage with a small head phage phi.

Large-headed phages AR1, AR2, and AR3 differ from phages No. 1 and N19 of *B. mycoides* only in the structure of their end plate, which is much wider than the tail. The end plate of intact phage particles is rough in appearance (Figs. 72 and 73). During contraction of the sheath the end plate is drawn up along with the contracted sheath and its rough projections become more rigid and pointed. They arise from the proximal transverse disc and are joined together by the distal transverse disc. The end plate on the contracted sheath also projects considerably beyond its limits (Figs. 73 and 74). The head of these phages is an isometric polyhedron, most probably an icosahedron. The head capsid consists

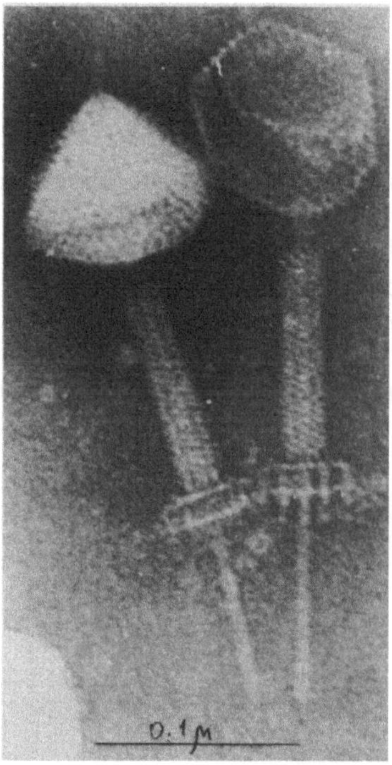

Fig. 74. Particles of phage AR3 of *Bacillus subtilis* with a contracted tail sheath. PTA. 220,000×.

of separate capsomeres, which have the appearance of hollow tubes (Fig. 74).

Other phages of *B. subtilis* have the same type of structure of their head, tail, and end plate: SP8 described by Davison [143], and SP50 studied by Eiserling and Boy de la Tour [157]. These workers point out that the head of phages of *B. subtilis* which they studied is most probably an icosahedron. They also state that the head capsid consists of hollow capsomeres about 70 Å in diameter. According to calculations given in the paper by Eiserling and Boy de la Tour [157], the head capsid of phage SP50 consists of 492 capsomeres.

Phage SP3 of *B. subtilis*, described by Eiserling and Romig [158], differs slightly from phages AR1, AR2, and AR3 and phages SP8 and SP50 in the structure of its end plate, which is similar in shape to the end plate of phage N19 of *B. mycoides* described above.

Despite similarity of general structural organization, phage AR1 differs slightly from phages AR2 and AR3 in the size of head and tail. Both the contracted and the stretched tail sheath of phage AR1 (Fig. 73) is shorter than the contracted and stretched tail sheaths, respectively, of phages AR2 and AR3 (Fig. 74), which are almost equal in size.

Phages AR1, AR2, and AR3 thus differ slightly from each other in the size of their structural elements. If phages AR1, AR2, and AR3, which I have studied myself, are compared with phages SP3, SP8, and SP50 of *B. subtilis*, described in the literature, it is clear that they also differ in size, concerning the considerable variation among natural forms of phages of similar structure.

Contraction of the tail sheath of phages AR1, AR2, and AR3 is accompanied by regrouping of its component morphological subunits, and the contracted sheath differs from the stretched in both structure and size (Figs. 73 and 74).

Partial contraction of the tail sheath has also been observed in phage AR3, just as in phage No. 1 of *B. mycoides*. Under these circumstances, the distal part of the sheath acquired the characteristic ultrastructure of the contracted sheath, while the proximal part still retained the structure of the stretched sheath (Fig. 65).

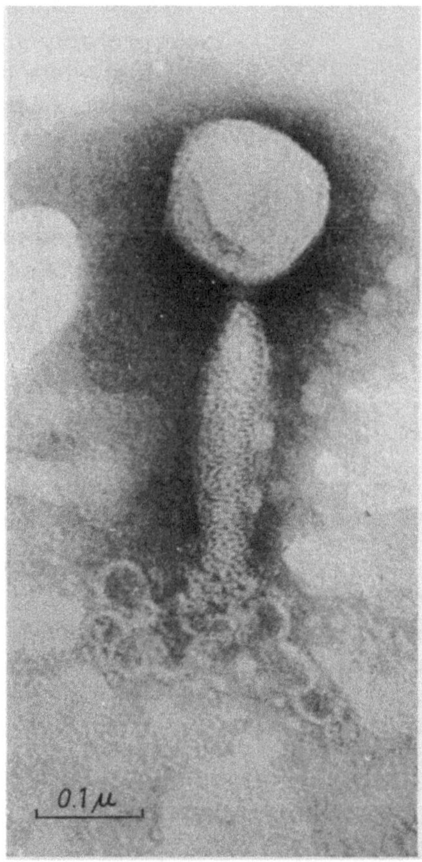

Fig. 75. Intact particle of phage AR9 of *Bacillus subtilis* with cigar-shaped tail formed by very thin fibrils attached to the collar at the base of the head. Thick, twisted fibrils are attached to the end plate. PTA. 150,000 ×.

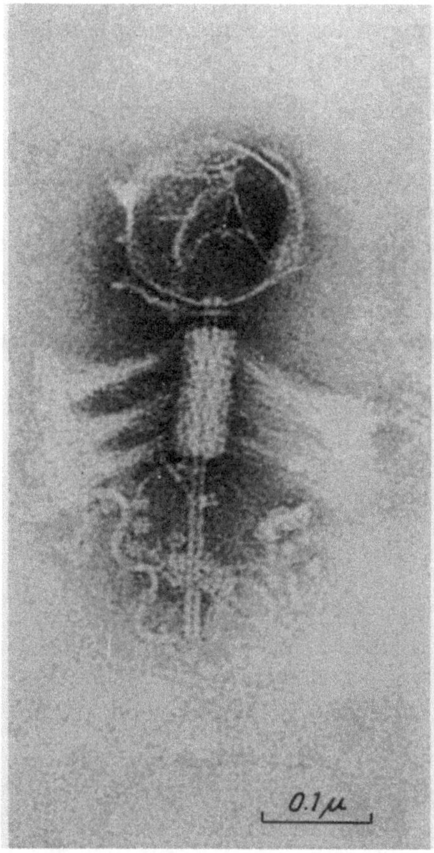

Fig. 76. Particle of phage AR9 of *Bacillus subtilis* with a contracted tail sheath which gives off thin fibrils grouped into bundles. The inner rod consists of morphological subunits. PTA. 150,000×.

The small-headed phage phi, as Azizbekyan and co-workers [3] showed, is liberated spontaneously and after induction by various lysogenic Marburg strains of *B. subtilis* and in its properties it is a defective phage. More detailed information about this phage will be given later in the description of the defective phages in Chapter 7.

Phage AR9, effective against Marburg strain SHgW of *B. subtilis*, has a distinctive morphology. The morphology of phage

AR9 has been studied by Belyaeva working at the laboratory of electron microscopy of the Institute of Molecular Biology, Academy of Sciences of the USSR [5, 6].

The head of phage AR9 is a polyhedron with easily distinguishable capsomeres, and most probably its shape is that of an icosahedron (Figs. 75 and 77). This phage is the largest of all so far studied. The diameter of its head is 1500 Å. Its tail has a contractile sheath. Inside the sheath is a hollow rod consisting of easily distinguishable subunits (Fig. 76). At the end of the tail is a small end plate, approximately equal in width to the tail sheath in its distal part (about 370 Å). Three powerful tightly twisting whip-like fibrils, composed of individual subunits, are attached to the end plate. Each fibril terminates in special structures resemb-

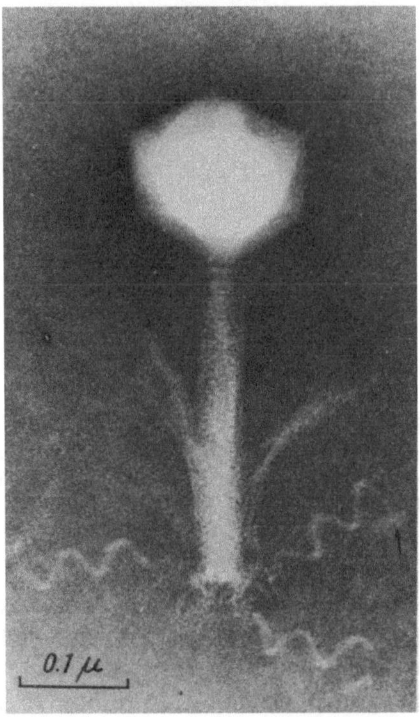

Fig. 77. Particle of phage AR9 of *Bacillus subtilis* with an uncontracted tail sheath giving off thin fibers. PTA. 150,000×.

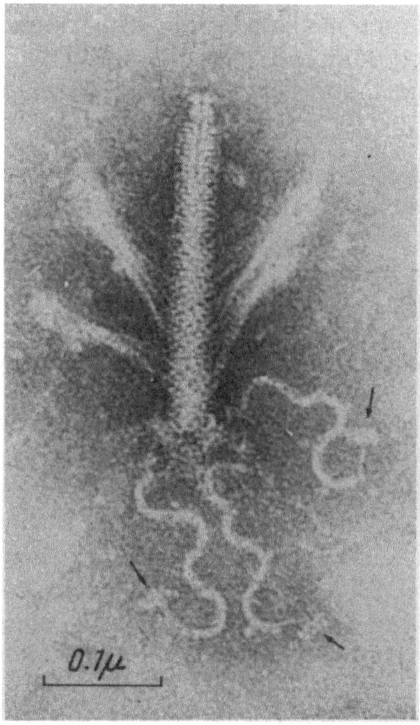

Fig. 78. Uncontracted tail of phage AR9 of *Bacillus subtilis* with clearly distinguishable details: sheath with crossed striation, end plate with twisted fibrils and suckers on their ends (shown by arrows), and bundles of thin fibers leaving the sheath. PTA. 150,000×.

ling suckers, consisting of four teeth which can be distinguished two-dimensionally (Figs. 77 and 78). The unique feature of phage AR9 is the presence of unusual additional structures associated with its tail, and in all probability these play an important role in interaction between the phage and the host cell.

The uncontracted tail sheath is cigar-shaped, as a result of the large number of very thin fibers apparently given off by the morphological subunits of the tail sheath. When the tail sheath is stretched these fibers run in a proximal direction and are attached to the collar on the rod at the base of the head (Fig. 75).

Sometimes on a phage particle with stretched sheath these thin fibers become detached from the collar and spread out in bundles away from the tail in a proximal direction (Figs. 77 and 78).

The direction of the fibers is changed when the sheath contracts and they leave the sheath in bundles running distally (Fig. 76). The change in direction of the bundles of fibers caused by contraction of the sheath may be taken as evidence that the fibers are connected with morphological subunits undergo regrouping, and this is responsible for the change in direction of the fibers.

The length of the uncontracted tail of phage AR9 is about 2700 Å. Its width varies, being 370 Å in the distal part and about 290 Å in the proximal part. Cross striation is clearly visible on the tail sheath. The uncontracted sheath consists of 54 transverse bands formed by morphological subunits. During contraction of the tail sheath it shortens by more than half (1200 Å) and becomes uniform in width throughout its length (570 Å). As a result of contraction of the sheath, the tail rod is exposed: its width is 140 Å and the diameter of its internal canal is 75 Å.

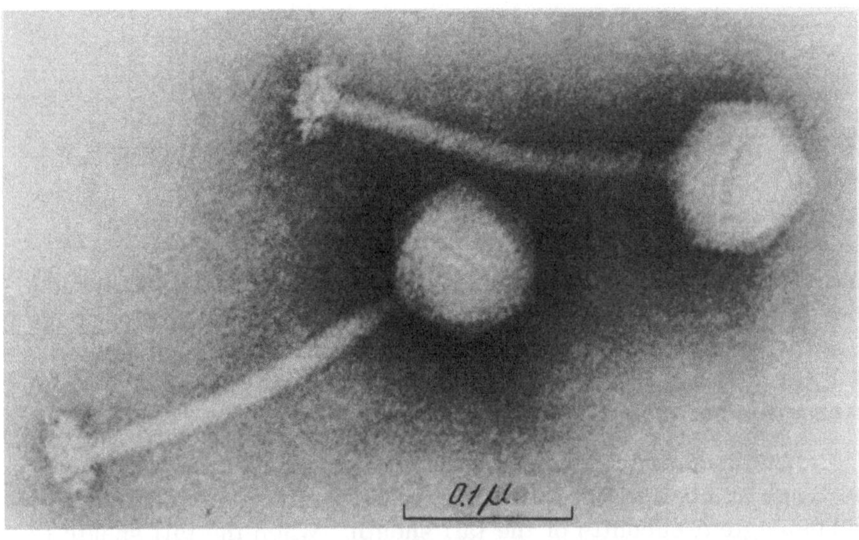

Fig. 79. Particles of phage P4 of *Staphylococcus aureus* with uncontracted tail and well-developed end plate. PTA. 220,000×.

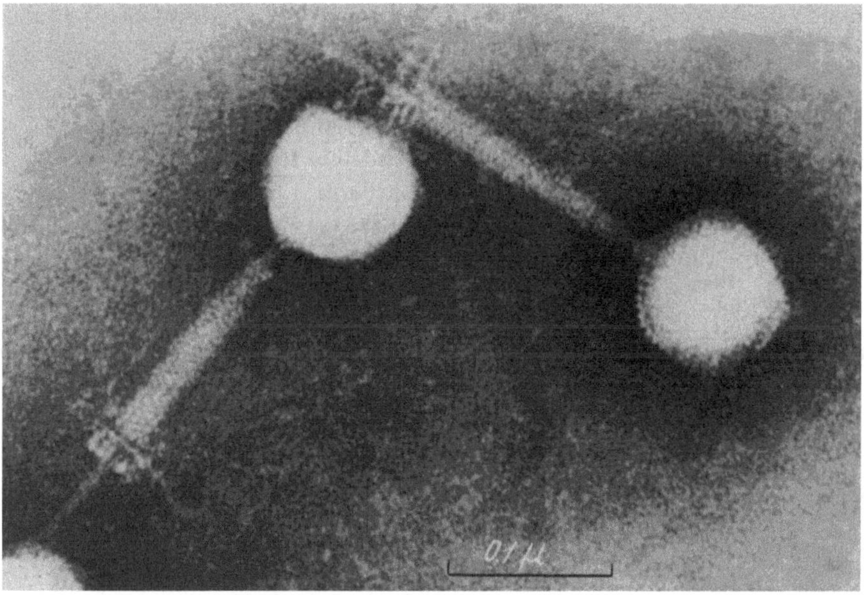

Fig. 80. Particles of phage 1623 of *Staphylococcus aureus* with contracted tail sheath. PTA. 220,000×.

Recently, particles of unusual structure, similar in some details to phage AR9, have been described by Eiserling [156] in the case of phage PBS1 of *B. subtilis*. Early studies [178, 223] showed that phage PBS1 is adsorbed only on the flagella of *B. subtilis* cells. This may account for the complex structure of phage particles of the PBS1 and AR9 type.

STAPHYLOCOCCAL AND STREPTOCOCCAL PHAGES

The study of phages infecting cocci have shown that many of them have a tail with a contractile sheath.

I have studied 6 phages of *Staphylococcus aureus* strain 728 (P2, P3, P4, P8, P9, P10) (Fig. 79), phage 1623 of *Staphylococcus aureus* strain 1623 (Fig. 80), and phage RZh of *Streptococcus lactis* (Figs. 81a, b; Fig. 82), which are similar in structure and size to phage AR2 and AR3 of *B. subtilis*.

The head of these phages is an isometric polyhedron, the capsid of which is built from hollow capsomeres.

The tail consists of an outer sheath, which is a spirally coiled strand composed of morphological subunits. The helical sheath strand winds around the inner hollow tail rod, which is exposed when the sheath contracts. Contraction of the sheath is accompanied by regrouping of the subunits, leading to changes in the structure of the sheath and in its diameter.

On the segment of the rod lying next to the head of phage RZh is a collar-like structure such as is frequently found on other phages.

In the structure of their end plate, the staphylococcal and streptococcal phages which I have studied resemble phages AR1, AR2, and AR3 of *Bacillus subtilis*. They project considerably beyond the limits of the tail and have tangled projections (Figs. 79; 80; 81a, b; 82).

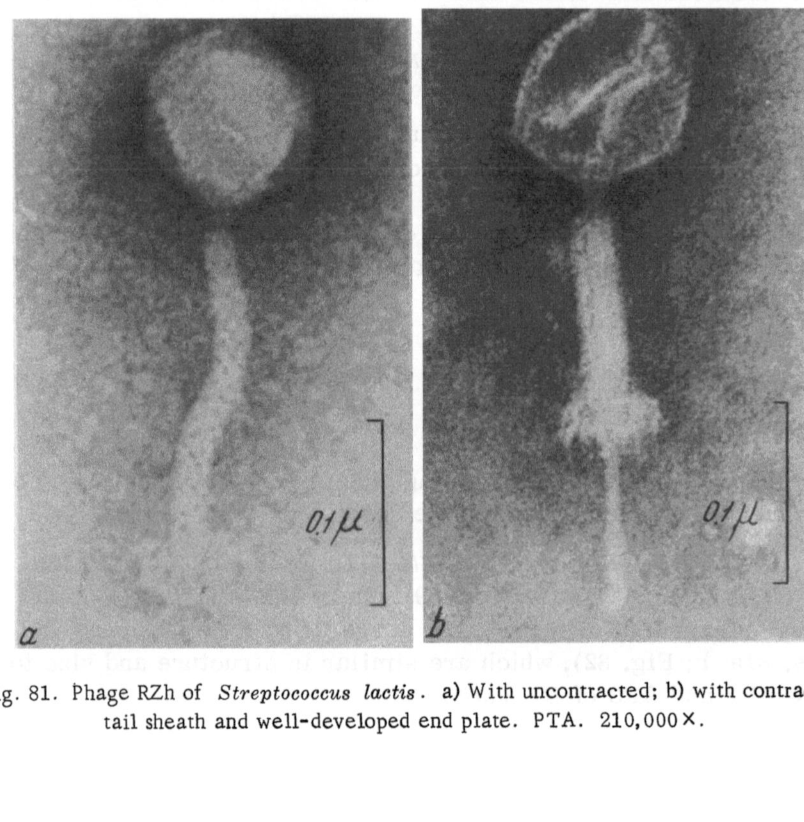

Fig. 81. Phage RZh of *Streptococcus lactis*. a) With uncontracted; b) with contracted tail sheath and well-developed end plate. PTA. 210,000×.

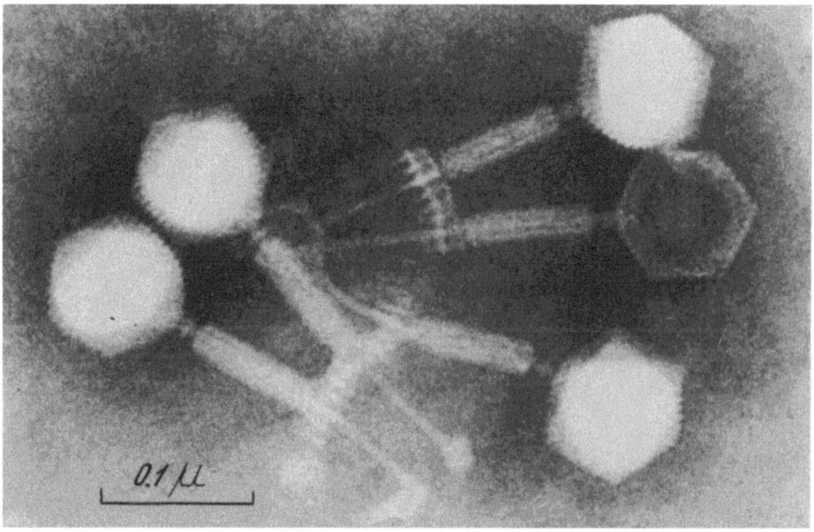

Fig. 82. Particles of phage RZh of *Streptococcus lactis* with contracted tail sheath and pointed projections from the end plate. PTA. 180,000×.

Staphylococcal phages P2, P3, P4, P8, P9, P10, and 1623 are identical in structure and size (Table 8). Staphylococcal phage Twort [259, 373, 374] is very similar in structural details and size to the other staphylococcal phages described above. The small variations in size of the head and tail of the staphylococcal phages can be explained either by slight morphological variations or by inaccurate calibration of the magnifications in the electron microscope. An example of this is given by reports published by many investigators in which the dimensions of the same phages differ slightly from each other although the order of size is generally the same. For example, in his various publications, Bradley gives slightly different sizes for the same phages [102, 106, 108, 277]. This factor must be taken into account when the dimensions of identical phages are compared.

Hence, the group of phages with a contractile tail sheath includes a number of members differing from each other in certain structural details of the tail and end plate and in the shape of their head.

Chapter 7

Defective Phages and Bacteriocins

During our study of phage No. 1 of *B. mycoides*, Tikhonenko and Bespalova [53] showed that among typical particles with a large head, other particles with a much smaller head are frequently found. Small particles appeared from time to time in a broth phage lysate of *B. mycoides* and quickly disappeared after several passages.

The study of plaques of phage No. 1 on solid media revealed that in some cases, among colonies of the usual type with transparent center and clearly outlined edges surrounded by an opaque halo of incomplete lysis, plaques appeared with a ring-like structure consisting of alternating opaque and transparent zones.

Electron-microscopic investigations showed that coexistence of phage particles with small and large heads occurs only in plaques of the latter type. However, more than 100 successive subcultures taken from one plaque of ring-like structure failed to produce complete separation of the different forms of phage contained in them. Only by special selection was it possible to obtain a high proportion of phage particles with a small head.

The study of the fine structural details of the two forms of phage particles present in one plaque showed that particles with a large head are phage No. 1 described above (Figs. 61 and 68). Particles of the other type have a hexagonal head when examined two-dimensionally, about 2.5 times smaller in diameter

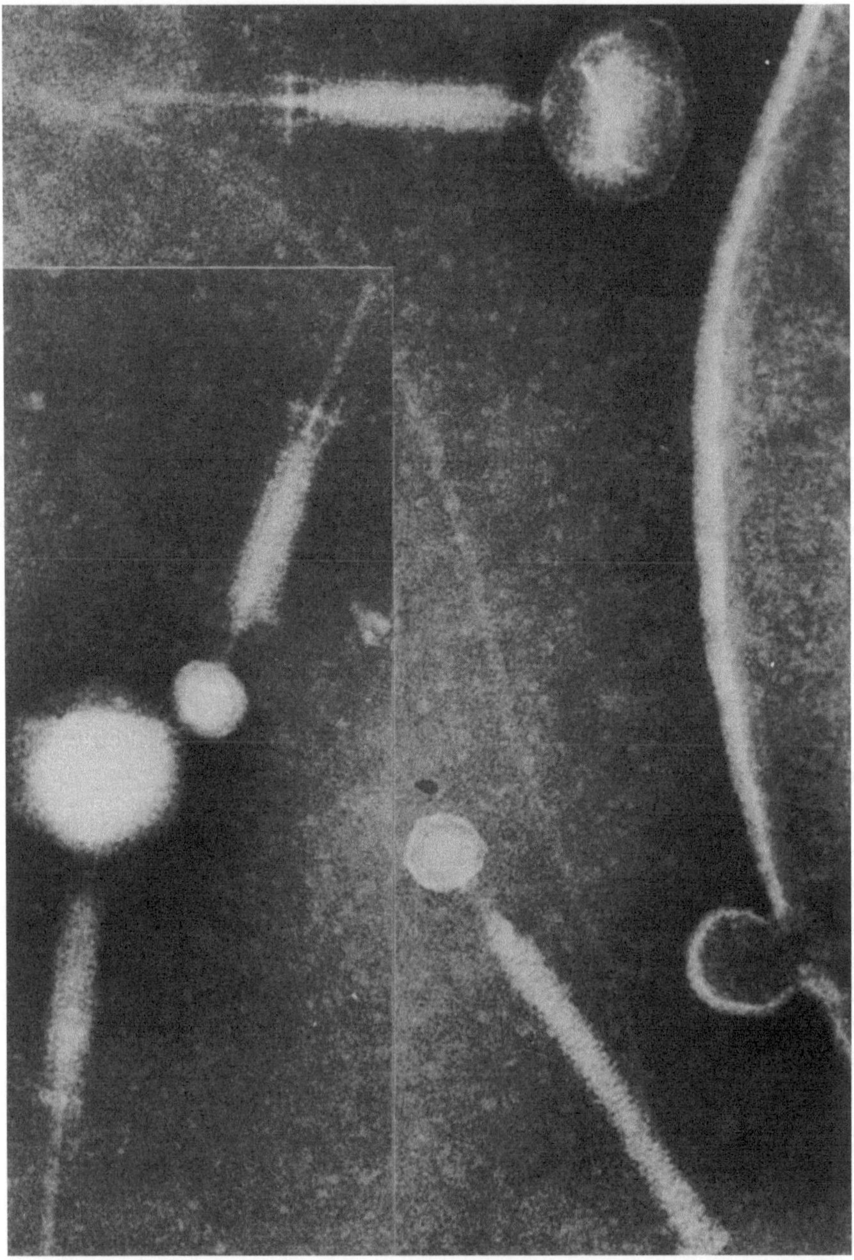

Fig. 83. Two forms of phage (No. 1 and No. 1M) of *Bacillus mycoides* with large and small heads and with uncontracted and contracted tail sheaths. PTA. 300,000×.

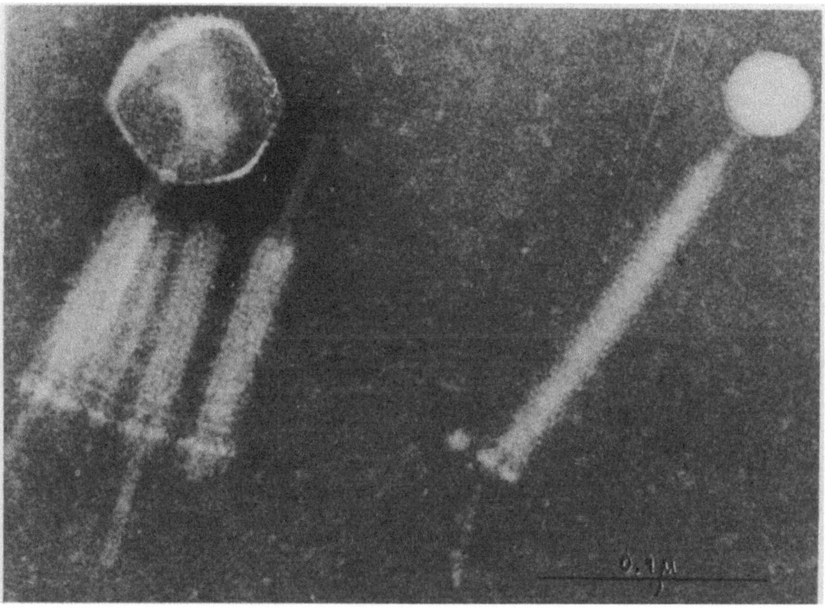

Fig. 84. Phage N17 of *Bacillus mycoides* with two types of particles. PTA. 300,000×.

than the head of phage No. 1, and 19 times smaller in volume than the head of phage No. 1, assuming that its head is of the same octahedral shape (Fig. 83). Particles with a small head were called phage No. 1M. The same phenomenon has been described for a new phage isolated from soil and active against the same strain of *Bacillus mycoides*, which I have called phage N17 [50, 55, 363]. This phage also contains two types of particles in the same plaque, i.e., particles with large and small heads (Fig. 84) similar in morphology and size to phage No. 1 and phage No. 1M [53]. The dimensions of the particles of these phages are given in Table 8.

Despite differences in the size of the heads of these phages, the tails of both forms are completely identical (Figs. 83 and 84). No differences were found in the structure of their end plate. Just as in the case of phage No. 1, the end plate of phage No. 1M and of particles of phage N17 with a small head possesses a single thin fiber (Fig. 84). If the end plate of phage No. 1M is seen endways, it is hexagonal in shape, with a hole in the center and six thickenings on each corner of the hexagon (Fig. 85). The tail sheath of phage No. 1M is contractile and its structure, both when stretched

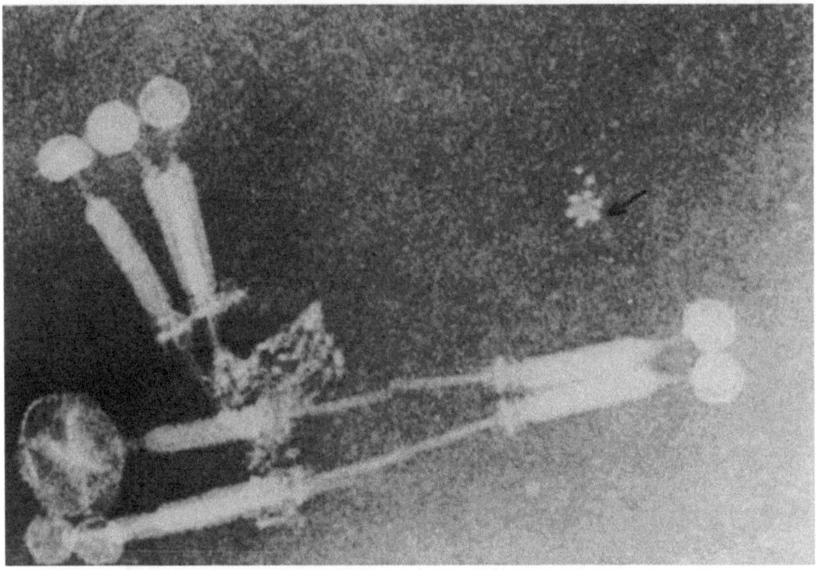

Fig. 85. Two forms of phage of *Bacillus mycoides* (No. 1 and No. 1M) with large and small heads and with a contracted tail sheath. An isolated hexagonal end plate can be seen (indicated by an arrow). PTA. 180,000×.

and when contracted, is identical with the structure of the sheath of phage No. 1 (Fig. 83).

As mentioned above, many repeated subcultures of a mixture of phage No. 1 and No. 1M failed to separate them. This led to the suggestion that strain No. 1 of *B. mycoides* may be lysogenic, and that the phage particles with a small head may be temperate phage liberated from the cells after their lysis by virulent phage. However, experiments to study induction of *B. mycoides* cells with ultraviolet radiation did not lead to liberation of phage with a small head.

It must also be noted that the small-headed phage accompanies only phage No. 1 and is not found during lysis of cells by other phages active against the same strain of *B. mycoides* [50], but differing from it in morphology: phages N5 (Fig. 44a, b) No. 2, N6II, and N19 (Figs. 70 and 71).

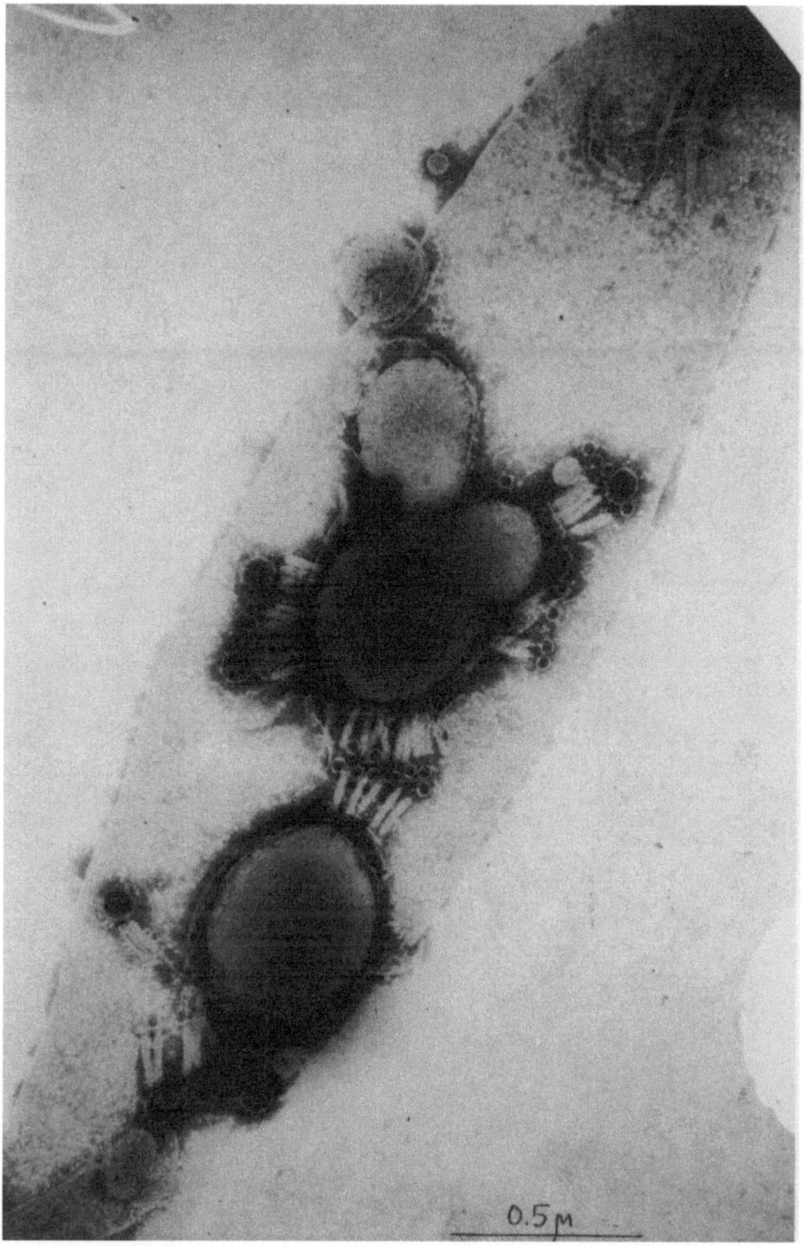

Fig. 86. Development of two forms of phage N17 in a *Bacillus mycoides* cell. PTA. 50,000×.

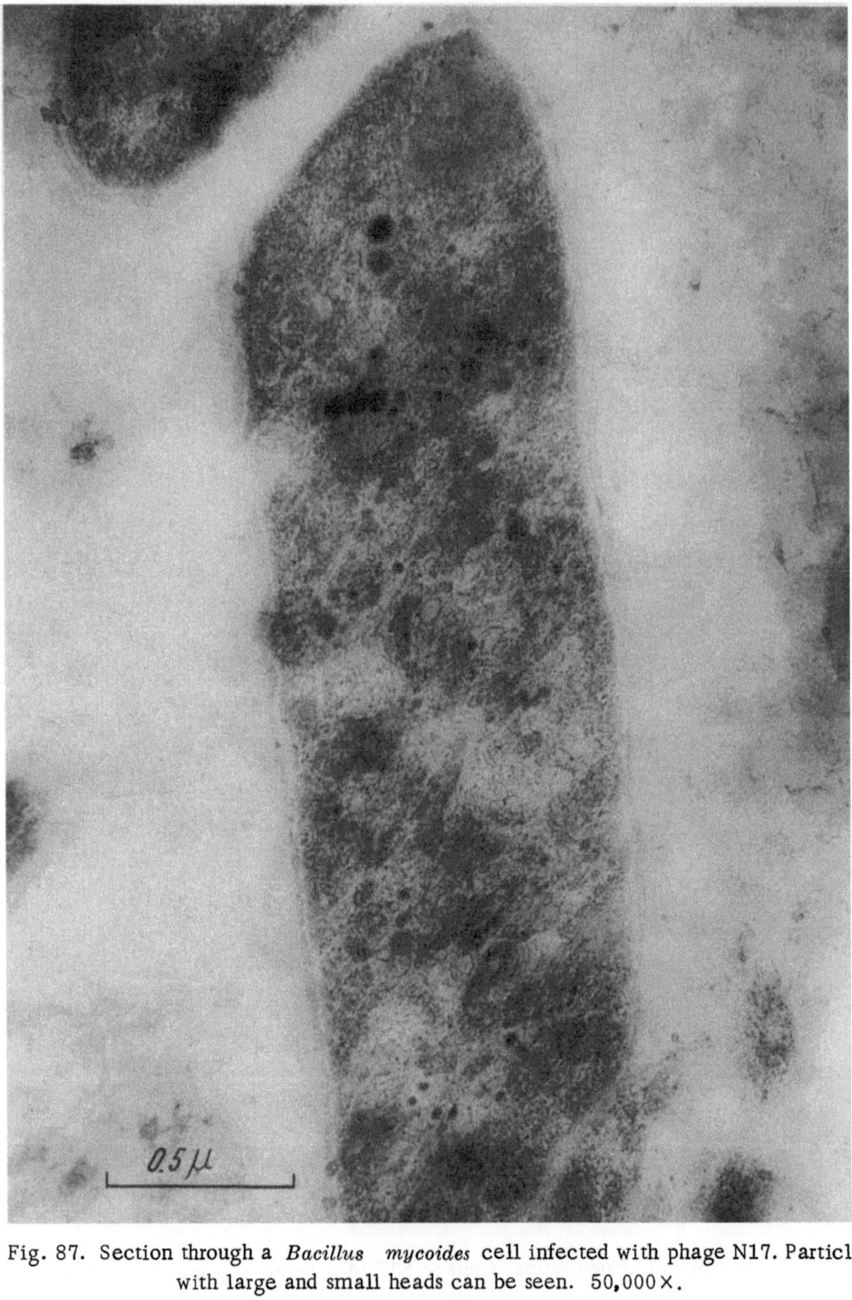

Fig. 87. Section through a *Bacillus mycoides* cell infected with phage N17. Particles with large and small heads can be seen. 50,000×.

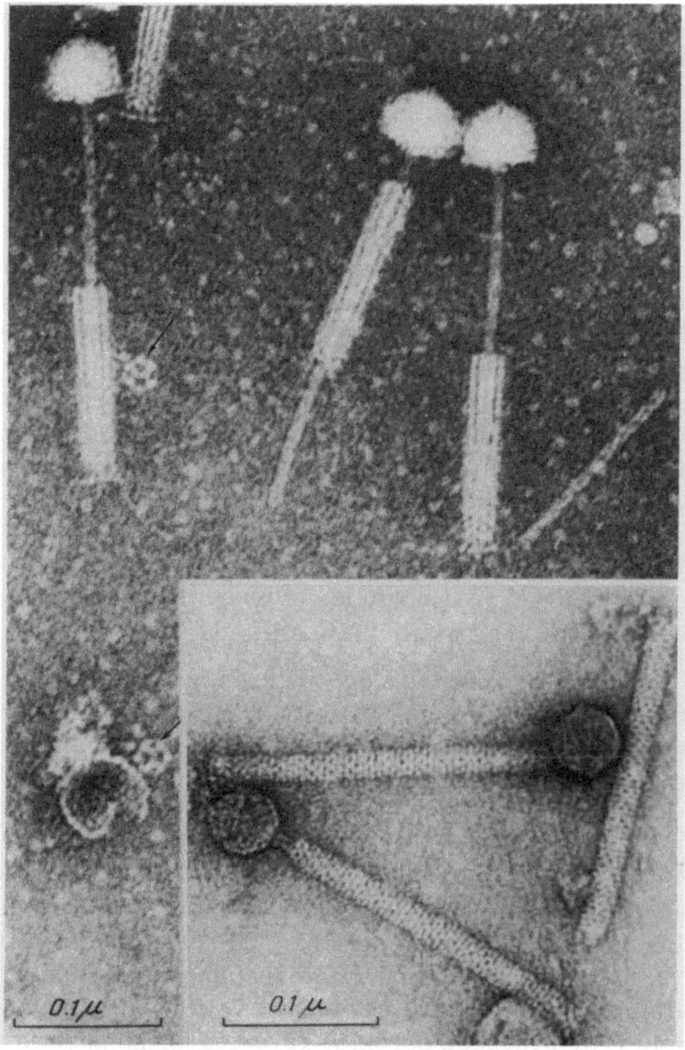

Fig. 88 Fig. 89

Fig. 88. Particles of phage ϕ of *Bacillus subtilis* obtained after induction with ultraviolet light, with a contracted tail sheath. Six fibers are present on the end plate. The arrows indicated isolated end plates. PTA. 240,000 ×.

Fig. 89. Particles of phage ϕ of *Bacillus subtilis*, with a stretched tail sheath. Uranyl acetate. 240,000 ×.

I conclude from these facts that particles of phage No. 1M, with a small head, may develop in a cell only through the action of virulent phage No. 1, and that the information required to form the tail of small-headed particles is evidently provided by the genome of the large-headed phage, because the tails of both types of particles are absolutely identical. It has also been found that phages against the same strain of *Bacillus mycoides*, but with different morphology, do not cause the formation of small-headed particles.

In all probability the small-headed phage is temperate but also defective, because the formation of a particle of this phage requires an assistant in the form of virulent phage of particular morphology. I therefore postulated that both types of phage must develop simultaneously in the same bacterial cell. By negative staining (Fig. 86) and in ultrathin sections (Fig. 87) [55, 363] it has been shown that one bacterial cell may contain particles of phage with large and small heads simultaneously. It is interesting to note that both small-headed and large-headed phages are readily absorbed on the surface of the bacterial cell. However, without the presence of phage No. 1, particles of phage No. 1M cannot develop in the cell.

The same phenomenon was encountered by Anderson [81], who isolated two forms of phage P1 of *Salmonella typhimurium* from the same plaque. These forms differed from one another only in the size of their head (Table 8).

The nature of the phenomenon described above is still incompletely understood and requires further study.

Recently, a number of investigators found that several Marburg strains of *B. subtilis* are lysogenic and produced defective phages [219, 336, 350]. Electron-microscopic examination of these cultures after induction with ultraviolet radiation or by the action of mitomycin C or hydrogen peroxide revealed phage particles which these workers described as phage μ and PBSX.

Defective phage designated phage ϕ (Fig. 88) has also been found by Azizbekyan and co-workers [3] in 7 Marburg strains of *B. subtilis*. Phage ϕ is always found in plaques formed by lysis of cultures by phages AR1, AR2, AR3, and AR9, the morphology of which was described in Chapter 6, and it differs sharply from them in the size of their head and the structural details of the tail. In its morphology, phage ϕ resembles the phages μ and PBSX described by Ionesco and co-workers [219] and by Seaman and co-workers [336].

The diameter of the head of phage ϕ particles is about half that of the head of phages AR1, AR2, and AR3 among which they are found (Table 8). The tail of phage ϕ also differs from that of phages with a large head in its size and in the structure of its end plate. The end plate of phage ϕ has no attached projections and its diameter is equal to the diameter of the sheath (Fig. 88). When seen endways, the end plate resembles a hexagonal nut from which six thin straight fibers radiate like a whisk (Fig. 88).

The tail sheath of phage ϕ is contractile, but unlike the phages described above, when contracted it may lie in different segments of the rod, being found both in its proximal and its distal part (Fig. 88). Contraction of the sheath of phage ϕ, just as in the case of other phages, is accompanied by regrouping of the morphological subunits. This can be seen clearly on the photomicrographs with the sheath stretched and contracted (Figs. 88 and 89). As the phage sheath contracts, it becomes wider and shorter by about half its length when stretched.

The phenomenon of simultaneous existence of two types of phage particles in the same plaque was described above for phage No. 1 of *B. mycoides*. However, the two forms of phage with large and small heads active against *B. mycoides* have tails which are identical in size and in fine structure, whereas the structural details and size of the tail of phage ϕ differ significantly from those of tails of *B. subtilis* phages with a large head, among which they are found. Furthermore, phage ϕ can accompany any phage of *B. subtilis* with a large head, regardless of differences in their morphology. The small phage of *B. mycoides* is found, as was mentioned above, only among particles of phage No. 1 with a large head. This suggests that the small and large forms of phage of *B. subtilis* are not genetically connected, unlike the two forms of phage of *B. mycoides*. The appearance of phage ϕ in a plaque during lysis of cultures of *B. subtilis* by other virulent phages is attributed to the fact that the cells of *B. subtilis* are lysogenic and can liberate temperate phage ϕ.

Irradiation of *B. subtilis* cells with ultraviolet light in the exponential phase of growth [3] showed that they liberate large numbers of phage ϕ particles. These particles are indistinguishable in size from the phage particles with a small head found in plaques along with phages AR1, AR2, AR3, and AR9. Phage isolated from cultures of the Marburg strain of *B. subtilis* after induction with ultraviolet light, if applied to an indicator plate culture, caused lysis of the bacteria, but did not reproduce, exhibiting what is known as the killing effect. These results suggest that phage ϕ is a defective phage. It must be pointed out in this connection that the heads of all phage ϕ particles, even with a contracted sheath, are filled with DNA contents, and I consider that this is additional confirmation of the defective nature of phage ϕ.

Ionesco and co-workers [219] also consider that phages liberated by lysogenic strains of *B. subtilis* are defective. Incidentally, phage ϕ can be liberated spontaneously by unirradiated cells also, but only in very small amounts. For instance, whereas from 10 to 15 phage particles per field of vision were found in a preparation made from irradiated material after ultracentrifugation, there were only 1-2 particles in the whole preparation made from unirradiated material.

What is the explanation for the appearance of large numbers of defective phage ϕ particles along with other phages possessing a large head? If we assume that phage ϕ cannot be liberated independently from lysogenic cells, the role of the large-headed phage is simply one of opening up the cell. However, experiments with lysozyme, which produces artificial lysis of bacteria not infected with phage, showed that under these circumstances no small phage is found. This fact suggests that the large-headed phages cause induction of phage ϕ in *B. subtilis* cells.

Comparing the morphology of phage ϕ liberated by 7 strains of *B. subtilis* [3] with previously described inducible phages μ [219] and PBSX [336], it can be concluded that most probably in all cases the phage is the same. Bradley [105] later described phage GA2, liberated by cells of *B. subtilis*, and also similar in its morphology with the defective phages described previously. The impression is created that all Marburg strains are lysogenic and liberate defective phage.

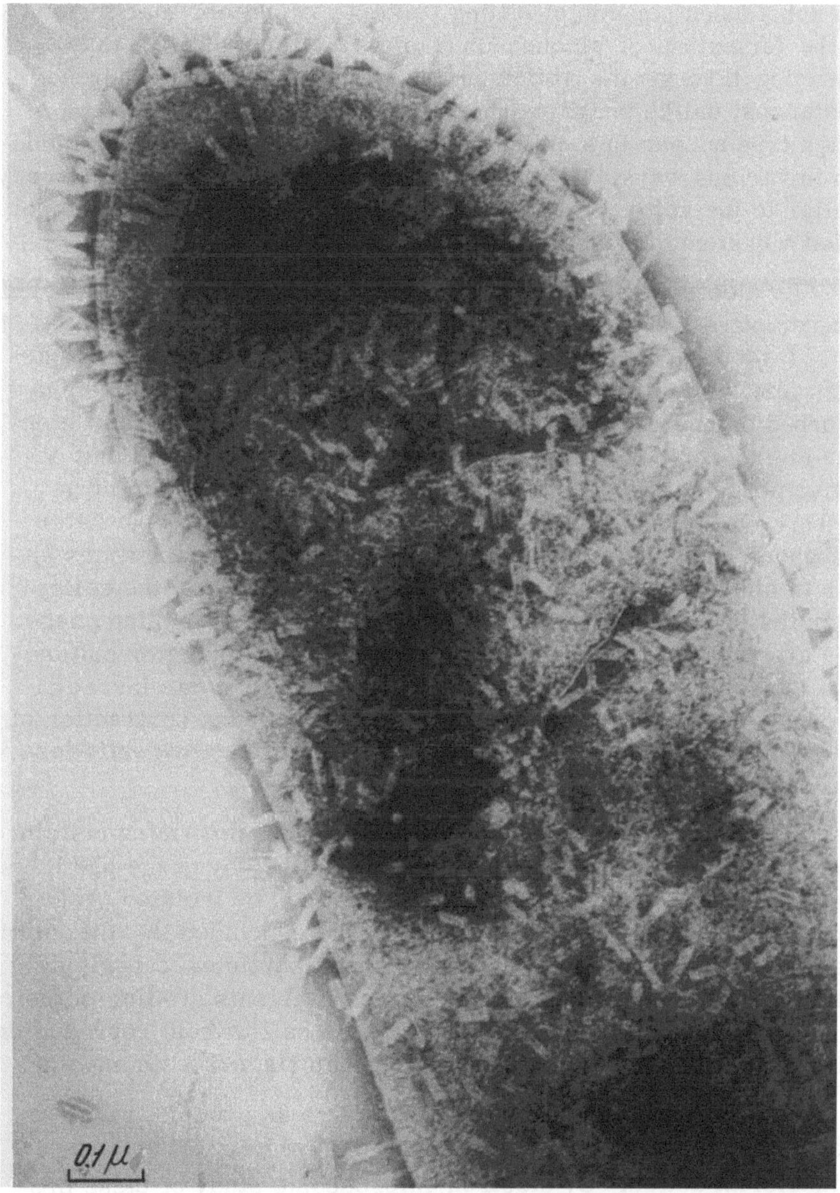

Fig. 90. Adsorption of particles of defective phage D52 on a cell. PTA. 90,000 ×.

Investigations have shown [35, 76, 176, 220, 281, 291, 326, 358] that many defective lysogenic strains of bacteria liberate special substances capable of killing bacteria, a process manifested by the formation of plaques on a plate culture, similar to those appearing through the action of phage. However, these lytic substances, unlike phage, cannot reproduce. Usually, lytic agents of this type appear in a culture either spontaneously or after induction in various ways. In its manifestations this phenomenon is very similar to the action of antibiotics, and such an agent is therefore called a bacteriocin (colicin, pyocin, and so on).

By electron-microscopic investigation of the agents liberated by a defective lysogenic strain of *Proteus mirabilis*, Taubeneck [358] showed for the first time that the killing effect is produced by particles similar in structure to the phage tail. These particles are adsorbed on and produce lysis of the bacterial cells. In joint electron-microscopic investigations, Taubeneck and I showed that defective phage particles, resembling tails, are adsorbed in large numbers on the bacterial cell, causing its death (Fig. 90). Later, Taubeneck and Zickler [359] found that inactivating substances appear in old filtrates containing agents causing death of the cells, under the influence of which defective particles resembling phage tails are rendered incapable of absorption on an indicator culture or of causing death of the cells. Electron-microscopic investigation showed that these inactivating substances cause contraction of the outer sheath of such tails, and in this state they evidently lose their ability to destroy the cells.

Later investigations of cells of *E. coli* 15 producing colicin showed that death of the cells is produced either by phage particles consisting of a head without DNA and a tail, or by isolated phage tails [76, 176, 281, 326]. Therefore, it was concluded that the colicin effect is due to incomplete, defective phage particles, capable of killing the cell but not of reproducing in it. Agents similar in their morphology to phage, capable of killing the cell without reproducing in it, are produced by many species of bacteria and actinomycin.

High-molecular weight proteins known as pyocins, which are liberated by some strains of *Pseudomonas aeruginosa*, also possess antibacterial action. By electron-microscopic study of these proteins, Ishii, Nishi, and Egami [220, 291] and Bradley [107] showed that they are very similar in structure to the tails of the T-even

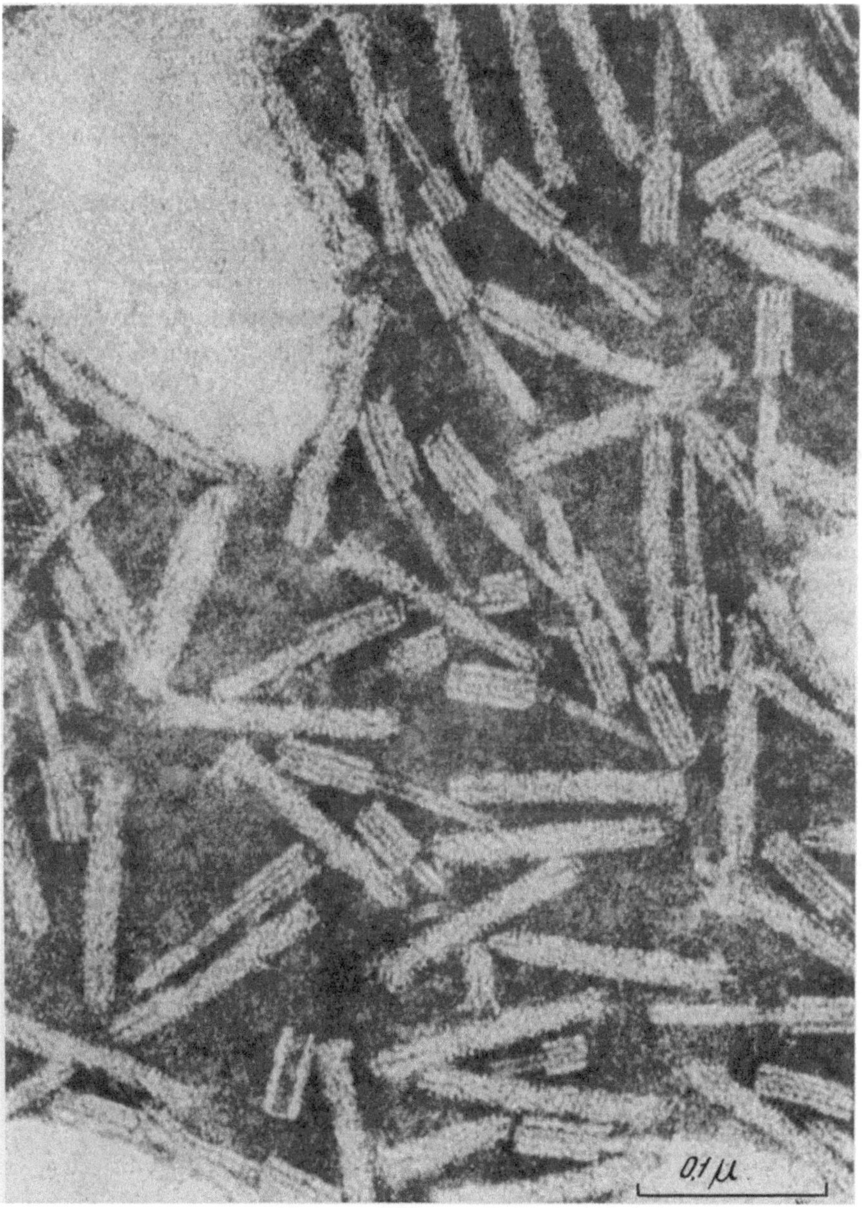

Fig. 91. Pyocin particles. 250,000 × [220].

phages. The pyocins are tails 1200 Å long and 150 Å wide, consisting of a contractile outer sheath and a hollow inner rod (Fig. 91). At one end of the tail is an end plate with fibers. The tail sheath is formed of a spirally coiled strand enveloping the inner rod. If pyocin is treated with 0.1% sodium dodecylsulfate solution, the sheath contracts and the helix forming the sheath unwinds, thus deepening their resemblance to the tails of the T-even phages. In this case, the isolated phage tails possess bactericidal action.

Pyocin P28, with a different structural organization, was isolated from *P. aeruginosa* cells by Takeya, Minamishima, and Amako [357] after induction of the cells with mitomycin C. This lytic agent consists of curved rods with an internal canal. They measure 90 Å in diameter and between 1000 and 4000 Å in length. However, rod-like structures about 1000 Å in length are more common. These workers consider that this agent resembles in its structure the rod-shaped phage PS of *P. aeruginosa* containing single-stranded DNA [355], but they point out that the cross striation on particles of pyocin P28 is more clearly defined than on phage PS. In my opinion, pyocin P28, which causes death of sensitive cells, is a defective phage consisting only of tails which, in structure, resemble the noncontracting tails of phages of morphological group IV.

It must be assumed that defective phages possess definite enzyme activity, concentrated at the end of the tail and capable of producing death of the cell only, without the reproduction of new phage particles in it, because these particles either do not possess the genetic principle or, for some reason or other, cannot be transmitted to the cell.

Chapter 8

Action of Chemical and Physical Agents on Various Phages

The intimate mechanism of interaction between phage and bacterium cannot be understood without knowledge of the physiological role of the structural phage proteins. Although the role of the nucleic acid as infective principle has been precisely established [201], the role of the individual protein structures of the phage is still not clear. The relatively complex structure of the tail and the presence of at least four different proteins in the phage particle suggest that the role of its protein components is not limited purely to the function of protecting the nucleic acid against external agents. The study of the function and ultrastructure of the protein elements of phage is interesting, both from the point of view of a further understanding of the mechanism of phage infection and also from the point of view of elucidation of the general principles governing formation of these proteins in the cell.

It has now been established that the phage particle contains various enzymes, such as phosphatase [60, 61, 155] and an enzyme of the lysozyme type [12, 91, 113, 187, 247, 279, 287, 311, 338]. There is reason to believe that these enzymes are connected with the structure of the tail, but their precise localization has not yet been determined. It is therefore not quite clear what part the individual structures play in the process of transmission of the infective principle to the bacterial cell.

This problem can be studied by the method of dividing the phage particle into its component structural elements and then studying their properties, or by investigating the injuries caused to individual structures through inactivation of the phage by various external agents.

Early studies, before the use of the electron microscope, yielded only general information on the inactivating action of various agents on phage particles. However, the mere establishment that an inactivating action is in fact present does not answer the question of how the phage particle is damaged and on which structural elements of the phage particle various agents act. Inactivation of phage can be expected to be accompanied by injury either to its protein structure or to its nucleic acid or to both components together.

The high resolution of the electron microscope can shed considerable light on these matters, and in combination with other methods of investigation it has assisted the development of the functional-morphological approach in virology.

Winkler and co-workers [392], for example, who studied the morphology and other properties of phage T4 after exposure to ultraviolet radiation, found that if a wavelength of 265 mμ was used, mainly DNA was damaged. A wavelength of about 235 mμ had a strong action on phage protein. Electron-microscopic investigation of phage particles damaged by ultraviolet radiation showed that inactivation of phage is accompanied by destruction of the head envelope with liberation of DNA and by a change in the tail structure, in which either the tail passes into a contracted state or the sheath is broken up into fragments. On the basis of these investigations it was postulated that phage can cause death of the cell by means of two independent factors. One is the injection into the cell by the phage of certain substances (most probably DNA), which are damaged at 265 mμ. The other is determined by the function of the tail, whose structure is damaged at 235 mμ, possibly as the result of a disturbance of its enzyme activity. Evidence in favor of this view is given by these workers' findings, indicating the ability of phage particles with injury only to the head and with an intact tail structure to cause death of the host cell.

Valuable information on the mechanism of inactivation of structural elements of the phage particle by various physical and chemical agents, accompanied by morphological data, have been obtained by other workers, but unfortunately few such investigations have yet been carried out, and these mainly on the T-even phages of *E. coli* B.

A series of investigations by Anderson and co-workers [78, 79, 80, 83] showed that the T-even phages lose their infectivity when damaged by osmotic shock (e.g. when a suspension of phage in concentrated glycerol solution or in 4 M NaCl is diluted quickly with distilled water). These experiments enabled Anderson et al. to show for the first time that the head of the T-even phages has a semipermeable envelope by rupture of which the internal contents are liberated. Fraser and Williams [181] later confirmed Anderson's findings and observed a particle of phage T6 with a ruptured head envelope surrounded by DNA filaments. This discovery acted as the starting point for many subsequent experiments shedding light on the functional role of individual components of the phage and on their structural details.

The DNA liberated from the phage head becomes accessible to the action of deoxyribonuclease, the action of which can result in only a "ghost" of the protein cover of the phage particles, i.e., the empty head envelope with the tail being left in suspension. According to Hershey [199], these ghosts account for 95% of the total protein of phage T2. They can be adsorbed onto sensitive *E. coli* cells and can even kill them, but no new phage particles are produced in the cell under these circumstances [96, 183, 198]. The defective phages mentioned in Chapter 7 have a similar action on the cell.

Electron-microscopic investigations [80, 132] have shown that phage particles attach themselves to the bacterial cell by their tail. Consequently, the phage tail can be regarded as the organ of adsorption, and it must possess structures enabling the phage to interact specifically with the bacterial cell. In the same way it has been shown [383, 395] that the tail of phage T5 can attach itself reversibly to spherical bodies liberated from the bacterial membrane, which are evidently isolated cell receptors.

Jesaitis and Goebel [221] showed that the effect of a lipocarbohydrate isolated from phase II cells of *Shigella sonnei* is to release the DNA from phage T4, thus showing that the material of the bacterial cell membrane can act on the phage particle. This reaction is highly specific, because it takes place between the receptors of the phage particle and phagoreceptors which were isolated from the bacterial membrane [185, 381].

By means of physical and chemical agents capable of breaking up the particles of T-even phages into structural components, and using an electron-microscopic control, a number of investigators [111, 225, 233, 237, 390] have established that the tail fibers have the most marked adsorptive properties. Of all the structural elements of the tail, it is they which carry out the specific interaction between the phage particle and the host cell.

Unfortunately, no information is yet available concerning the role of the phage end plate in adsorption. Perhaps it is the site of the phage enzymes producing lysis of the bacterial cell wall. Indirect evidence in favor of this suggestion is given by the work of Taubeneck and Zickler [359], showing that defective phages, consisting of isolated tails, lose their ability to cause death of bacterial cells after inactivation, expressed morphologically as contraction of the tail sheath and, in all probability, as partial destruction of the end plate. This work clearly confirms the importance of a study of the action of inactivating agents on phage structure to elucidate the functions of each particular structure in the process of infection.

The work of Williams and Fraser [390], Kellenberger and coworkers [237, 238], and Brenner and co-workers [111] has yielded valuable information on the fine structure of the component elements of phage T2, whose proteins differ in their antigenic properties and react differently to physical and chemical agents.

It is also been demonstrated in work on other phages by Tikhonenko [45] and Tikhonenko and Kuimova [59] that the structural elements respond differently to the destructive action of different physical and chemical agents. These facts indicate heterogeneity of the proteins of the phage virion.

A very important discovery was made by the use of electron microscopy. It was found that the tail of the T-even phages possesses a contractile organ, which later was found to be present in many phages infecting different species of bacteria. If T-even phages were treated with hydrogen peroxide, zinc cyanide, or cadmium salts, by freezing and thawing, and by many other agents, the phage tail sheath shortened by 30%, and this shortening was due not to destruction but to contraction [86, 111, 229, 251, 252, 253, 255, 390]. Similar contraction of the phage tail sheath also occurs when phage particles interact with isolated membranes of bacterial cells [231, 253].

On the basis of their observations, Kozloff [249] and Brenner and Horne [110] put forward the following hypothesis to explain the mechanism of infection of the bacterial cell by T-even phages: the phage particle is adsorbed by means of the tail fibers onto the bacterial cell wall. Zinc-containing proteins present in the bacterial membrane hydrolyze the end of the phage tail, causing contraction of the sheath and liberation of the inner rod which, like a syringe, pierces the cell wall enabling the phage DNA to pass from the head through the rod canal into the interior of the bacterial cell.

This hypothesis of the mechanism of infection can perhaps be accepted, but only for phages with a contractile tail sheath. The mechanism of infection of bacterial cells by phages whose sheath does not contract still remains completely unknown. It is to be expected that the more intensive research at present being conducted on the study of the structure and function of individual elements of different phages will help to give a more complete picture of the mechanism of infection of the bacterial cell by phage particles with different structural organizations and to elucidate the general principles governing this complex process.

In order to understand the functional role of each structural element in the process of infection, it is first necessary to isolate each in a pure form and to study the various properties of proteins contained in the phage virion.

I have used various procedures in an attempt to discover the conditions permitting stepwise degradation of phage particles to be produced in order to isolate their structural elements in a pure form.

In the course of these investigations, I also counted on obtaining additional information concerning the fine structural organization of the structural elements of the phage particle, because the information to be gained by studying the structure of the intact particle confirming the structure of these elements is to some extent limited.

The objects chosen for these investigations were concentrated and purified suspensions of three morphologically different phages.

1. Phage No. 1 of *B. mycoides*, possessing a tail of complex structural organization (group V).

2. Phage T2 of *E. coli* B for comparison with phage No. 1 of *B. mycoides* (group V).

3. Phage s_d of *E. coli* SK, possessing a tail which, despite its small size, nevertheless shows signs of structural differentiation (group III).

The study of certain biochemical and physicochemical properties of the protein structures and of their morphological changes, resulting from treatment with various chemical and physical factors, was carried out principally on these three phages.

ACTION OF pH

Phages exhibit considerable resistance to changes in pH of the medium. As Adams [1] points out, phages are resistant to pH changes within the range from 5.0 to 8.0, and at low temperature from 4.0 to 9.0-10.0.

The work of Herriott and Barlow [197] showed that phage T2 can be precipitated at pH 4.0 without loss of infectivity. This property was used by these workers to obtain concentrated phage suspension. However, different phages have different limits of resistance to changes in the pH of the medium, and sensitivity to pH must therefore be established individually for each phage.

Van Vunakis and co-workers [371] showed that the action of alkali causes destruction of phage T2 ghosts. They found that alkali causes gradual degradation of phage proteins. It was shown by ultracentrifugation that ghosts of phage T2 break up into small structural units with a molecular weight of about 80,000 and components of higher molecular weight, resistant to concentrated solutions of alkali. According to these workers, the low-molecular-weight protein represents individual subunits of the head envelope, and the high-molecular-weight component represents the phage tail. This indirect evidence of the existence of subunits forming the protein head envelope of phage T2 was subsequently confirmed by electron-microscopic investigations studying the macromolecular organization of various phages [9, 44, 143, 157] and, as already mentioned above, they are a common feature of the capsid structure of all phages.

Brenner and co-workers [111], by strong acidification of a suspension of phage T2 to pH 2.0 followed by treatment with proteolytic enzymes (trypsin, chymotrypsin), succeeded in breaking up particles of phage T2 into separate structural components: the protein envelope of the head, the sheath, the rod, and the tail fibers. Separation of the phage particle into its structural elements enabled these workers to study the fine morphological details of their structure, and some of the physicochemical properties and the amino acid composition of the proteins forming these elements.

By an electron-microscopic study of the action of trimethylphenylammonium, possessing the properties of a strong alkali, on various phages, I showed [45] that this agent produces gradual degradation of the phage particles, different phages reacting differently to it. When phage T6 was treated with high concentrations of trimethylphenylammonium, the tail sheaths remained intact in the preparations, while the sheaths of phage No. 1, on the other hand, were quickly broken up leaving the tail rods intact.

These preliminary investigations showed conclusively that phage particles can be broken up into individual structural elements by treatment with alkalies at different pH values. It was therefore decided that, in order to avoid the introduction of proteolytic enzymes into the system, it is best to use the method of gradual alkalification of the phage suspension for this purpose.

Stepwise fragmentation of the phages was carried out with NaOH or KOH, which was added to the phage suspension up to pH values ranging from 8 to 12.5.

Using an electron-microscopic control, it was possible to determine which structural elements of different phages remain intact or are destroyed during treatment with alkali at specified pH values.

Phage T2

As described above, the normal particles of phage T2 (Figs. 52 and 57) consist of a head filled with DNA, an outer sheath, and an inner tail rod. The inner rod of normal phage T2 particles can be seen only next to the head as a thin neck joining the head to the tail. The tail terminates in an end plate which has six thin fibers.

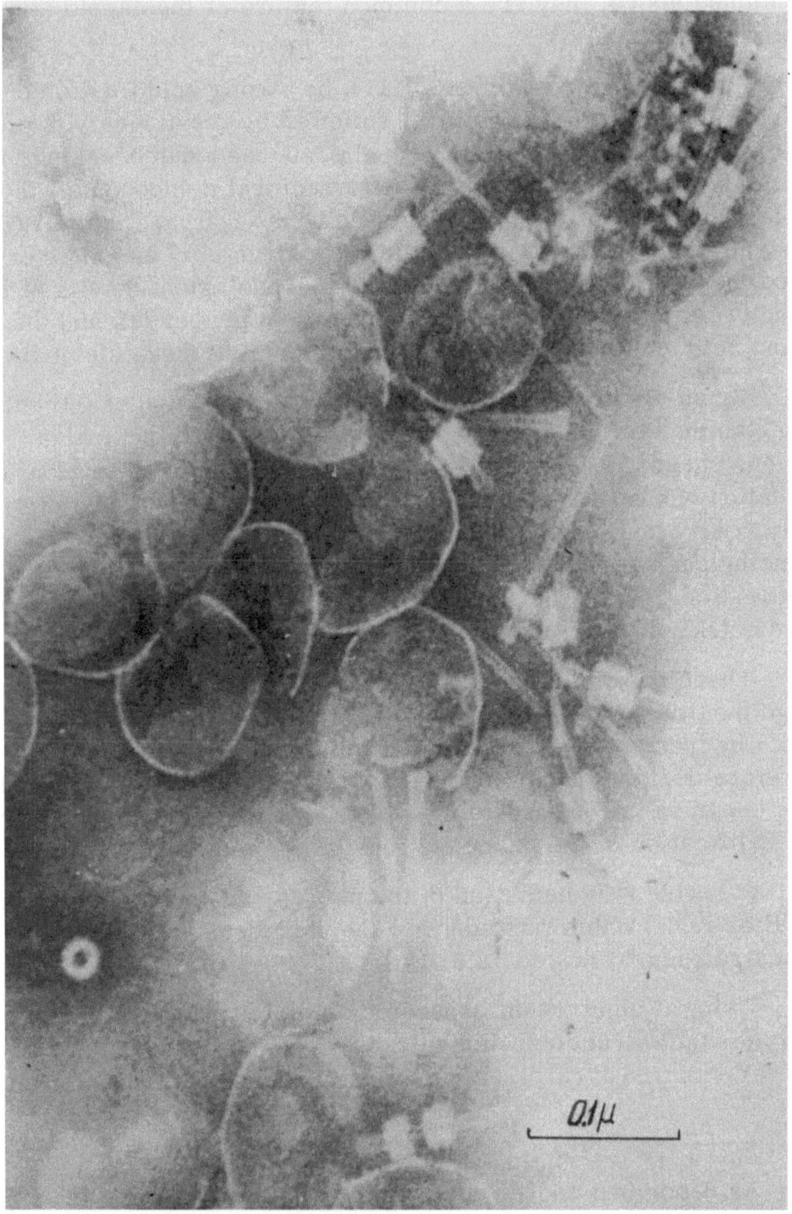

Fig. 92. Phage T2 treated with alkali (pH 11.0). Empty capsids and detached tails with a contracted sheath, isolated end plates, and the uncoiled strand of a tail sheath can be seen. PTA. 200,000×.

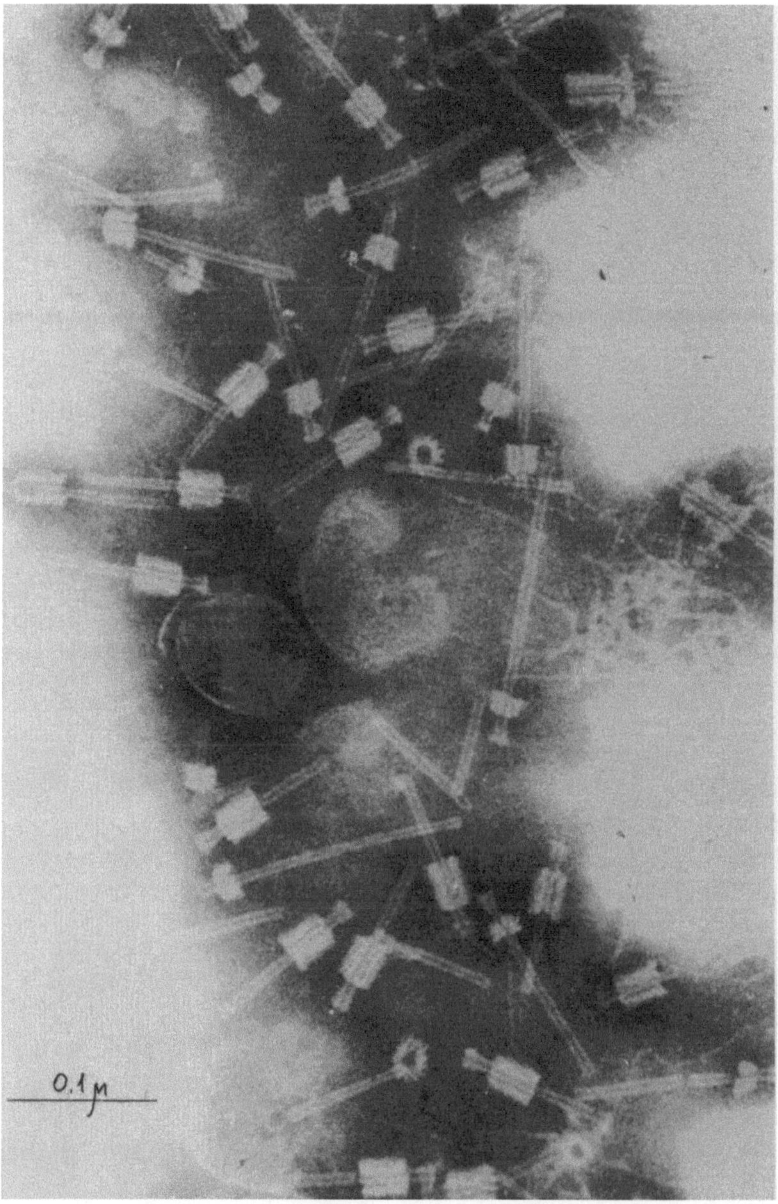

Fig. 93. Phage T2 treated with alkali (pH 11.5). The specimen contains mainly isolated tails with a contracted sheath. PTA. 200,000 ×.

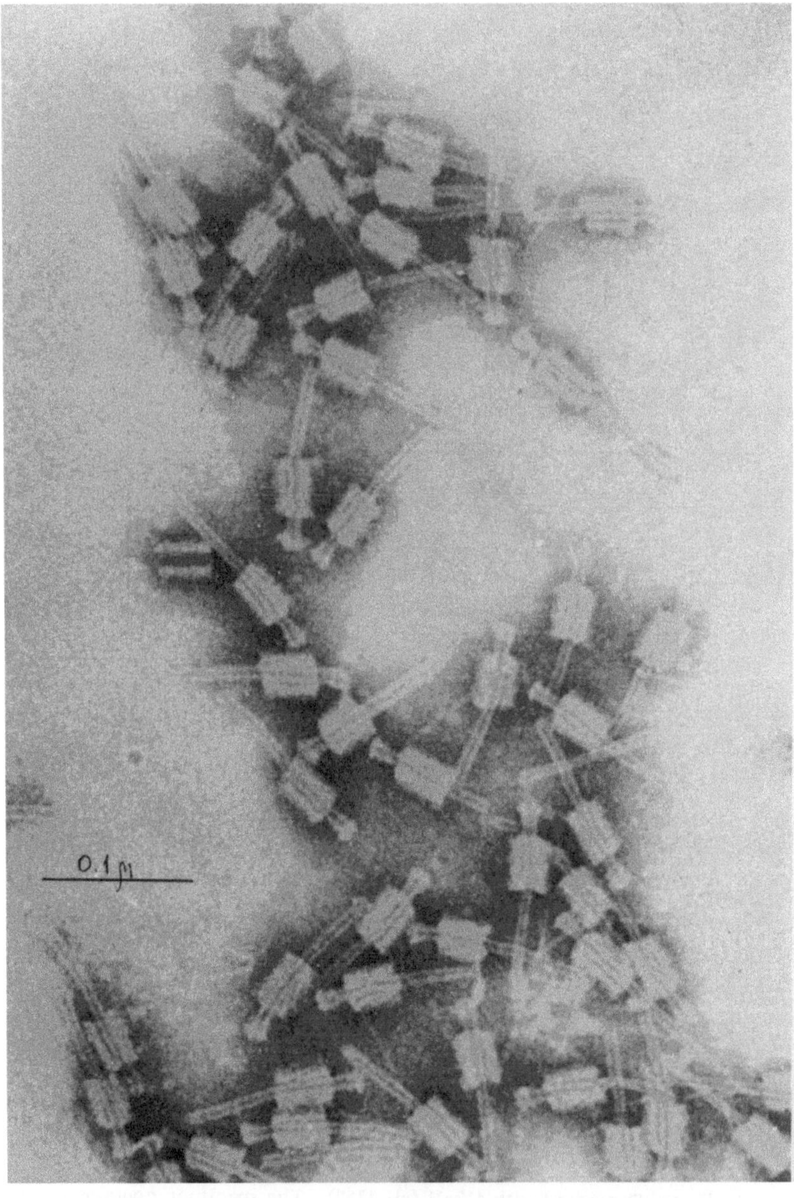

Fig. 94. Phage T2 treated with alkali (pH 11.8). Only contracted sheaths with a rod have been preserved. PTA. 200,000 ×.

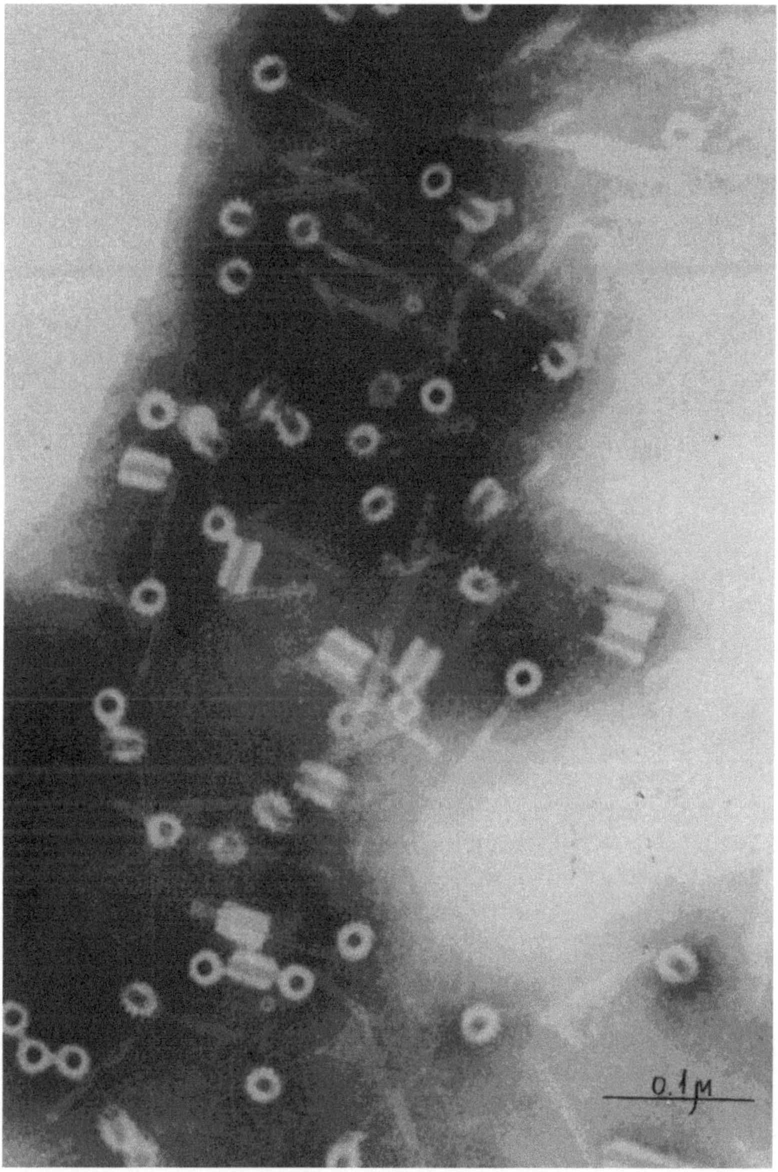

Fig. 95. Phage T2 treated with alkali (pH 12.0). Disconnected tail sheaths and rods can be seen. PTA. 200,000 ×.

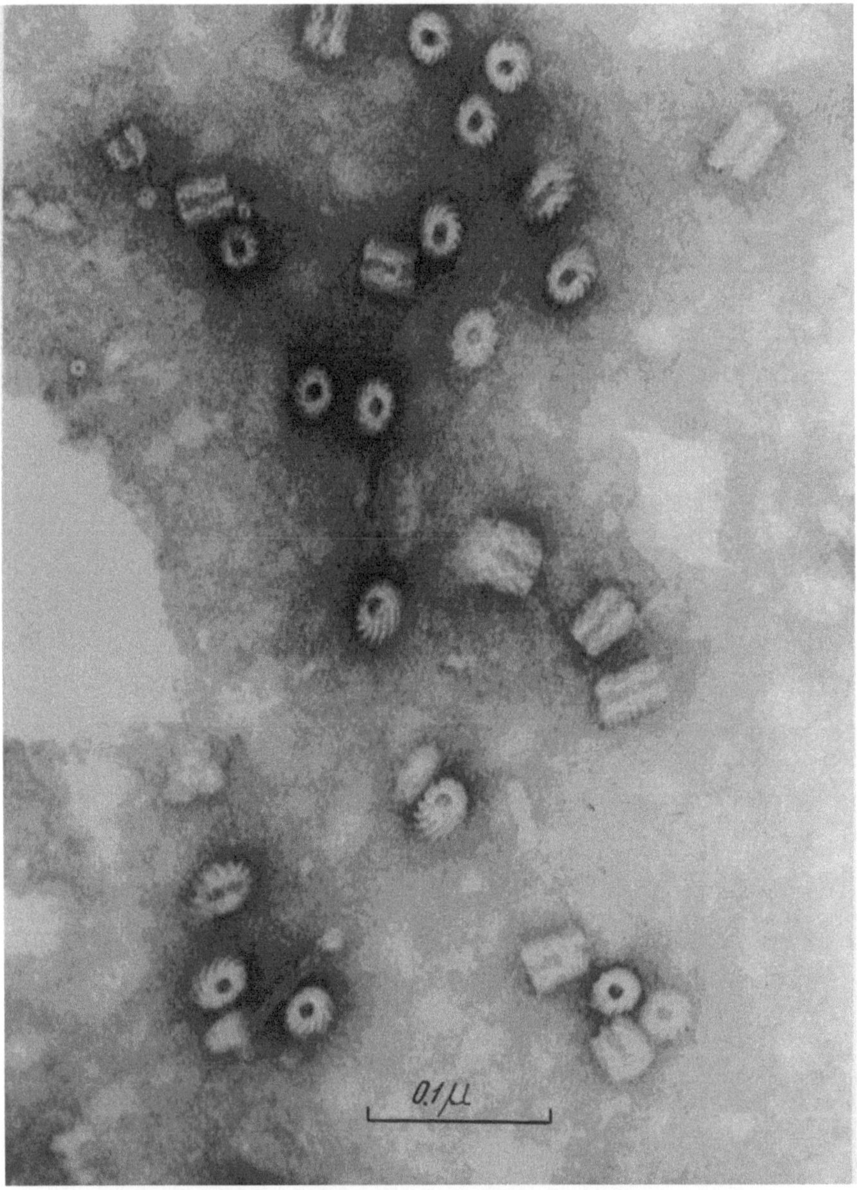

Fig. 96. Phage T2 treated with alkali (pH 12.4). Contracted tail sheaths without rods remain. PTA. 240,000 ×.

Tikhonenko and Poglazov [61] showed that phage T2 particles break up with a change of pH from 10.0 to 11.5. Fragmentation begins with rupture of the phage capsid and discharge of the inner contents of the head into the external medium (Fig. 92). This is accompanied by an increase in the viscosity of the test suspension.

As the pH rises the capsid begins to break up, and the tail separates from it. The sheath on tails separated from heads is in a contracted state. At these same pH values, separation of the end plate and tail fibers is also often observed. End plates separated from the sheaths, when lying on end, appear like a six-pointed star (Figs. 92 and 93). Some particles retain their tail fibers on a half-fragmented end plate attached to the contracted tail sheath (Fig. 93).

It was shown by treatment of phage T2 with alkali that in some cases the spirally coiled strand forming the tail sheath begins to uncoil and to resemble a stretched spring (Figs. 73, 74, 112). (A detailed account of the structure and some properties of the sheaths of phage T2 will be given below.)

Anderson and Stephens [94] also found that solutions of weak alkalies can not only cause contraction of the sheath of phage T6, but also uncoiling of the helix of the tail sheath.

In all probability the appearance of uncoiled helices is due to rupture of the bonds between adjacent turns of the coiled strand. The presence of these bonds holds the tail sheath in a tightly coiled state.

In a suspension of phage T2 treated with alkali in the pH range from 11.5 to 12 the capsid is completely fragmented and only the contracted tail sheaths remain, surrounding the inner hollow rod. Under these circumstances, the end plate is completely destroyed (Fig. 94).

Stronger action with alkali (pH 11.8-12.5) causes rupture of the bond attaching the outer sheath of the tail to the rod, and these two structural elements become disunited (Fig. 95). Under these conditions rods and sheaths can easily be separated into fractions by ultracentrifugation.

The tail sheaths are most resistant to the action of alkali. Whereas fragmentation of the rods can be observed at pH 11.8, the contracted sheaths remain intact in suspensions alkalified to pH 12.0 or higher (Fig. 96).

This unequal resistance of the various elements of the phage particle to different pH values of the medium during alkalification can be used to fractionate the protein structures of phage particles. Centrifugation of a phage suspension alkalified to pH 11.5 or slightly higher, when complete lysis of the phage capsid is observed, leads to sedimentation of the tails and to retention of the dissolved capsid protein in the supernatant.

A slight difficulty in the way of centrifugation is the fact that the liberated DNA gives the solution high viscosity. Because of this, the suspension must be diluted a little and centrifugation carried out at 100,000 g for 1 h. Examination in the electron microscope of specimens prepared from the residue shows that it contains only contracted phage tails (Fig. 94). Groups of tail fibers can often be found in the supernatant.

When a suspension of phage treated with alkali at pH 12.0 or higher was centrifuged, only contracted tail sheaths without the rods were sedimented (Fig. 96). The fragmented protein of the rod and capsid and the tail fibers mainly stayed behind in the supernatant.

The suggested method of fractionation of phage into its structural components [61] is fairly simple, but requires constant electron-microscopic control because the pH values at which the heads and rods undergo lysis may vary slightly depending on the phage concentration. The fractions thus isolated can be used for biochemical and physicochemical investigations.

Phage No. 1 of *Bacillus mycoides*

Compared with phage T2, phage No. 1 is more labile and can be easily damaged not only by many different agents, but even during preparation of the electron-microscopic specimens. The main result of this damage is that the tail sheath becomes contracted.

Elevation of the pH to 9.0 causes no significant changes in the structure of phage No. 1. Empty heads are found in only a very small number of virions and the sheath of some tails becomes contracted, although the overwhelming majority of particles are completely indistinguishable from the control.

A further increase in pH to 9.0–10.0 causes emptying of the capsid and contraction of the tail sheath of nearly all virions. In

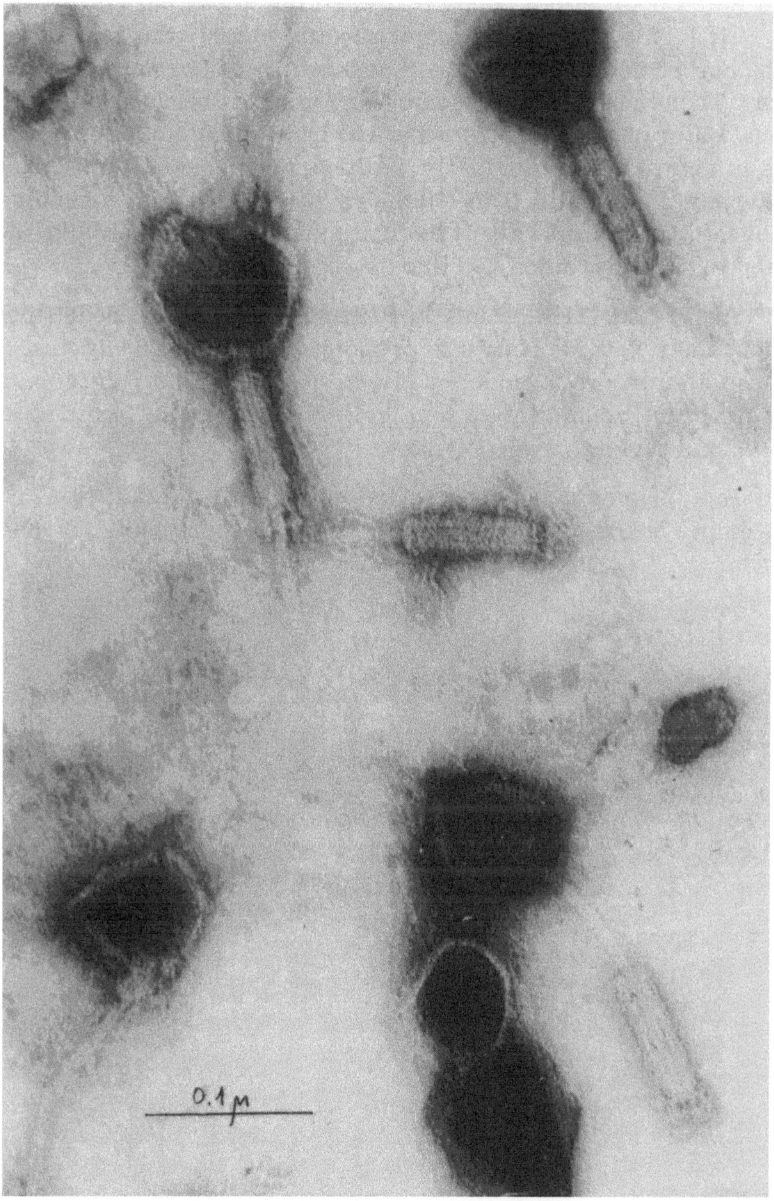

Fig. 97. Phage No. 1 of *Bacillus mycoides* treated with alkali (pH 10.0). Emptying of the head and contractions of the tail sheath are taking place. Uranyl acetate. 220,000 ×.

some cases the tail is broken off the head, the sheath separates from the rod or slides along it toward the distal part of the tail (Fig. 97). This photomicrograph reveals clearly the fine structure of the contracted sheath and rod consisting of morphological subunits. These specimens become very viscous because of massive liberation of phage DNA from the head into the external medium. This is shown morphologically by the appearance of empty phage heads and of very thin DNA filaments in electron-microscopic specimens. At these pH values the end plate as a rule remains attached to the contracted tail sheath.

At pH 11.0-11.5, empty head envelopes and tail rods, mostly without their sheaths, begin to predominate in the specimens. The tail rod also shows a tendency toward aggregation by the formation of a structure consisting of long hollow tubes, equal in diameter to the rod, but much longer (Fig. 98).

In a phage suspension treated with alkali at pH 12.0-12.5 only empty head envelopes remain, many of them partially de-

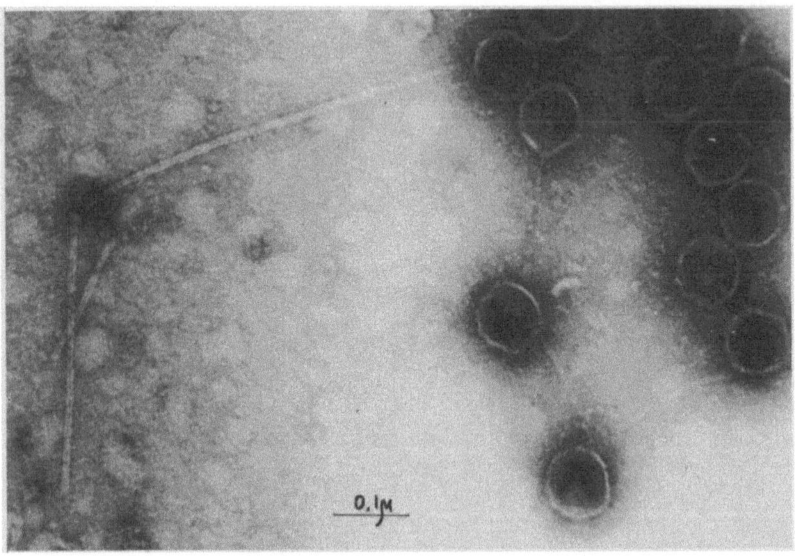

Fig. 98. Phage No. 1 of *Bacillus mycoides* treated with alkali (pH 11.5). The capsid and tail rod are preserved but the tail sheath is destroyed; long rod-like structures (polyrods) are appearing. PTA. 100,000 ×.

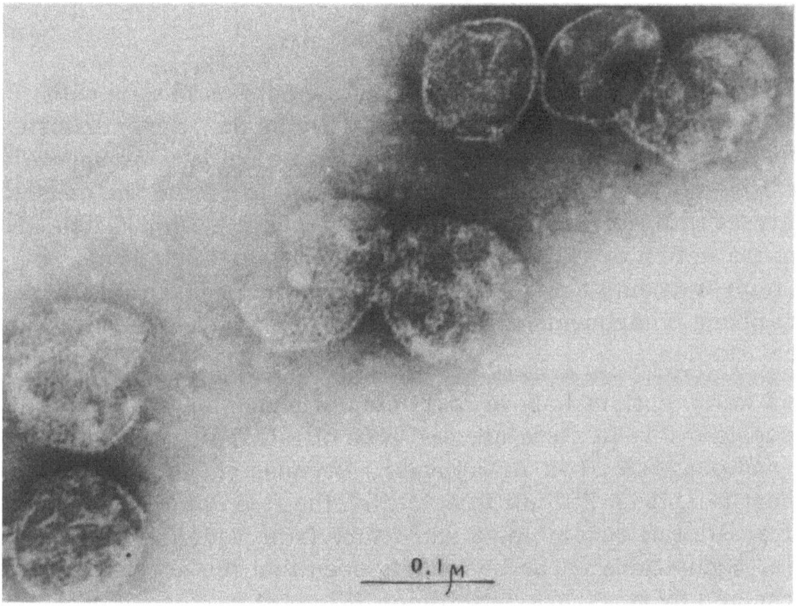

Fig. 99. Phase No. 1 of *Bacillus mycoides* treated with alkaline (pH 12.0). The capsids remain but the tail sheath and rod are destroyed. PTA. 180,000 ×.

stroyed and broken up into their component morphological subunit (Fig. 99). It can be seen in Fig. 99 that the capsomeres of the capsid resemble short hollow polyhedral tubes.

Under these conditions, the tail sheath and rod are probably broken up into small, component, morphological subunits.

The structural element of phage No. 1 most resistant to alkalies is thus the head capsid, followed by the tail rod; the least resistant structure is the tail sheath, which begins to be hydrolyzed at comparatively low pH values.

The stepwise destruction of the various phage elements depending on pH values indicates qualitative differences between the structural proteins forming these various elements of the phage particle. These properties of the proteins make it possible to subdivide phage particles into individual fractions consisting of particular structural elements.

Phage s_d

The effect of chemical and physical agents on phages with short tails has received comparatively little study. Nevertheless, the investigation of this matter would help to elucidate the specificity of phage action on the bacterial cell and to reveal the causes of the structural individuality of particular phages. In addition, the study of the action of various agents on phage particles would result in improvement of methods of isolation and preparation of individual phage components for further biochemical and physicochemical studies.

As was mentioned above, particles of phage s_d of *E. coli* SK differ considerably in structure and size of tail from phage T2 of *E. coli* and phage No. 1 of *B. mycoides*. Because phage s_d has a very short tail, it is difficult to establish the fine details of its structure. Its tail resembles a short tube from which a thin rod projects. Sometimes it can be clearly seen that the short tail tube is intersected by two transverse discs (Fig. 26).

The work of the author, Velikodvorskaya, and Belykh [57] has shown that the action of alkali on phage s_d at pH 9.0-10.0 causes emptying of the head of some particles. The tails mostly remain attached to the empty phage heads. In some cases, the tails also begin to break up, liberating separate structural elements. Free-lying hollow structures with a hole in the center can then be seen. These are liberated tail rods consisting of short hollow tubes, appearing endways as hollow rings (Fig. 28). The discovery of these structures confirms the complex organization of the tail of phage s_d, indicating that its short tail possesses a hollow inner rod as well as an outer sheath.

At pH 10.7 emptying of the heads of most phage particles takes place, accompanied by an increase in the viscosity of the suspension and by fragmentation of the tail. Empty capsids and pieces of the fragmented tail can be seen in such specimens in the form of short, filamentous structures (Fig. 100).

The action of alkali causes emptying of the phage head, probably by rupturing its capsid, followed by gradual hydrolysis of tail protein, and at pH 11.0, the tails are completely fragmented. The protein forming the capsid is more resistant to the action of alkali, the structure and polyhedral shape of the capsid persisting even at pH 12.0 (Fig. 101).

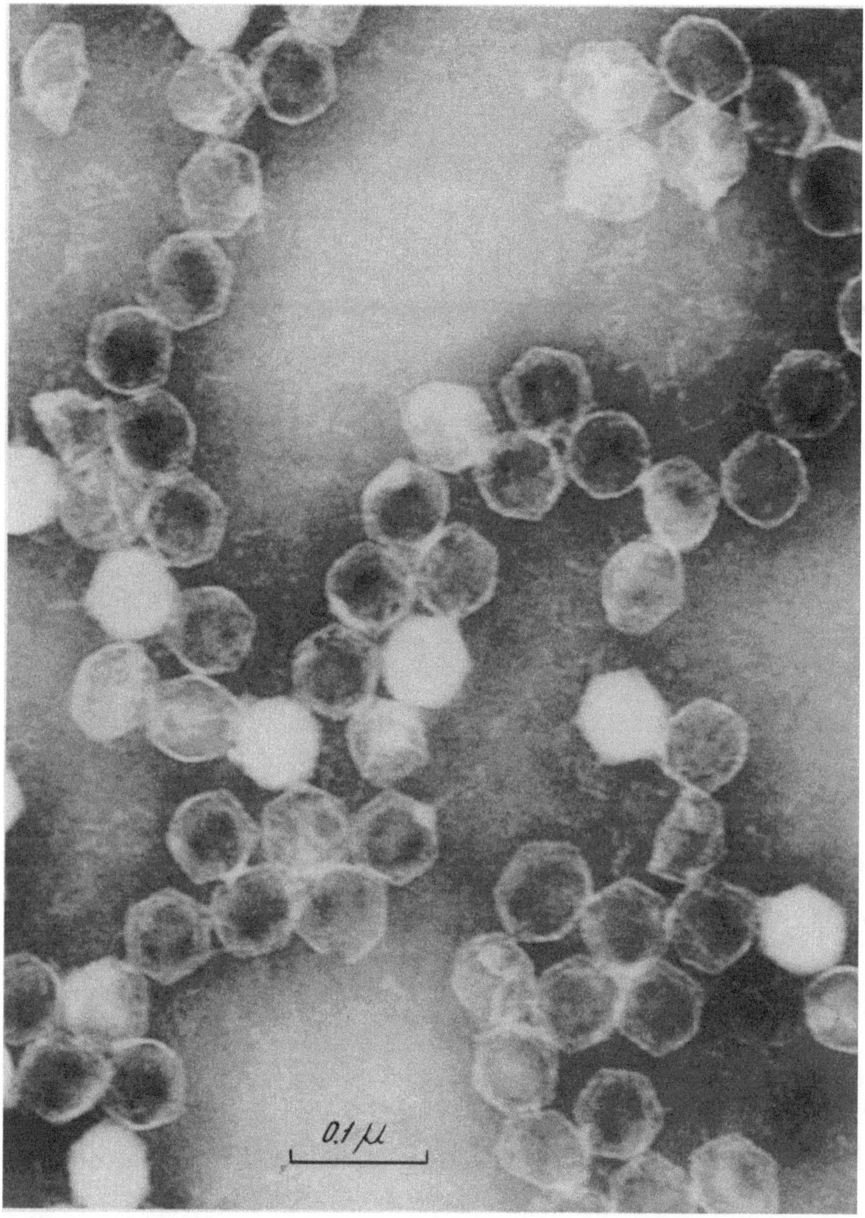

Fig. 100. Phage s_d of *Escherichia coli* SK treated with alkali (pH 10.7). Emptying of the head and destruction of the tail are taking place. PTA. 180,000 ×.

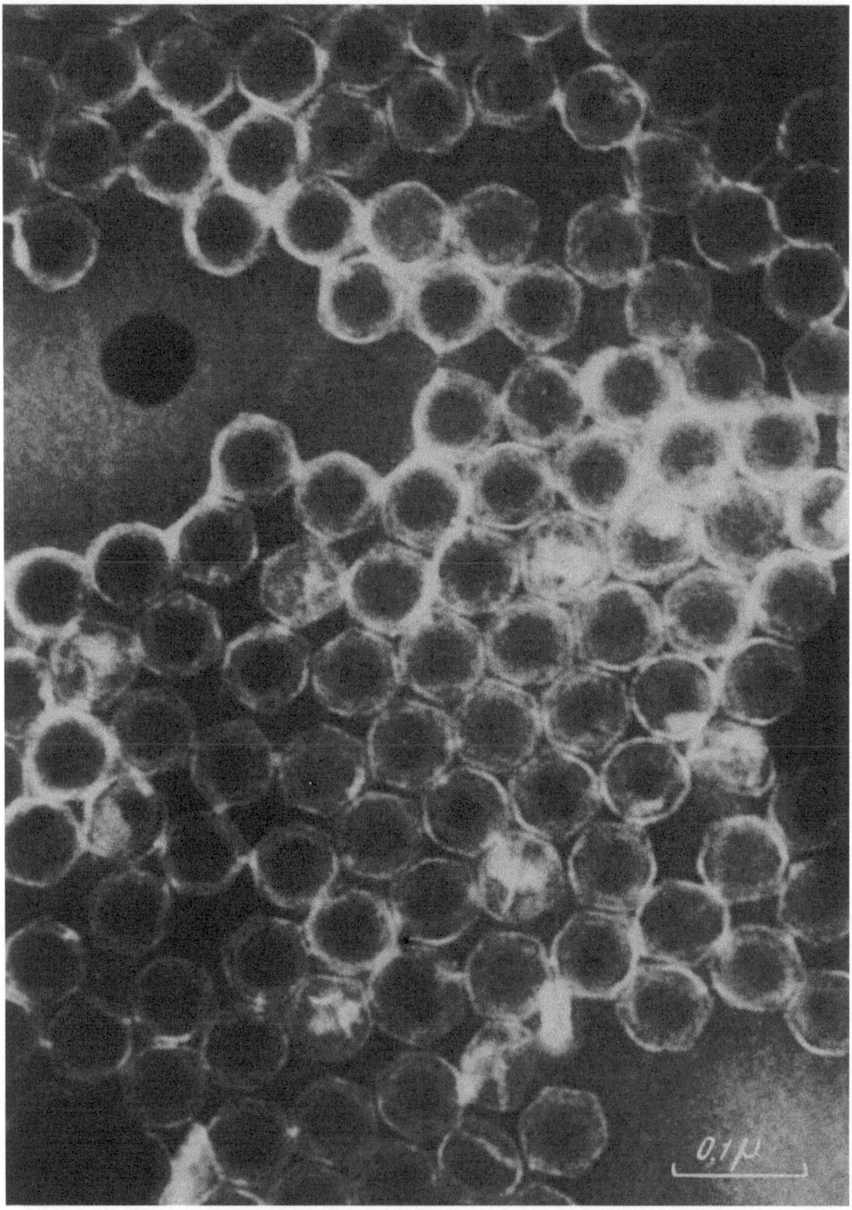

Fig. 101. Phage s_d of *Escherichia coli* SK treated with alkali (pH 12.0). Empty phage heads without tails remain. PTA. 180,000 ×.

In the pH range from 11.0 to 12.0, a pure fraction of phage s_d capsids can be obtained. Unfortunately, the use of alkali to isolate the tail fraction introduces considerable difficulties, because at pH 9.0 the connection between individual structural elements of the tail itself is broken. Furthermore, at pH 9.0, many phage particles still remain intact. By the use of more gradual changes of pH within the range from 9.0 to 10.7 it is possible to obtain conditions under which individual tail structures of phage s_d can be isolated. However, they are extremely difficult to identify morphologically, because of their very small size.

UREA AND OTHER AGENTS BREAKING HYDROGEN BONDS

The inactivating action of urea on phage particles has been known for a long time. As long ago as 1933, in his investigations of the classification of coli — dysentery phages, Burnet [117] used their sensitivity to urea as a differential character and found considerable differences in the rate of inactivation of different phages. Sato [330] found that urea has an inactivating action on phage T4.

Urea has also been used for extraction of the nucleic acid from phage particles [130, 180]. A phage suspension treated with urea became highly viscous, indicating release of nucleic acid from the phage head. By using an 8 M solution of urea, Fraser and co-workers [180] isolated DNA from phage T2, and this was then used to infect the protoplasts of *E. coli* cells.

Phage T2

During an electron-microscopic study of phage T4 treated with urea, Daems and co-workers [139] found that most particles have emptied heads, although a few still have heads filled with nucleic acid; the tail sheath of all the phage particles are contracted. The end plate of the tail is drawn upward together with the sheath. On the basis of their investigation, they concluded that urea disturbs the structure of the tail leading to contraction of the sheath and to rupture of the capsid. Similar observations were made by Hofschneider and Müller-Jensen [208, 286].

I obtained similar results by treating a suspension of phage T2 with 4 M urea solution [49]. Figure 102 shows that urea causes

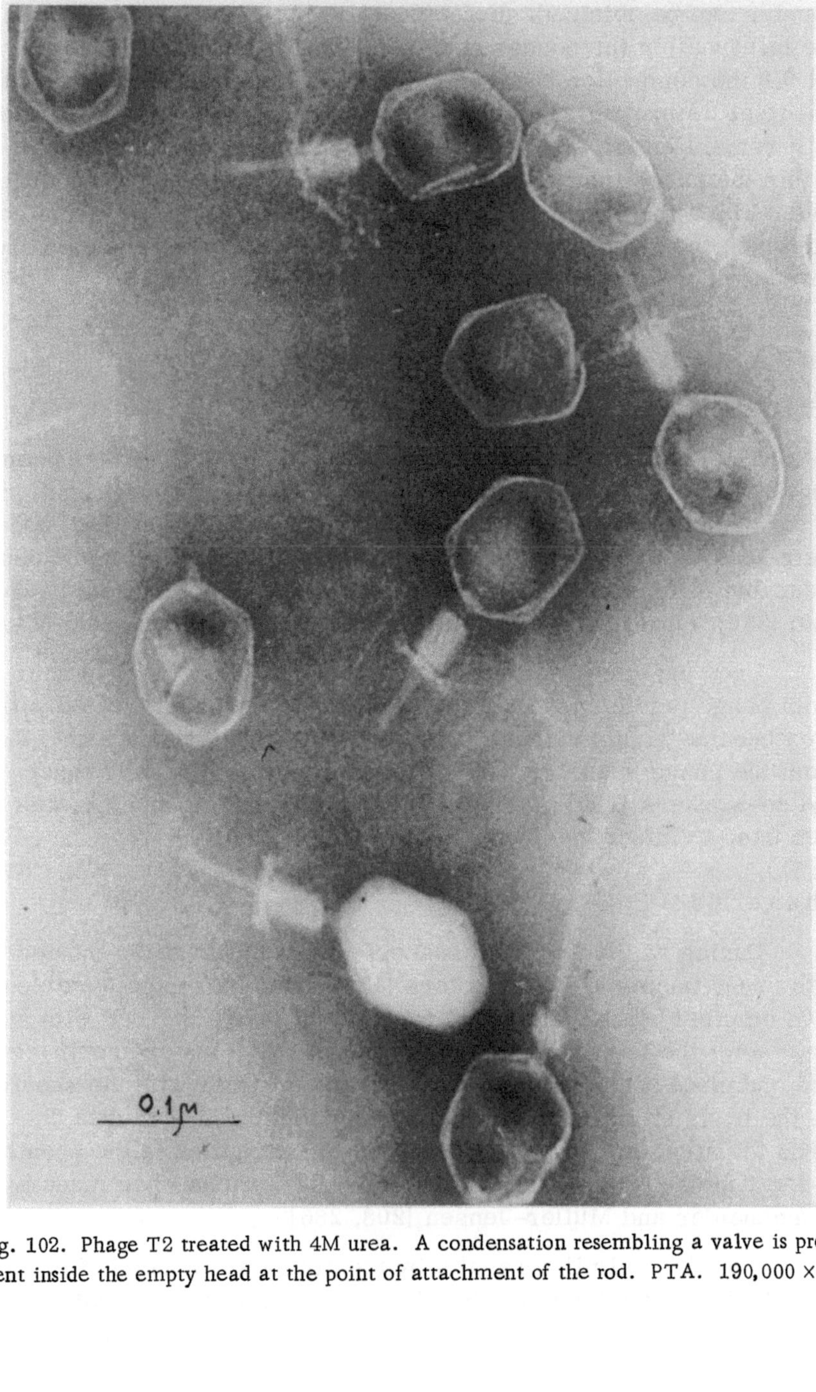

Fig. 102. Phage T2 treated with 4M urea. A condensation resembling a valve is present inside the empty head at the point of attachment of the rod. PTA. 190,000 ×.

contraction of the tail sheath and emptying of the head of most phage particles. Particles with a contracted tail sheath but still containing DNA in their heads, tails with a contracted sheath but without a head, and tail rods without a sheath are also found.

In my opinion, DNA is liberated from the head of phage T2, because of rupture of the capsid. The polymorphic picture observed during fragmentation of phage T2 by urea does not permit the isolation of the structural units of the phage particle in a pure form. However, the work of Müller-Jensen and Hofschneider [286] gives some idea of the functional role of the tail in the infection process. These workers showed that phage T2 particles treated with urea and containing DNA in their head and a contracted tail sheath cannot produce infection of normal *E. coli* cells, but can infect only cells which have been washed in water or in tris-sucrose, thus producing certain changes in the bacterial cell wall. This finding suggests that when the tail sheath contracts, its ability to produce hydrolysis of the cell wall is lost, and in that case the sole function of the contracted tail is mechanical perforation of the weaker bacterial cell wall by the rod, thereby making infection of the cell possible.

Phage s_d

Phages with a simpler morphological organization, i.e., possessing short tails and a smaller head, are more resistant to certain agents. For example, the T-odd phages are resistant to osmotic shock [78], although some of them, phage T7 for example, are easily inactivated by cationic detergents [309].

Phage s_d is no exception in this respect. It is highly resistant to many agents to which other phages are susceptible. For example, whereas 4 M urea causes liberation of DNA from the head of phage T2, it has no action whatever on phage s_d.

It has been shown that phage s_d, likewise, is resistant to osmotic shock [64]. This feature of phage s_d makes it difficult to obtain "ghosts" in a pure form for the study of their protein component. The author, Velikodvorskaya, and Belykh [57] hoped to obtain a positive effect by increasing the urea concentration, but even 8 M urea produced no morphological changes in phage s_d. The phage particles remained intact in these urea concentrations.

Urea ruptures hydrogen bonds. It might be supposed that the basis of the resistance of phage s_d to urea is that the stability of its capsid is determined by the existence of other bonds. To verify this suggestion, the action on phage s_d by two other agents which likewise rupture hydrogen bonds, namely formamide and ethylene chlorhydrin, was studied.

Experiments showed that formamide, in 20% concentration, liberates the contents of the heads of some phage particles into the surrounding medium, accompanied by an increase in viscosity of the suspension. At the same time, fragmentation of the tail and, in some cases, its separation from the head begins to occur. On the detached tail, the end plate, shaped like a six-pointed star, becomes clearly distinguishable (Fig. 27).

An increase in the concentration of formamide to 30% causes a further increase in the viscosity of the suspension. Electron-microscopic studies showed that the heads of most particles are emptied and their DNA liberated into the surrounding medium. However, some phage particles remain intact. The tail of most particles is detached from the head and is apparently partially fragmented (Fig. 103).

Higher concentrations of formamide (40–50%) cause emptying of the heads of all the phage particles. Empty head envelopes with fragments of the tail are visible in the specimens.

The action of ethylene chlorohydrin on phage s_d was studied in the same concentration as formamide.

The action of ethylene chlorohydrin was found to be similar to that of formamide, but its action on phage s_d is stronger. The lowest concentration of ethylene chlorohydrin (10%) has the same effect on phage s_d as formamide in the highest concentration used. A 50% solution of ethylene chlorohydrin causes complete breakdown of the phage s_d protein, leaving only phage DNA in the specimen.

As mentioned above, urea has no destructive action on phage s_d, whereas formamide and, in particular, ethylene chlorhydrin fragments phage particles vigorously. This fact suggested that certain substances, preventing rupture of the bond and stabilizing its protein structure, are present in the capsid of phage s_d. Formamide and ethylene chlorohydrin evidently remove these substances. Both formamide and ethylene chlorohydrin are known to be readily

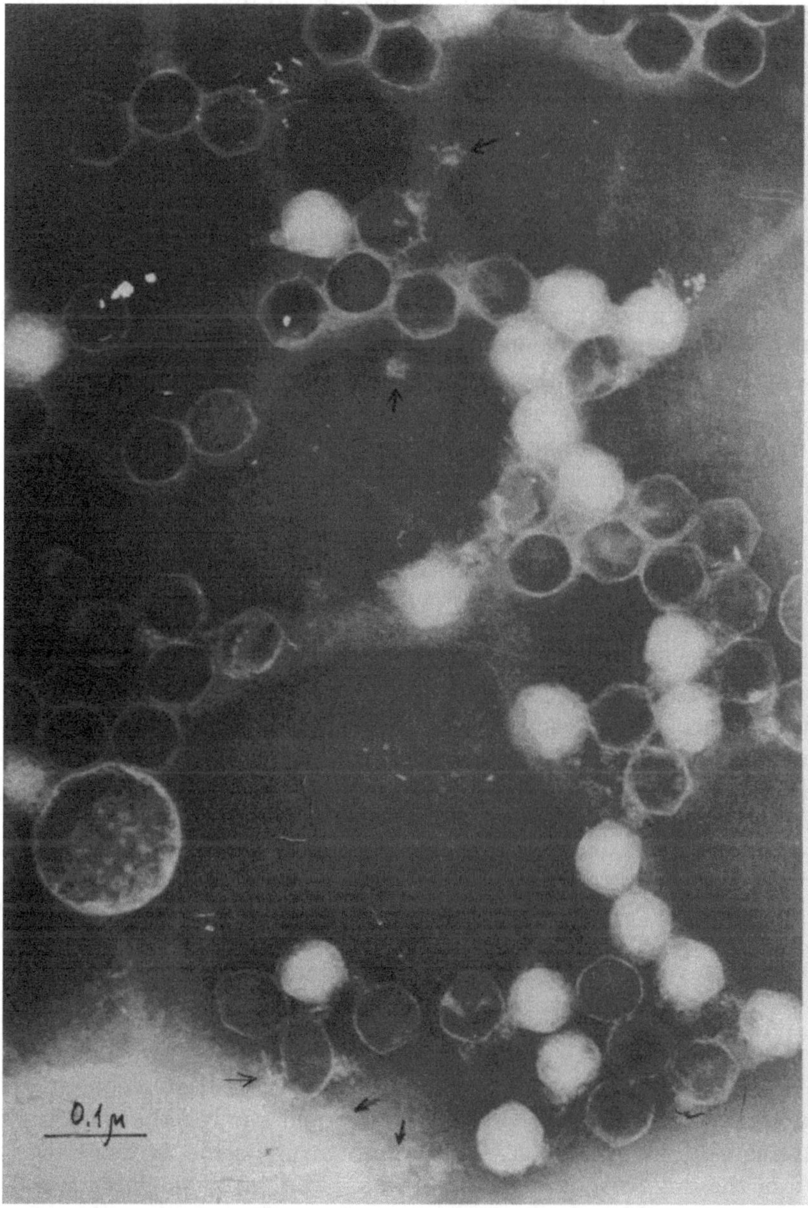

Fig. 103. Phage s_d of *Escherichia coli* SK treated with 30% formamide. Most particles have empty heads with detached tails (indicated by arrows). PTA. 130,000×.

soluble in lipids. It was therefore postulated that formamide and ethylene chlorohydrin can disturb a lipoprotein complex possibly existing in the envelope of the phage s_d head. After removal of the lipoprotein complex, the phage capsid becomes more accessible to the action of formamide and ethylene chlorohydrin as agents breaking hydrogen bonds, causing rupture of the head envelope, liberation of its DNA, and detachment of the tail. The possibility is not ruled out that other agents dissolving lipids may also disturb the bonds determining the stability of the phage s_d capsid.

This suggestion was verified as follows. Before the addition of urea, a suspension of phage s_d was treated with substances dissolving lipids, i.e., diethyl ether, petroleum ether, and chloroform, for 1 h with continuous agitation. These substances themselves have no action on the phage structure. Particles of phage s_d treated with diethyl and petroleum ethers and chloroform are indistinguishable morphologically from controls.

When added to a phage suspension treated with diethyl and petroleum ethers, 6 M urea does not disturb the integrity of the phage structure and there is no change in the viscosity of the suspension. However, the addition of 6 M urea to a phage suspension treated for 1 h with chloroform with continuous agitation leads to a sharp increase in viscosity of the suspension. Control electron-microscopic examination showed that the overwhelming majority of phage particles become empty. Preparations of phage s_d treated with 6 M urea alone, despite continuous agitation for 1 h at room temperature, are indistinguishable from controls.

It was concluded from these experiments that the resistance of the protein envelope of phage s_d to various agents compared with the T-even phages of *E. coli* B is due to the fact that it contains a substance extractable with chloroform, but insoluble in diethyl and petroleum ethers.

Velikodvorskaya, Chikova, and Lysenko [10] subsequently established the nature of this substance and showed that phage s_d contains a large quantity of lipids amounting on the average to 2.4% of the dry weight of its particles. The same workers found a small content of lipids (0.4%) also in phage T2. Neither phosphorus nor cholesterol was found in the composition of the lipid fraction, suggesting that phage lipid belongs to the group of neutral lipids.

The capsids of phage s_d and phage T2 thus differ quantitatively in their lipid content. The high lipid content in the capsid of phage s_d makes it highly resistant to the action of various chemical agents. This may be the reason why phage s_d is extremely specific against only one strain of *E. coli* SK and is inactive against other strains of bacteria of the coli — dysentery group.

DETERGENTS

To inactivate viruses and phages, investigators have for a long time used surface-active substances or detergents. Klein and coworkers [241] showed that many cationic and anionic detergents inactivate various phages. Phage T2 is an exception to this rule. However, sodium dodecylsulfate, in high concentrations, was used by Mayers and Spizizen [271] to isolate the nucleic acid from phage T2. The same detergent acts differently on different phages. For example, the cationic detergent dodecyltrimethylammonium inactivates phage T7 rapidly but has no action on phage T6 [309]. However, phage T6 is quickly destroyed by other detergents (benzyldodecylmethylammonium chloride) and more slowly by sodium dodecylsulfate [310].

The work of Fraenkel-Conrat [173] showed that detergents separate the protein and nucleic acid of the tobacco mosaic virus. This enabled him to reconstruct virus particles experimentally from their separate components. However, little if any work has been done to study the action of detergents on phages accompanied by morphological control.

Japanese workers [220] have recently shown that 0.1% sodium dodecylsulfate causes unwinding of the sheath helix of pyocin particles, which are similar morphologically to the tail of the T-even phages.

I have made an electron-microscopic study of the effect of sodium dodecylsulfate on the structure of certain phages [45]. I found considerable difference in the reaction of different phages to this agent. Phage s_d, for instance, when treated with 0.5-1% sodium dodecylsulfate solution releases its nucleic acid, leading to the appearance of empty phage capsids and to the accumulation of numerous DNA filaments. Phage T6 is highly resistant to the action of this detergent, remaining undisturbed with its morphology

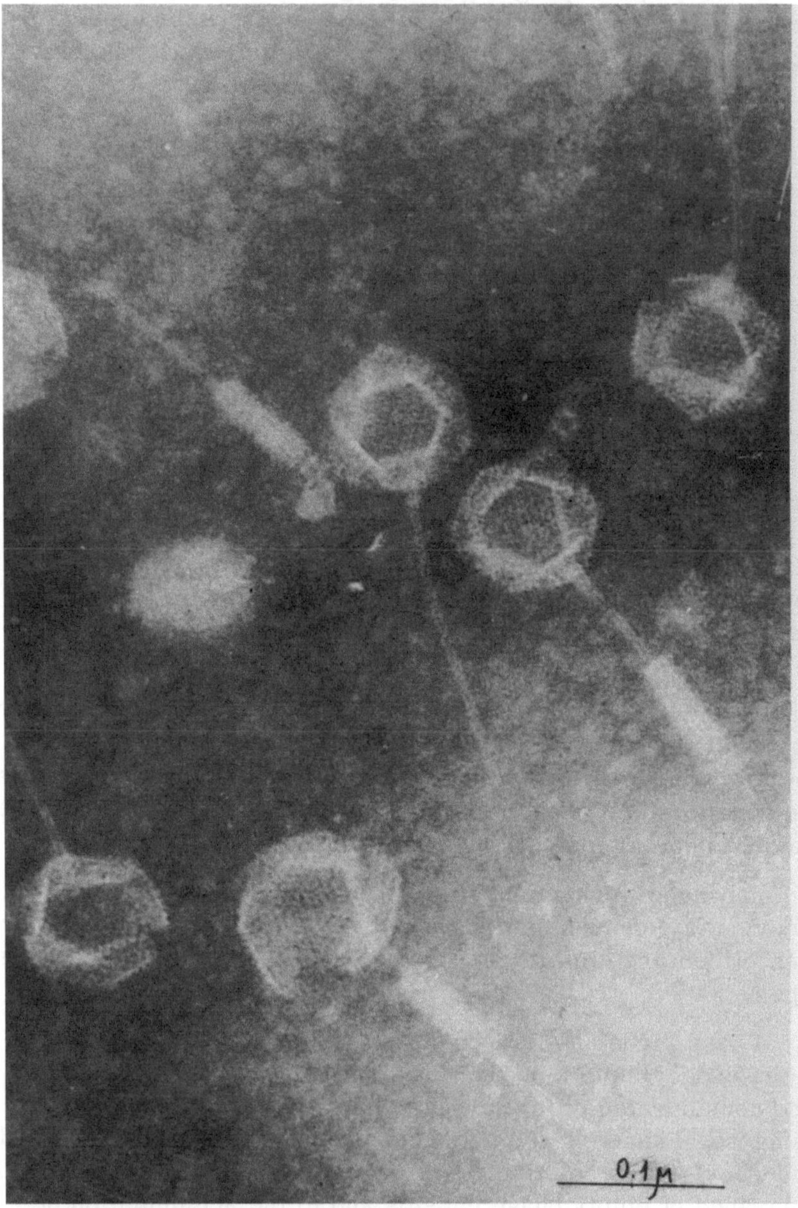

Fig. 104. Phage No. 1 of *Bacillus mycoides* treated with 0.1% sodium dodecylsulfate for 1 h. Emptying of the head and destruction of the tail sheath are observed. PTA. 220,000 ×.

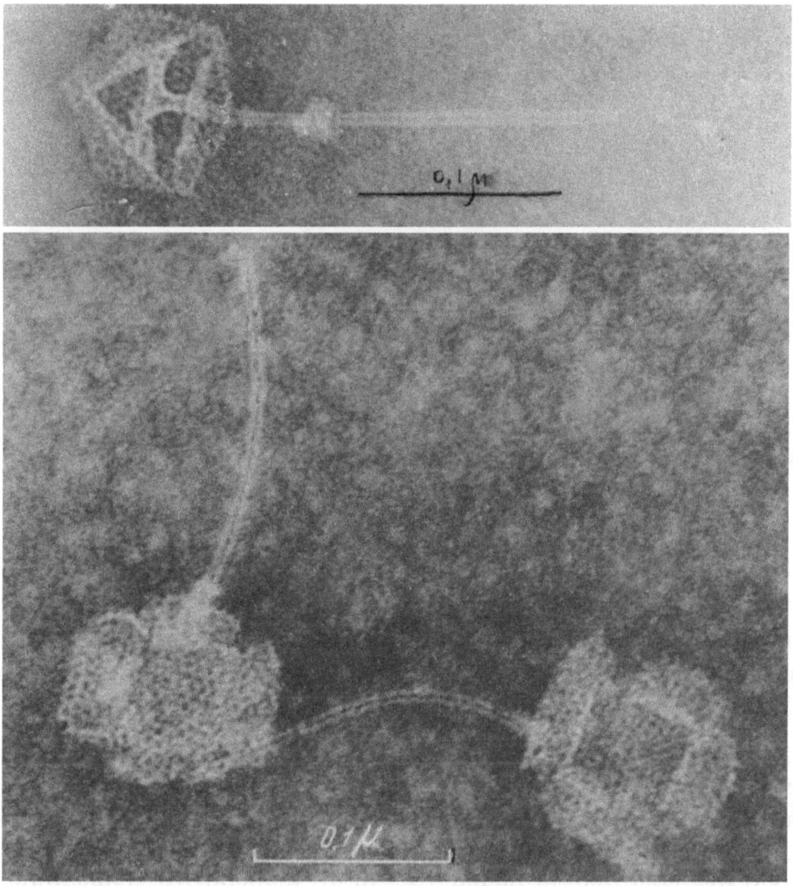

Fig. 105. Phage No. 1 of *Bacillus mycoides* treated with 0.1% sodium dodecylsulfate for 24 h. Complete destruction of the sheath and liberation of the inner tail rod are taking place. A phage particle with a small fragment of sheath can be seen above. PTA. 260,000 ×.

unchanged even after exposure to a 2% concentration of the detergent. Phage No. 1 of *B. mycoides*, on the other hand, is easily broken up even by the action of low concentrations (0.1%) of sodium dodecylsulfate.

However, these electron-microscopic investigations were carried out with the use of shadowing methods, which did not permit the fine details of the structure of the phage elements to be determined in the course of fragmentation of the particles [45].

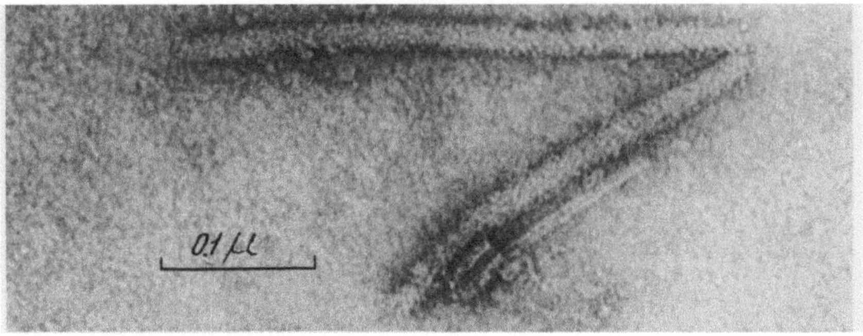

Fig. 106. Phage No. 1 of *Bacillus mycoides* treated with 0.1% sodium dodecylsulfate for 1 h. Polysheath formation can be observed. PTA. 200,000 ×.

By the negative shading method I was able to obtain more precise information concerning the character of the damage done to the phage structure by the detergent [47, 49].

Phage T2

Like phage T6, phage T2 is very resistant to the action of sodium dodecylsulfate. Its particles remain intact even in a 2% concentration of the detergent and are indistinguishable morphologically from controls.

In some cases, admittedly very rarely, the detergent causes rupture of the protein envelope of the phage T2 head followed by release of the DNA into the external medium as a compact, irregular ball. However, the same phenomenon is sometimes observed in control preparations of phage T2. In all probability, it develops under the action of forces of surface tension, breaking up the phage particles lying on the edge of the drying drop of contrast stain and unprotected by the contrast material.

Phage No. 1 of *Bacillus mycoides*

In contrast to the T-even phages, phage No. 1 of *B. mycoides* is extremely sensitive to the action of sodium dodecylsulfate. A relatively low concentration of this detergent (0.1%) causes emptying of the phage head accompanied by discharge of the DNA into the external medium. A suspension of phage No. 1, treated with detergent, immediately becomes highly viscous. At the same time, sodium dodecylsulfate causes contraction of the tail sheath with its gradual fragmentation. The destructive action of the detergent increases with an increase in the time of exposure. The sheath can often be seen to have moved nearer to the distal end of the tail or to be completely separated from the rod (Fig. 104). In addition, the tail sheath shows a clear tendency toward fragmentation of the turns of its helix into morphological subunits, thereby becoming shorter in length. Only a small fragment of sheath remains on the rod of some particles after their destruction. Most particles retain the bare rod attached to the empty head (Fig. 105).

When separated from the rods, the sheaths show a tendency toward aggregation. In such cases the length of the aggregated sheaths is much greater than the length of one contracted sheath (Fig. 106). The possibility is not ruled out that these long aggregates of sheaths are formed by self-organization of the disintegrated morphological subunits along small fragments of the sheaths which, in this case, act as "centers of crystallization," just as is found during reconstruction of the tobacco mosaic virus capsid [173].

When the sheath is completely destroyed, the inner hollow rod of the tail is exposed and its structure is very resistant to the action of this detergent. It remains connected to the empty protein envelope of the head.

The empty capsid of the head often appears burst, as a result of which it loses its polyhedral shape. However, its structural organization still remains. The individual capsomeres forming it can be clearly distinguished as short, hollow polyhedral tubes (Fig. 105).

Higher concentrations of sodium dodecylsulfate (0.3-0.5%) cause complete destruction of the tail sheath, which disappears as a morphological entity. The head capsid and the tail rod remain intact. Not even an increase in the concentration of the detergent to 1% can break up the rod and head capsid into separate subunits.

The most labile protein structure of phage No. 1 during exposure to sodium dodecylsulfate is thus the tail sheath.

FREEZING AND THAWING

In the one investigation reported in the literature, carried out in 1956 by Williams and Fraser [390], an electron-microscopic study was made of morphological changes produced in phage T2 by the action of rapid freezing and subsequent thawing. These workers showed that the particles of phage T2 become fragmented after freezing and thawing. As a result of this destructive action, DNA is liberated from the head and the tail sheath contracts. In addition, detachment of the complete tail from the head of the phage particle is frequently observed. To increase the contrast of their electron-microscopic specimens, the technique of shadowing with metal also was used, so that the fine structure of the individual structural elements of the phage particle could not be properly established.

In my own experiments for subdividing phages into their separate structural units and to study their reaction to freezing followed by rapid thawing, I used suspensions of phages T2 of *E. coli* B and No. 1 of *B. mycoides*.

The procedure was as follows. A concentrated suspension of phage in physiological saline, 1 ml in volume, was quickly frozen in a mixture of dry ice with 96% ethyl alcohol and quickly thawed in warm water. Freezing and thawing were repeated five times, samples being taken every time for examination in the electron microscope. Before making electron-microscopic specimens, the phage suspension was purified by drop dialysis. In some cases, dialysis was not carried out and specimens were made from unpurified phage suspension.

Phage T2

The results obtained by freezing and thawing a suspension of phage T2 were similar to those described by Williams and Fraser [390]. Phage T2 proved comparatively resistant to this procedure. After the first three successive freezings and thawings, most of the phage T2 particles remained intact, retaining the morphology of normal phage. However, a few particles were broken up. Rupture of the head capsid and detachment of the tail were observed in the broken particles. Some detached tails had a contracted sheath, others still had a stretched sheath.

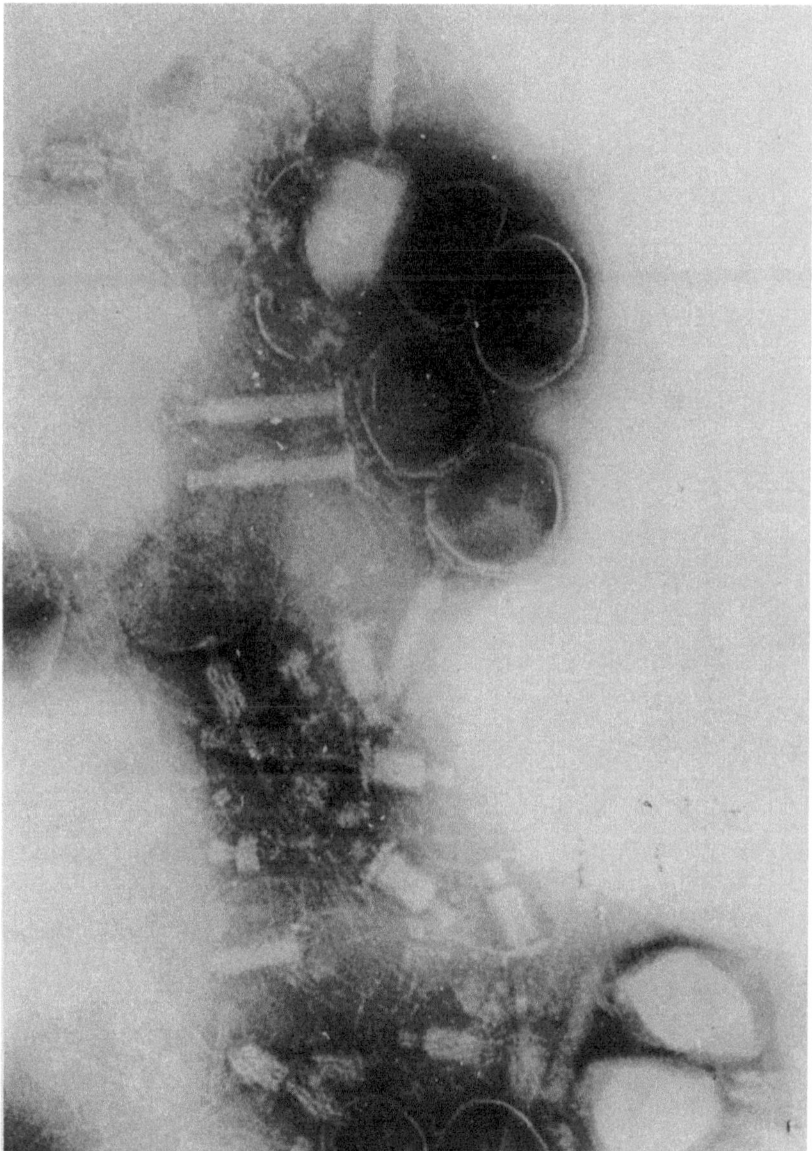

Fig. 107. Phage T2 after freezing and thawing 5 times. PTA. 200,000 ×.

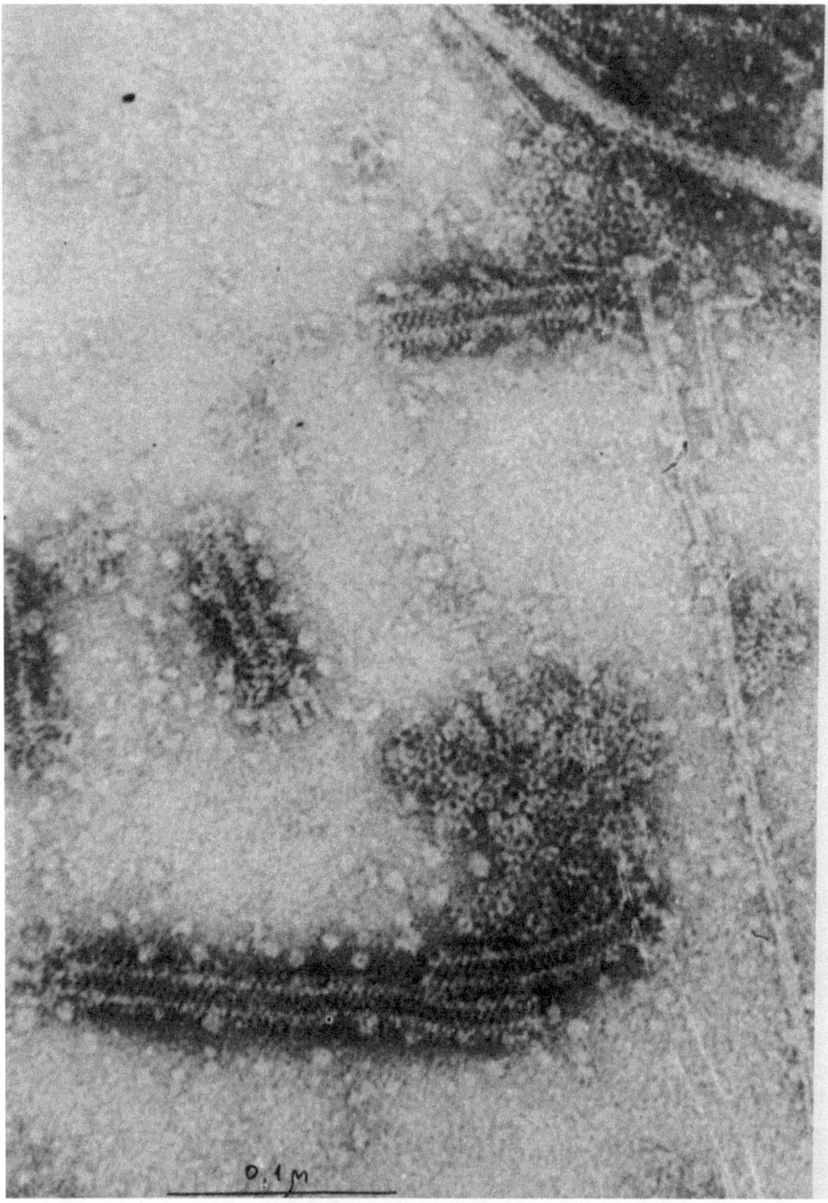

Fig. 108. Phage No. 1 after freezing and thawing three times. Disintegration of the capsid into capsomeres and of the sheath into morphological subunits and the formation of polysheaths and polyrods are taking place. PTA. 300,000 ×.

The most demonstrative picture of disintegration of phage T2 as a result of this procedure was observed after freezing and thawing for 5 times. In that case, nearly all the phage heads had lost their DNA. Some head envelopes appeared burst. Numerous detached tails were found in the specimens, with a contracted or uncontracted sheath (Fig. 107). After this procedure, the end plate of the phage tails with the thin fibers arising from it are comparatively well preserved.

Phage No. 1 of *Bacillus mycoides*

Phage No. 1 of *B. mycoides* proved less resistant to this procedure. Immediately after the first freezing and thawing, destruction of the phage particles takes place with liberation of DNA from the head and contraction of the tail sheaths. Particles in which the sheath has slid away from the rod are often seen.

After three freezings and thawings, most phage particles are highly fragmented into their component parts: the head capsid breaks up into individual capsomeres, while the tail separates from the head and, in turn, breaks up into sheath and rod. In addition, during freezing and thawing, the sheaths break up into separate morphological subunits. In cases when only part of the anterior wall of the sheath is destroyed, the inner cavity of the sheath is exposed where the subunits are detached, but is hidden in the neighboring segment by the subunits still preserved. The anterior wall of some tail sheaths is completely destroyed and the structure of its inner cavity can be clearly seen along its entire length (Fig. 60).

Short fragments of the broken sheaths and longer structures may be seen consisting either of several contracted sheaths joined together or newly constructed contracted sheaths (polysheaths) formed from dissociated morphological subunits. In length they considerably exceed the normal contracted sheath, but are exactly equal to it in width (Fig. 108).

The tail rods also undergo profound changes during freezing and thawing. They are either broken up into smaller fragments or they become longer. The structure of the lengthened rods is similar to normal, and like the normal rods they have an inner canal. In some cases it can be clearly seen that the rods are built of morphological subunits. Possibly in this case also, as a result of freezing and thawing, the rod structure breaks up into separate morphological subunits, which are then reconstituted, but into longer structures or polyrods (Fig. 108).

The end plates on the tail of phage No. 1 are well preserved after freezing and thawing. They mostly remain attached to the contracted sheaths, even in cases when the sheath has lost its rod (Fig. 60).

It is clear from the photomicrograph (Figs. 60 and 108) that the tail sheath is composed of separate morphological subunits arranged to form a helix. The arrangements of the subunits of the contracted sheath differs from that of the stretched sheath. The morphological subunit of the contracted sheath appear longer. In all probability, contraction of the tail sheath is accompanied by changes in the conformation of its morphological subunit.

The structure of the head capsid after fragmentation by freezing and thawing is very interesting. Most capsids are highly fragmented. In some cases they are broken up into separate capsomeres (Figs. 60 and 108). The structure of the individual capsomeres thereby becomes clearly distinguishable and they can be seen to be short, hollow tubes, hexagonal in section, built of separate structural units.

Fragmentation of the phage particle by freezing and thawing has thus given accurate information on the structure of individual capsomeres of the capsid and has shed some light on the properties of the protein of the sheath and rod, with their manifest tendency toward aggregation.

THE EFFECT OF TEMPERATURE

Thermal inactivation of phages has been studied in some detail. Many investigators have found that phages are considerably resistant to the temperature factor. As long ago as 1926, d'Herelle [196] observed that some phages are inactivated by heating to 75°C only after an exposure of 30 min, while others quickly die at 70°C.

The kinetics of thermal inactivation of different phages has been the subject of much investigation [73, 257, 305].

The results show that thermal inactivation of phages is a kinetic reaction of the first order. However, phages differ in their degree of thermostability. Phages of the thermophilic bacteria, which are inactivated only at 100°C, have the highest observed resistance to heat [388].

Many investigators have found that the sensitivity of phages to heat depends on the chemical composition of the medium. In a saline medium, phages are more sensitive to the temperature factor than in broth [73, 188, 260, 289]. Pottinger and Bachofer [306] have shown that the rate of thermal inactivation of phages is sharply reduced if bivalent cations are added to the medium, Mg^{++} and Ca^{++} ions being most effective in this respect. These workers postulated that protection of the phage against the action of heat by bivalent cations is based on their ability to combine with phage DNA. In Gol'dfarb's opinion [11], thermal inactivation cannot be due to action on nucleic acid along. He considers that thermal inactivation may be the result of a disturbance either of the adsorption function of phage or of other properties of the phage protein, notably its lytic activity, which is localized in the protein structures of the phage tail. To confirm this argument, Gol'dfarb and Avdeeva [12] showed that ghosts of phage T4 lose their ability to form a protoplast, i.e., do not destroy the bacterial cell wall, at temperatures at which thermal inactivation of phage takes place.

Lark and Adams [260] have given a detailed description of the physical and chemical aspects of thermal inactivation of phage T5 of *E. coli* B. They found that inactivation of phage is accompanied by liberation of nucleic acid into the solution, and the remaining protein phage ghosts lose their ability to become adsorbed onto bacterial cells.

Despite the many investigations of the action of temperature on phages, there is little or no information available on morphological changes taking place in the phage particle during exposure to heat.

It seems to me that observations on changes in phage morphology during thermal inactivation could provide valuable information on the functional role of the structural components of the phage particle and on the structure of the denatured proteins, because values of the temperature coefficient of thermal inactivation of phages, details of which are given in Gol'dfarb's monograph [11],

Table 9. Effect of Temperature on Infectious Activity of Phages

Temperature, °C	Titers of phages		Temperature, °C	Titers of phage No. 1
	s_d	T2		
50	$4 \cdot 10^{12}$	$5 \cdot 10^{11}$	50	$1 \cdot 10^{10}$
60	$3.5 \cdot 10^{9}$	$3 \cdot 10^{11}$	52	$1 \cdot 10^{10}$
70	$2 \cdot 10^{8}$	$1 \cdot 10^{6}$	54	$3 \cdot 10^{9}$
80	$2 \cdot 10^{7}$	0	56	$2 \cdot 10^{7}$
90	0	0	58	$3 \cdot 10^{3}$
100	0	0	60	0
Control	$5.5 \cdot 10^{12}$	$6 \cdot 10^{11}$	Control	$7 \cdot 10^{10}$

indicate that thermal inactivation is largely associated with denaturation of phage protein. Since the structural proteins of different phages are not identical, it is to be expected that the morphological changes resulting from exposure to heat likewise must vary.

Tikhonenko, Velikodvorskaya, and Belykh [57] made an electron-microscopic study of changes in the morphology of phage s_d during heating. Similar investigations have also been carried out later by the author and Belyaeva on phages T2 of *E. coli* and No. 1 and N19 of *B. mycoides* [51].

A suspension of the phages was heated under standard conditions. A phage suspension in 0.9% NaCl solution was heated for 10 min at a temperature of between 50 and 100°C, with a resulting gradual loss of infectious activity (Table 9).

As Table 9 shows, inactivation of different phages begins at different temperatures.

Phages s_d and T2 were most resistant. A sharp decrease in the titer of phage T2 is observed at 70°C, and it falls to zero at 80°C. Phage s_d begins to undergo appreciable inactivation at 60°C and its infectivity completely disappears at 90°C.

Phage No. 1 is highly sensitive to the action of the temperature factor, its titer falling at 54–56°C and reaching zero at 60°C.

Phage s_d

I have studied changes in the ultrastructure of phage s_d during exposure to heat [57]. Heating phage s_d to 50°C for 10 min causes certain morphological changes in the phage particle compared with the control picture. The integrity of the capsid of some phage particles is disturbed, and release of the contents of the head into the external medium begins. The tail remains attached to the head, but its structure changes slightly, in all probability, due to the initial stages of destruction of the end plate.

Heating a suspension of phage s_d to 60° and 70°C for 10 min causes the release of DNA from the overwhelming majority of phage particles. In the specimens, deformed empty heads are found surrounded by filaments of DNA escaping from them. The short tails, consisting principally of an end plate, still remain on some phage particles, but their integrity is evidently disturbed and they are rough in appearance. In addition, detached tails can be seen in such preparations, appearing as discs surrounded by a halo of fibers and with a hole in the center.

Further heating to 80–100°C for 10 min completely destroys the protein structure of the phage. In such preparations, only strong strands of DNA, consisting of separate filaments, are present.

Heating a suspension of phage s_d from 50 to 90°C thus causes gradual destruction of the protein component of the phage particle until its structure completely disappears.

The temperature factor, causing gradual destruction of phage s_d, could be used to isolate the structural components of this phage. However, since fragmentation begins at fairly high temperatures (70°C), there is the risk of possible denaturation of the phage protein. Nevertheless, the morphological study of phage structure during its fragmentation has shown that the short tail of phage s_d possesses an end plate which is similar in structure to the end plate of long-tailed phages.

Phage T2

Rapid release of DNA from phage T2 begins at a temperature of 60°C. In such preparations, the phage particles lie among a dense network of DNA filaments. The heads of most particles become empty. Meanwhile, the tail sheath contracts, although some particles

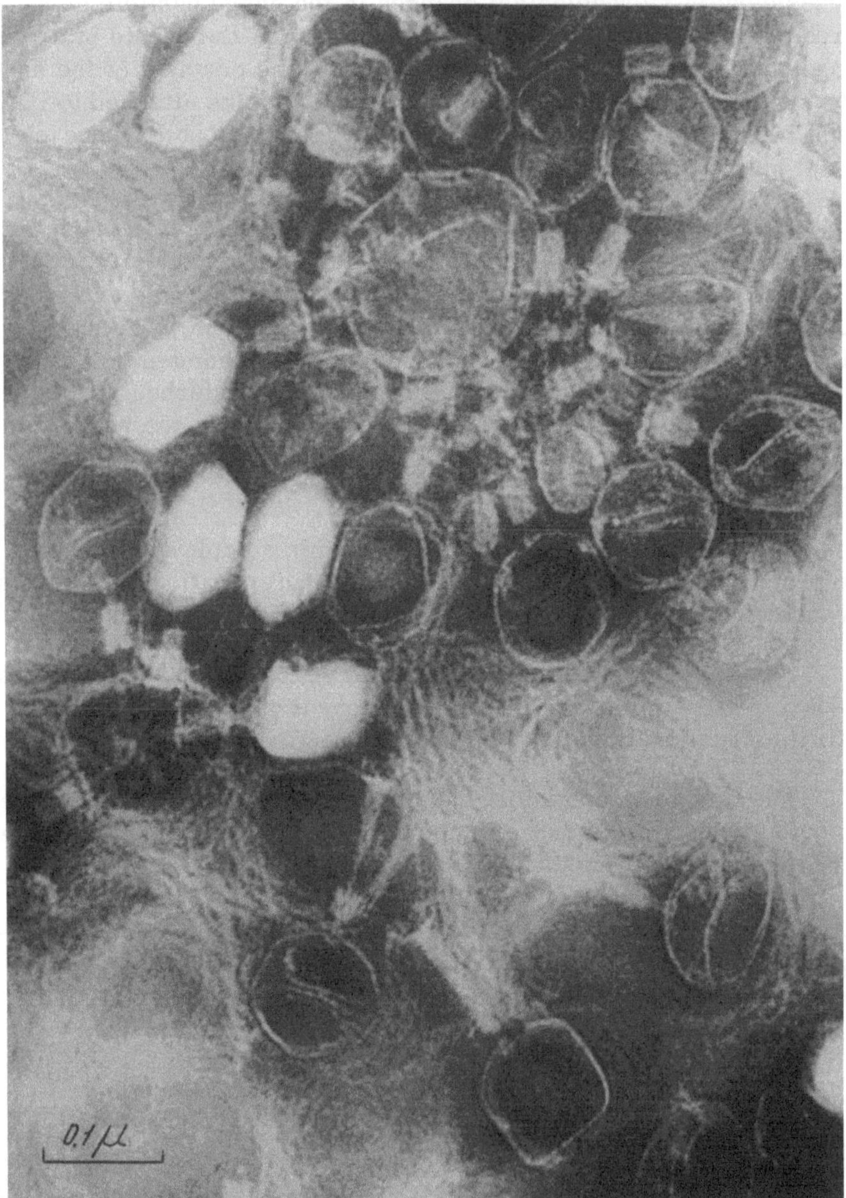

Fig. 109. Phage T2 after heating to 60°. PTA. 160,000 ×.

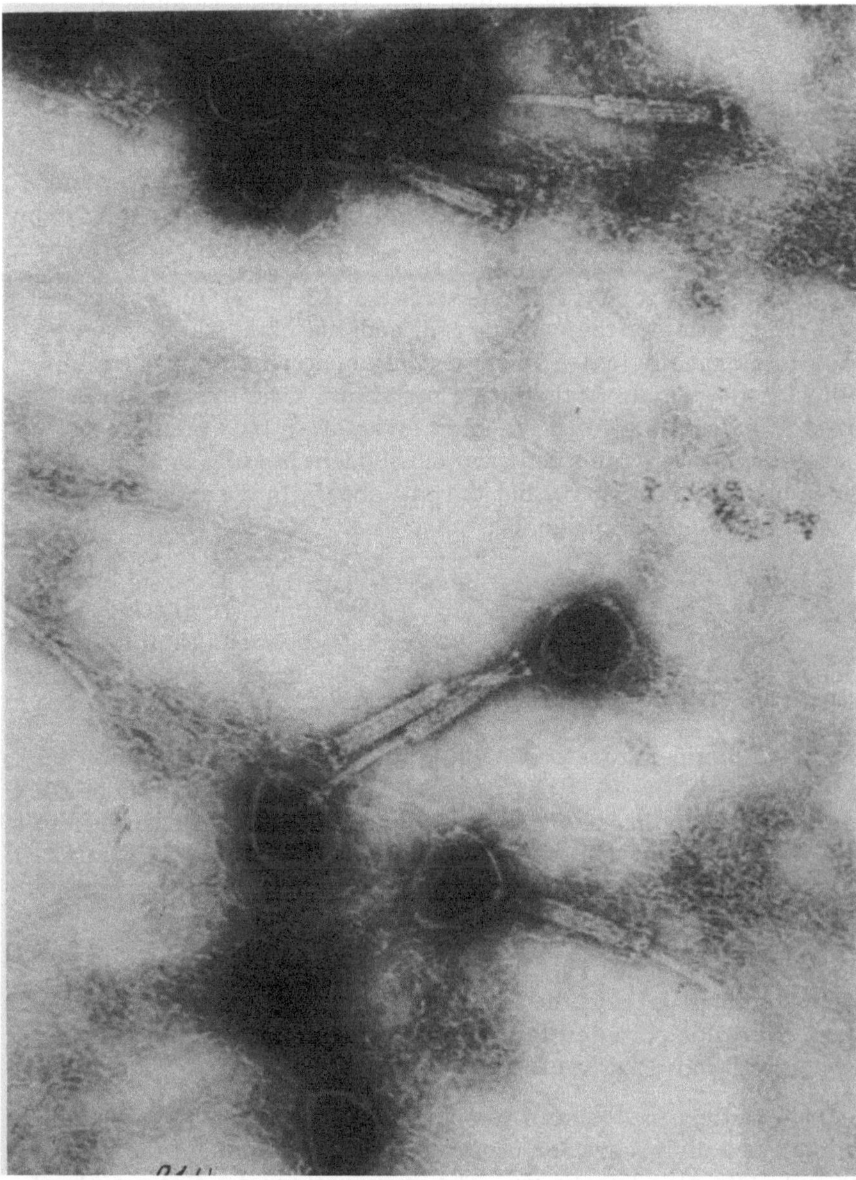

Fig. 110. Phage No. 1 of *Bacillus mycoides* after heating to 70°. PTA. 140,000 ×.

are found with an empty head and an uncontracted tail sheath. While some particles are undergoing morphological changes as a result of heating, intact phage particles also are relatively numerous (Fig. 109).

Raising the temperature to 70°C results in emptying of the head of all particles and contraction of their sheath. Such particles show a tendency to join together by their tails, forming rosette-shaped figures. At this temperature the end plates still remain attached to the contracted sheaths with the tail fibers arising from them.

A further increase in temperature (80-90°C) leads to complete destruction of the capsid, rod, and end plate which cease to exist as morphological elements. Only contracted tail sheaths without rods remain of the phage particles. The tail sheath of phage T2 persists, it will be noted, even after treatment of the phage suspension with alkali and subsequent heating to 100°C. These observations show that the tail sheath is the most resistant protein structure of phage T2.

Phages No. 1 and N19 of *Bacillus mycoides*

Phages No. 1 and N19 of *B. mycoides* respond in a distinctive manner to high temperatures [51]. These phages are both thermosensitive.

At a temperature of 50-60°C intensive fragmentation of the particles of phage No. 1 begins, accompanied by liberation of DNA into the surrounding medium. Slender DNA filaments woven into a network can be seen in the specimen. The tail sheath of all particles is contracted and the heads appear empty. Similar changes are observed in particles of phage N19.

At 70°C the tail sheath of phage No. 1, as a rule, begins to slide spontaneously off the rod and to break up gradually. Some phage particles completely lose their sheath and consist of a capsid and tail rod (Fig. 110).

A further increase of temperature to 80°C is accompanied by intensive disintegration of the tail sheath. Besides the sheath, the end plate also breaks up. The preparations consist mainly of deformed or half-disintegrated capsid and rods of phage particles (Fig. 111).

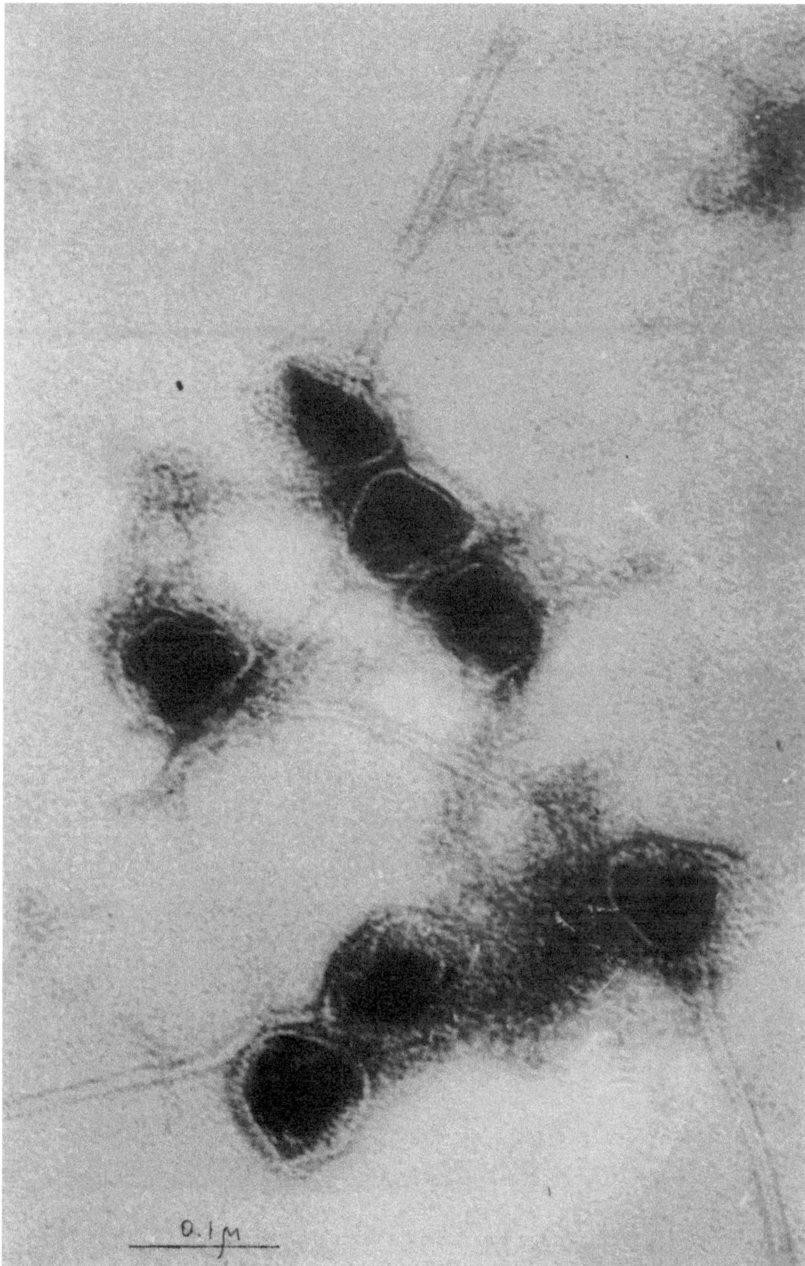

Fig. 111. Phage No. 1 of *Bacillus mycoides* after heating to 80°. Destruction of the tail sheath can be observed. PTA. 200,000 ×.

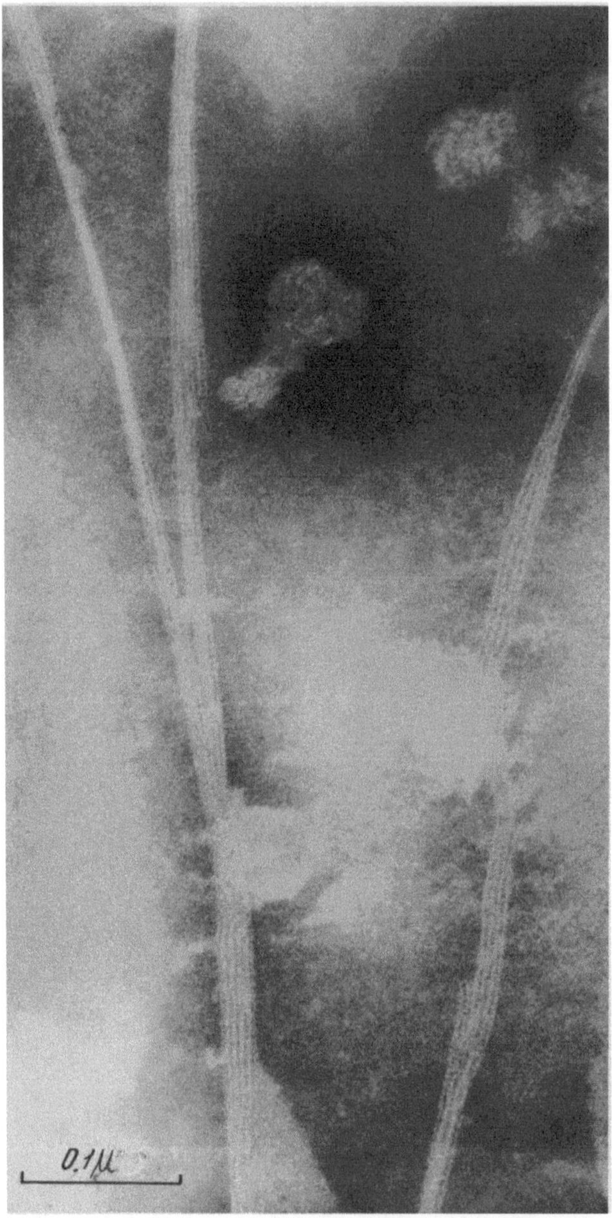

Fig. 112. Phage No. 1 of *Bacillus mycoides* after heating to 100°C. Long rod-like structures (polyrods) have appeared. PTA. 200,000 ×.

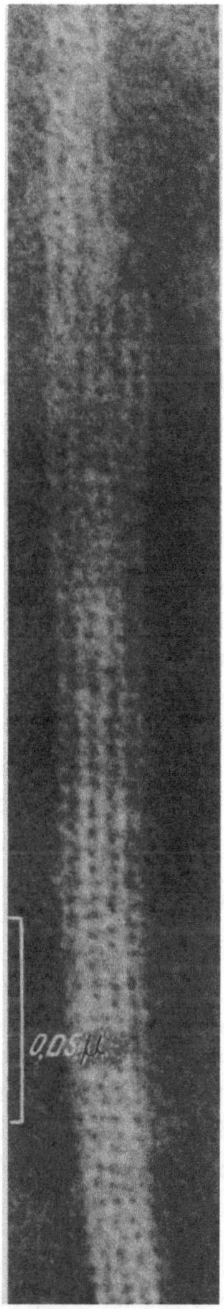

Fig. 113. Magnified fragment of Fig. 112. Morphological subunits forming polyrods can be seen. 500,000 ×.

An increase of temperature to 90°C causes more intensive fragmentation of the head capsid. Intact heads are no longer present in the preparation, whereas the rods still persist. However, in the course of further exposure, the rods undergo profound changes, seen most clearly in suspensions of phages No. 1 and N19 heated to 100°C. At a temperature of 90–100°C the structure of the rod not only is not destroyed but, on the contrary, it begins to lengthen gradually. The effect of lengthening the structure of the rod is seen at its maximum in phage No. 1. Whereas in specimens of a suspension of phage No. 1 heated to 90°C, structures corresponding in their morphology and diameter to the phage rod, but twice as long as the normal rod, appear, at 100°C the rod-like structures become very much longer, sometimes reaching several microns. These structures also show a tendency to aggregate, side by side, forming bundles (Fig. 112). In the enlarged fragment of this photomicrograph (Fig. 113) it can clearly be seen that the rod-like hollow tubes consist of individual subunits. The subunits of the rod-like structures appearing in the phage suspension after heating are more clearly distinguished than the subunits of the normal rod. In the rod-like structures aggregated into bundles the subunits form a cross striation which is distinguishable throughout the width of the bundle. In all probability the subunits of the rod join together in a helix to form the structure of the hollow tube. Sarkar and co-workers [329] consider that the hollow tube of the tail rod of phage T2 is formed by five strands, each consisting of identical polypeptide chains or subunits.

When a suspension of phage No. 1 or phage N19 is heated to 90-100°C, the rod breaks up either into short fragments or into separate subunits. As the suspension cools, the morphological subunits of the rod apparently organize themselves spontaneously into hollow tubes of different lengths (polyrods), identical in structure and diameter to the tail rods. The differences in length of the rod-like structures thus produced are very probably due to the uncontrolled process of self-organization, which is determined by electrostatic and thermodynamic properties of the identical subunits, or, according to Casper [122, 123], due to their polymerization or crystalization.

Structures in the form of long, rigid filaments were discovered by Kriss and me [24, 25] in 1953 and 1955 after exposing a suspension of phage No. 1 to a high hydrostatic pressure of the order of 5000 atm. Similar filaments appeared in a suspension of phage No. 1 after ultrasonic irradiation [62]. However, in these investigations the filaments were not identified with the structure of the tail rod, because the degree of contrast obtained by the shadow-casting method used in the early experiments did not enable the precise structural details of these filaments to be determined. All that could be deduced from the use of this method was that the filamentous structures formed by the action of high pressures consist of small subunits, but it was impossible to demonstrate that these filaments were hollow and were, in fact, aggregates of phage tail rods. By shadow-casting phage preparations after heating them to 100°C, it was found that the filamentous structures thus formed were morphologically identical with the filamentous structures appearing in a suspension of phage No. 1 after exposure to a high hydrostatic pressure.

On this basis it can be concluded that the long filamentous structures appearing in a suspension of phage No. 1 after exposure to a high hydrostatic pressure or to heating to 100°C are identical in origin, i.e., that they are rod-like structures.

Both heating and a high pressure cause disorganization of phage particles. In all probability, after the end of exposure, only the protein subunits of the rod still remain capable of self-organization.

Hence, in contrast to phages s_d and T2, phages No. 1 and N19 react distinctively to the temperature factor. The early reaction, expressed as separation of the nucleic acid and protein component, is similar in them to that taking place in other phages. The elements of phages No. 1 and N19 most sensitive to high temperatures are the tail rod and capsids; the rod is more resistant, because it shows ability to aggregate during exposure.

Destruction of phages No. 1 and N19 can be prevented if the phage suspension is fixed with 4% formaldehyde before heating.

Tikhonenko and Kuimova [59] showed that fixation of a phage suspension with 4% formaldehyde increases its resistance to the destructive action of the forces of surface tension arising during drying of electron-microscopic preparations in the air. As Staehelin [348] points out, treatment of tobacco mosaic virus with formalin makes it more resistant to the destructive action of detergents and heating. In all probability the same mechanism is brought into play when phages are fixed with formalin, increasing their resistance to various procedures.

During heating of suspensions of phages No. 1 and N19 preliminarily fixed with formalin, it was found that the morphological changes in the phage particles differ sharply from those observed when unfixed phage suspensions are heated [51].

Particles of phages No. 1 and N19 heated to 60-70°C retain in their general features the morphology of normal particles. In this case, not even liberation of DNA from the head takes place on heating. The tail sheath, as a rule, remains stretched, although its structure differs from that of the normal stretched sheath. It becomes coarsely granular in appearance and in some cases it appears riddled with holes (Fig. 114). Particles of phage No. 1 and N19, fixed in formalin, whether unheated or heated to 50°C, have the characteristic structure of normal unfixed control particles. Fixation in formalin also helps to preserve the slender tail fiber of the phage, which usually is easily damaged. It is well preserved not only on unheated particles, but also on particles heated to 50°C.

After heating of suspensions of phages No. 1 and N19, fixed with formalin to 80-100°C, besides coarse denaturation of the tail

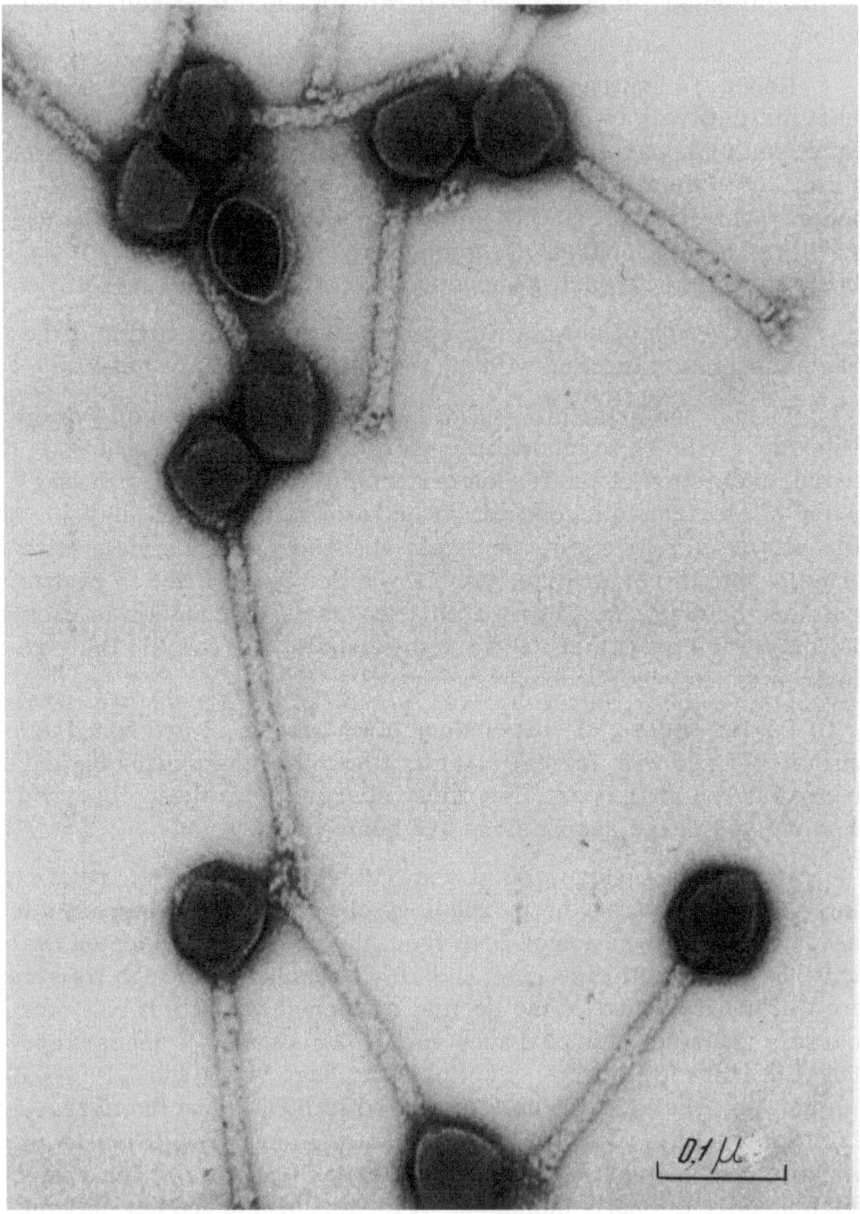

Fig. 114. Phage No. 1 of *Bacillus mycoides* fixed with 4% formaldehyde and then heated to 70°. Uranyl acetate. 170,000 ×.

sheath protein, marked deformation of the phage heads is also observed, most of them appearing empty. The heads become irregular in outline and either blurred in appearance or much smaller in size. Some phage heads shrink to about half their normal size when heated to 80-100°C, when the capsid walls appear condensed and thickened (Fig. 115a, b). Heating even to 100°C does not break up particles of phages No. 1 and N19, fixed with formalin, into separate structural elements. Naturally, no lengthened rod-like structures are formed in such preparations.

These results indicate that during fixation with formalin stronger bonds are, in all probability, formed, preventing breaking up of the phage particles either into structural components or into morphological subunits. No aggregates of rods are thus formed under these conditions.

ACTION OF ADENOSINETRIPHOSPHATASE ON PHAGES

As was mentioned above, the tail of some phages has a special structure which renders it contractile. The elementary act of contraction carried out by the tail sheath may be based on mechanisms similar to the contractile function of the muscle fiber. In muscle the reaction of splitting of adenosinetriphosphate (ATP) is the source of energy for muscular contraction, and, at the same time, the protein possessing ATPase activity itself modifies its mechanical properties under the influence of ATP (mechanico-chemical effect).

Experimental data [60, 61, 155] demonstrate that phage protein, like the contractile protein of muscles, can split ATP, i.e., it possesses the properties of phosphatase enzyme.

Preparations made from muscles or other contractile biological objects contract on the addition of ATP [29].

On this basis, Poglazov, Engel'gardt, and the author [33] decided to investigate whether similar phenomena are found in phages when treated with ATP solution. Under these circumstances it might be expected that the phage tail sheath would change into a contracted state. However, the experiments revealed a different and completely unexpected effect.

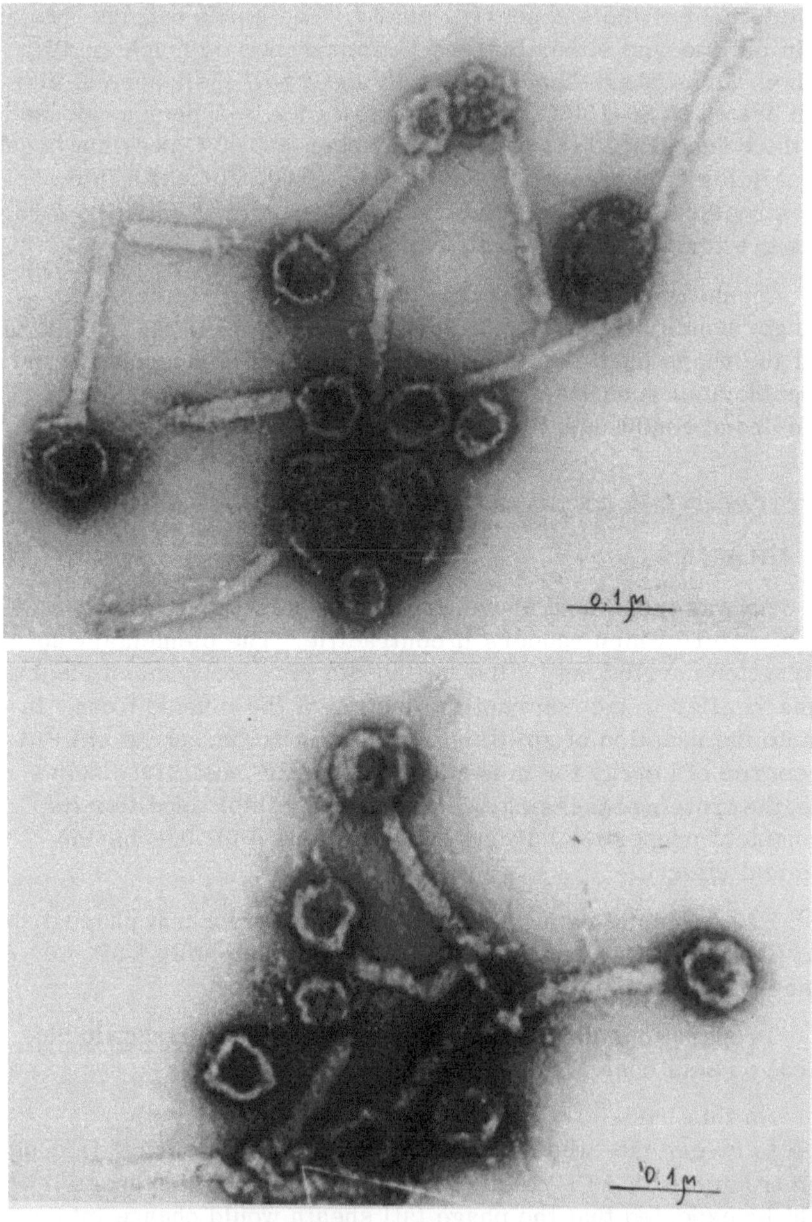

Fig. 115. Phages No. 1 (a) and N19 (b) of *Bacillus mycoides* fixed with 4% formaldehyde and then heated to 100°. Marked contraction of the capsid and deformation of the tail. Uranyl acetate. 140,000 ×.

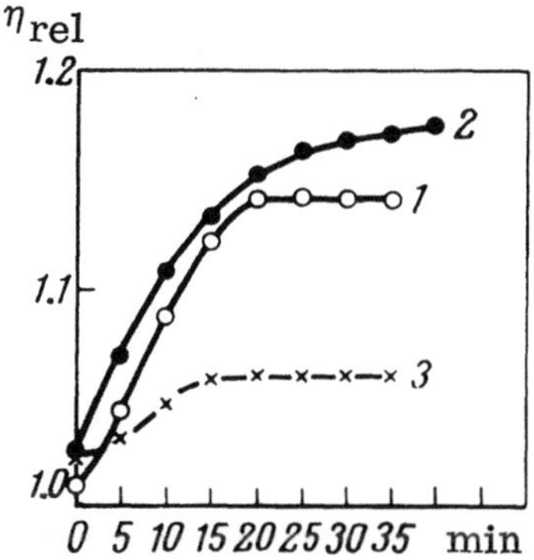

Fig. 116. Changes in viscosity of phage suspension after addition of 0.01 M ATP 1) Phage T2 of *Escherichia coli* B; 2) phage No. 1 of *Bacillus mycoides*; 3) phage s_d of *Escherichia coli* SK.

Experiments were carried out on concentrated suspensions of phages T2 of *E. coli* B, No. 1 of *B. mycoides*, and s_d of *E. coli* SK in 0.9% NaCl solution at 20°C. ATP solution, in the form of the sodium salt, was made up in 0.9% NaCl. The final concentration of ATP in the reaction mixture varied from 0.005 to 0.05 M. Viscosity was determined in an Ostwald viscosimeter. DNA was determined by the method of Webb and Levy [380] with p-nitrophenylhydrazine.

It was found that addition of ATP to a suspension of any of the investigated phages causes a sharp increase in the relative viscosity of the solution. The greatest increase in viscosity is observed with phage No. 1 of *B. mycoides* (Fig. 116). The viscosity of phage s_d showed the least increase. The optimal ATP concentration for a phage suspension containing 10^{11}–10^{12} phage particles/ml is 0.01–0.05 M. When working with a phage suspension of higher titer, more concentrated ATP solutions are required.

The maximal increase in viscosity takes place during the first 15–20 min. Subsequently, the increase in viscosity either stops, as in the case of phage s_d, or it continues to increase slowly, as with phage No. 1. If a phage suspension of high titer is kept with ATP for a long time, the solution thickens very considerably. The viscosity of such a solution may be 7 times higher than the initial viscosity of a phage suspension with a titer of $3.5 \cdot 10^{12}$. The phage titer under these circumstances falls by more than one order ($2.5 \cdot 10^{11}$ phage particles/ml).

The only substance composing the phage particle which can give rise to such an increase in viscosity is DNA. It was natural to suppose that under the influence of ATP, liberation of DNA from the phage must take place. Accordingly, the amount of DNA appearing in the medium during treatment of phage with ATP was investi-

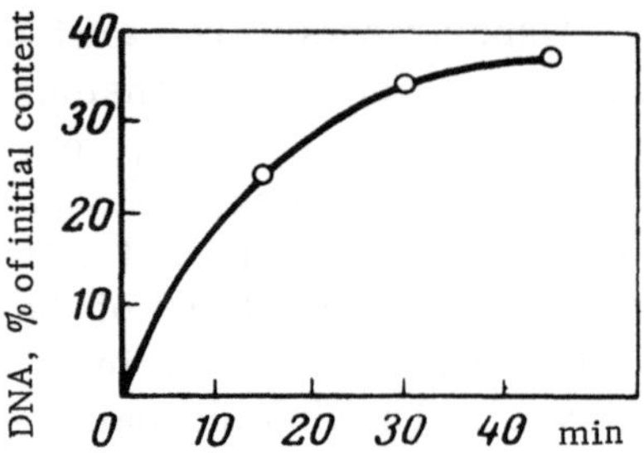

Fig. 117. Change in quantity of DNA liberated after addition of 0.01 M ATP to a suspension of phage No. 1 of *Bacillus mycoides*

gated. The preparation was divided into two samples. ATP was added to one (experimental sample) and the corresponding volume of 0.9% NaCl to the other (control sample). After specified time intervals small portions of suspension were taken from these samples and centrifuged for 1 h in the cold at 30,000 g. In the process of centrifugation the phage particles were sedimented. DNA liberated from the phage was determined in the supernatant.

As a result of the investigation it was discovered that much more DNA was present in the supernatant from the experimental samples than from the control. After incubation with ATP for 1 h about 30–40% of the particles of all investigated phages liberated DNA into the surrounding medium. As Fig. 117 shows, the increase in the amount of liberated DNA is parallel to the increase in viscosity of the solution.

Electron-microscopic investigations showed that phage preparations treated with ATP contain an overwhelming majority of phage particles with empty heads. DNA passes from the heads into the surrounding medium, lying among the phage particles in tufts or balls.

Particular attention must be paid to the fact that the tails of phages No. 1 and T2 remain unchanged after treatment with ATP, even if its concentration is increased to 0.05 M. Most particles retain an uncontracted tail, whereas their heads are completely emptied (Fig. 118a, b). This fact indicates that liberation of DNA from the phage particle can take place not only as a result of contraction of the tail, but also by participation of the head envelope.

Interesting investigations in this connection were carried out by Cummings and Kozloff [135, 136, 137], who found that the head of phage T2 can shorten during a change in pH or ionic composition of the medium and during interaction between the phage particle and bacterial cell. These facts are in agreement with my

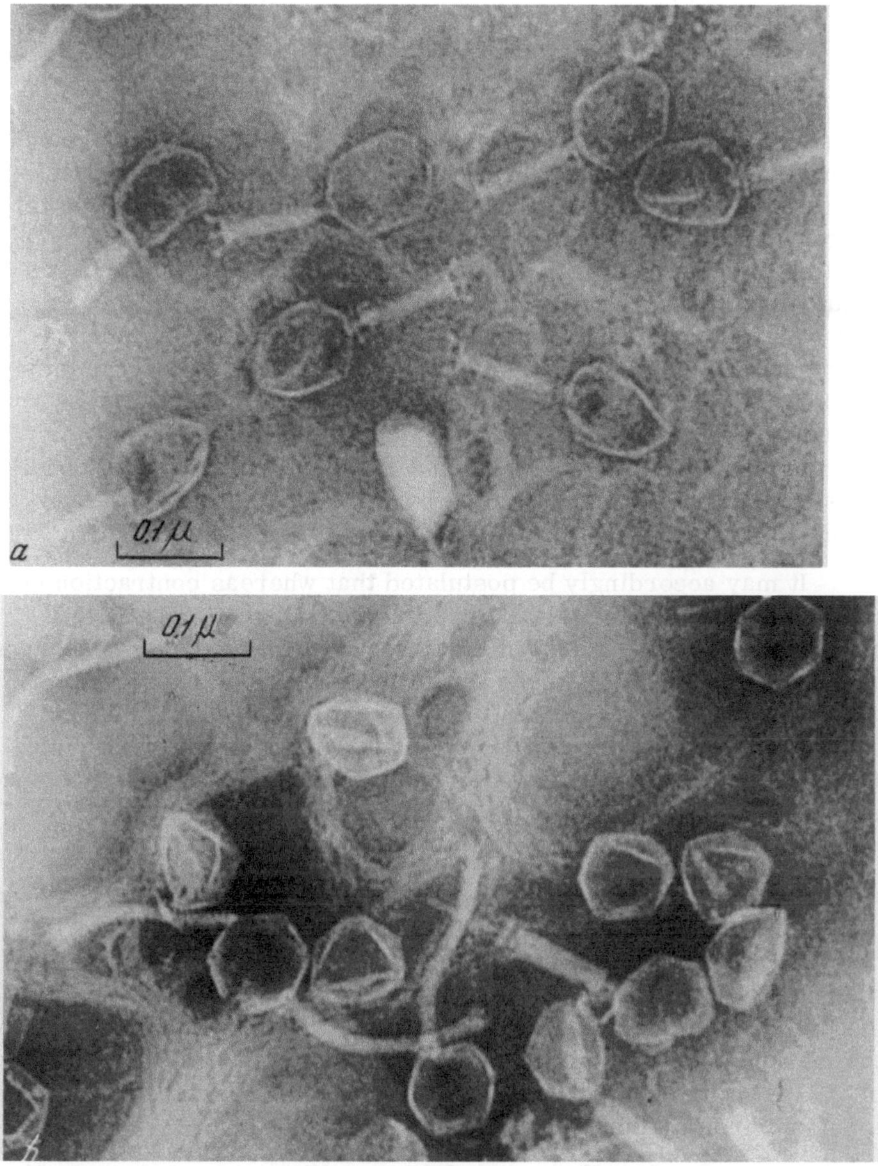

Fig. 118. Phages after treatment with ATP. PTA. 140,000×. a) Phage T2 of *Escherichia coli* B; b) phage No. 1 of *Bacillus mycoides* .

hypothesis of the important role of the structural protein forming the head capsid in the process of liberation of DNA from the head. The fact that shortening of the head can be produced under artificial conditions by the action of Ca^{++}, Mg^{++}, Zn^{++}, and Cd^{++} ions [137] also leads to the conclusion that the processes lying at the basis of contraction of the tail sheath and of shortening of the head of phage T2 are identical. In the latter case it is evident that conformational changes also take place in the subunits constituting the phage capsid. The work of Puck [308] and Adams [73] is worthy of mention in this respect. These workers showed that some phages require the presence of Ca^{++} in the medium in order to infect the host cell. The addition of citrate, EDTA, or ethylenediamine triphosphate has an inhibitory action on these phages [260]. Cummings and Kozloff [137] consider that before infection of the cell takes place, the head of phage T2 changes into the shortened form. Changes in the shape of the head under normal physiological conditions are caused, in their opinion, by components of the cell cytoplasm appearing as the result of phage — cell interaction.

It may accordingly be postulated that whereas contraction of the sheath taking place in the first stage of interaction between phage and cell is the result of disturbance of the integrity of the end plate, substances liberated from the cell during hydrolysis of the cell wall by the phage particle may act upon the phage capsid and facilitate liberation of DNA from it. It may be that *in vivo* ATP, which may be liberated from the cell after interaction with phage, may have some action on the structure of the head protein.

At the moment it is difficult to say how ATP acts on the phage particle. Is liberation of DNA from phage produced simply by the fact that ATP is present in the surrounding medium or does ATP play a role in the course of its hydrolysis by the phosphatase present in the phage particles ? This latter hypothesis is supported by the marked decrease in the velocity and completeness of liberation of DNA from the phage head in the presence of mercuric chloride, a poison strongly inhibiting phosphatase activity.

To some extent the action of ATP on liberation of phage DNA resembles the phenomenon of chemotaxis at the molecular level.

Van Vunakis and Herriott [372] found that pyrophosphate also liberates DNA from the T-even coliphages. They state that this reaction depends on the pH, temperature, and ionic composition of the medium and on the duration of exposure. The reaction can be inhibited by magnesium salts, putrescin, and spermidin. The mechanism of action of pyrophosphate is unknown. However, these workers suggest that pyrophosphate may act either as a chelating agent or as a coenzyme, or that it may act in some way on the phage particle to increase the tension in the phage head envelope. As a chelating agent, like Ca^{++} ions, it may also compete with metallic ions present in the protein component of the phage [254]. As a coenzyme it may catalyze the reaction stretching the phage head membrane. Finally, pyrophosphate may penetrate into the phage head and cause changes in the polyamine or cation bonds which, according to Ames and Dubin [77], stabilized the DNA. This last mechanism may rupture or stretch the compactly coiled DNA strand, thereby rupturing the head envelope.

I consider that there are good reasons for not accepting that contraction of the tail sheath of the phage particle alone can transmit nucleic acid into the bacterial cell. First, the tail sheath is not directly connected with the phage head, as can be seen from the numerous photomicrographs of phage particles with a contracted tail sheath. Second, phage particles with a contracted tail sheath, but whose head is filled with DNA, can often be observed. It is most probable, therefore, that the head envelope of the phage particle plays an important role in the physiological process of DNA liberation. It must be remembered that nearly all phage particles, although differing sharply in their tail structure, have a common structural detail in the head. This detail lies at the point of attachment of the rod or the whole tail to the head and has the appearance of an electron-dense disc or valve. Because of the very small size of this detail, it is difficult to determine its structure precisely. Nevertheless, it can be distinguished in phages with a short tail (Figs. 25c, 26, 30, 100) or with an uncontracting (Figs. 35b, c; 43a, b; 44b; 45; 47; 48; 49) or with a contractile tail sheath (Figs. 51, 68, 70, 74, 102). This universal structure, found in the head of different phages, possibly plays the role of a valve and is concerned in the process of transmission of nucleic acid along the tail canal to the host cell.

The process of transmission of the infective principle from phage to cell is complex. Further investigations are required to elucidate its successive stages. Presumably, not only the various structural components of the phage particle are concerned in it, but also substances present in the surrounding medium are liberated from the cell in the first stages of interaction with the phage particle. One such substance could be ATP. These substances may act specifically on the capsid protein, changing its shape and, thus, facilitating liberation of DNA from the head.

* * *

Various chemical and physical agents thus cause destructive changes in phage particles, expressed primarily by separation of the protein and nucleic acid components. This is followed by gradual destruction of the protein components of the phage particle. Some are destroyed by gentler procedures, while others require stronger treatment for their destruction.

Proteins sensitive to a particular procedure, in all probability, break up into small structural units, while resistant proteins break up into larger fragments. Later these fragments may act as centers of crystallization for the reconstruction of polysheaths and polyrods.

The irregular manner in which the phage particle breaks up suggests that it consists of a group of different proteins, heterogeneous in nature. The head capsid, the sheath, the rod, the end plate, and the tail fibers are all built of specific and different proteins. Meanwhile, it must be emphasized that even those elements of the phage particle which are morphologically identical in different phages react differently to the same procedures. This fact suggests that morphologically identical structures in different phages are built of a material which is specific for a particular phage.

Therefore, the property of phage particles of undergoing selective destruction during exposure to chemical and physical agents can be utilized for the isolation of fractions containing particular structural components of phage in a pure form.

The study of phage structure during destruction of the particle can also provide a basis for the identification of the functional role of its individual components in the process of infection.

Chapter 9

The Aggregative Properties of Phage Proteins

The study of the ultrastructure of bacteriophages at the current level has shown that their protein components are built from subunits arranged in a definite manner.

These investigations confirmed the hypothesis put forward initially by Watson and Crick in 1956 [22, 134], according to which the envelope of simple viruses must consist of similar protein subunits, because the nucleic acids of these viruses possess a comparatively small stock of information insufficient for synthesis of qualitatively different proteins. The uniformity of the protein subunit places limitations on the design of virus particles, as a result of which the capsids of simple viruses are represented either as rod-shaped structures with a helical arrangement of the subunits or as polyhedra with various types of cubic symmetry. Watson and Crick suggest that their ideas are applicable also to single components of the phage particle.

Identical subunits are aggregated in accordance with the principle of close packing, each subunit being surrounded by other subunits resembling it.

As Crick and Watson [22] claim, the increase in size of a protein structure is a process which can be called crystallization. The concept of crystallization of protein subunits is also accepted by Dulbecco (see the discussion to Crick and Watson's paper [22]). He considers that the crystallization principle can explain successfully some of the experimental data concerning phenotype combination in viruses. For example, the protein envelope of the phage particle formed in the cell during simultaneous infection by two phages may be a combination of the two parent forms. Furthermore, the composition of the proteins determined by this property is independent of the genetic characteristic of the DNA of the phage particle. In Dulbecco's opinion, this is proof that the protein components of phage are built from units which are made independently and are joined to the DNA only later.

Kellenberger [229, 230] postulates the existence of morphopoietic factors in the cell, which influence the final assembly of the phage virion.

The experiments of Schramm [332, 333] and of Harrington and Schachaman [193] showed that disintegration of particles of tobacco mosaic virus (TMV) into smaller protein units and nucleic acid can be produced *in vitro*. The protein units of TMV are capable of spontaneous aggregation into rod-like structures similar in their morphology to virus particles.

It was later shown [175, 334] that the separate components of a virus can be reassembled into active virus particles. According to Caspar [122], the TMV particle can be regarded as a crystal of limited size. Like a crystal, it can dissolve and recrystallize. Caspar claims that reconstruction of the virus particle is determined by the property of the protein subunits to aggregate into a helical structure, resembling the structure of a complete virus with nucleic acid. Interaction with nucleic acid determines the size of the virus particle and contributes to its stability.

After degradation of the TMV capsid in an alkaline medium, small aggregates consisting of a few subunits remain. Such aggregates are possibly centers of crystallization for reconstruction of the virus particle.

The mechanism of the spontaneous organization observed *in vitro*, in all probability, may also take place *in vivo*. Caspar accordingly suggests that there is no need for a special organizing factor for the union of individual virus particles during their synthesis.

The ability of virus proteins to organize themselves is evidently due to the presence of free energy bonds in some subunits. The stability of the aggregates is determined by geometrical affinity between individual subunits and by changes in the free energy bonds in the course of their interaction. A specific bond between identical subunits must result in symmetrical designs, because there is a very limited number of ways in which each unit can be connected to its neighbors, in order to provide for the maximal number of the most stable bonds between them. By virtue of these principles, identical subunits can join together spontaneously and quasi-equivalently as a result of the fact that the tendency toward the lowest level of energy is strong during the creation of protein structures [122, 123].

The biological importance of spontaneous organization of protein structures lies in the facilities which it provides for self control, presenting the incorporation of foreign subunits in these structures [124].

Despite the fact that bacteriophages have a more complex structure than TMV and contain proteins of several different types, the mechanism of self-organization of individual protein structures may also occur in phages.

POLYSHEATHS

In their study of concentrated phage T2 suspensions, Brenner and co-workers [111] discovered long helical structures which they took for the stretched helix of the tail sheath. However, their study of the morphology of these structures was incomplete.

Structures similar in diameter and morphology to isolated contracted sheaths and to unwound tail sheath helices of phage T2, yet attaining a considerable length much longer than a single sheath, were discovered by Poglazov and me [32] in a suspension of phage T2 treated with alkali.

I also found similar structures [48] when studying concentrated suspensions of phage T2 which had stood for a long time in a refrigerator. They are long aggregates consisting of thick, rigid filaments or coarse helices. The aggregates so discovered, at first sight, appear to differ in their fine structure. Some appear compact and resemble contracted tail sheaths (Fig. 119a). Others are fragmented in appearance, with the features of a coarse helix (Fig. 119b). Besides aggregates of the pattern described above, other structures are seen, one end of which consists of a stretched-out helix (Fig. 120). Sometimes, they are connected directly to the tail rod projecting from the phage head (Figs. 56a and 120).

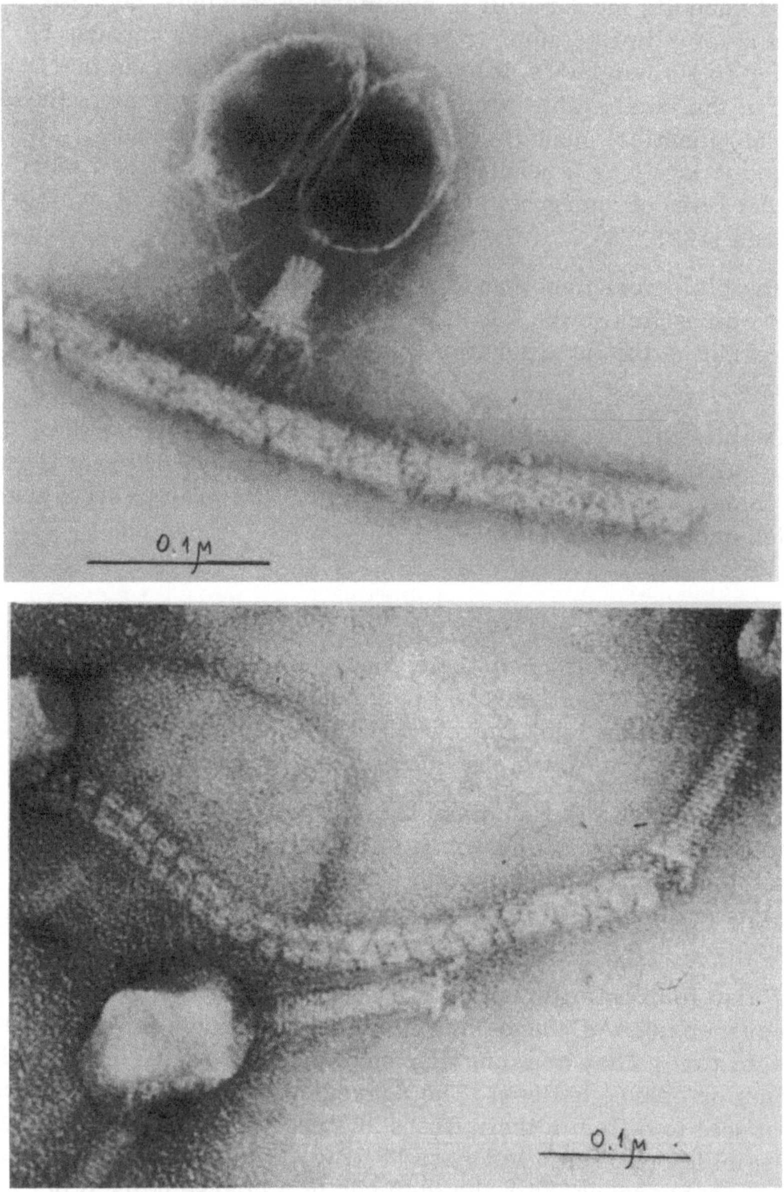

Fig. 119. Polysheaths of phage T2 of *Escherichia coli*. a) PTA. 240,000×; b) uranyl acetate. 200,000×.

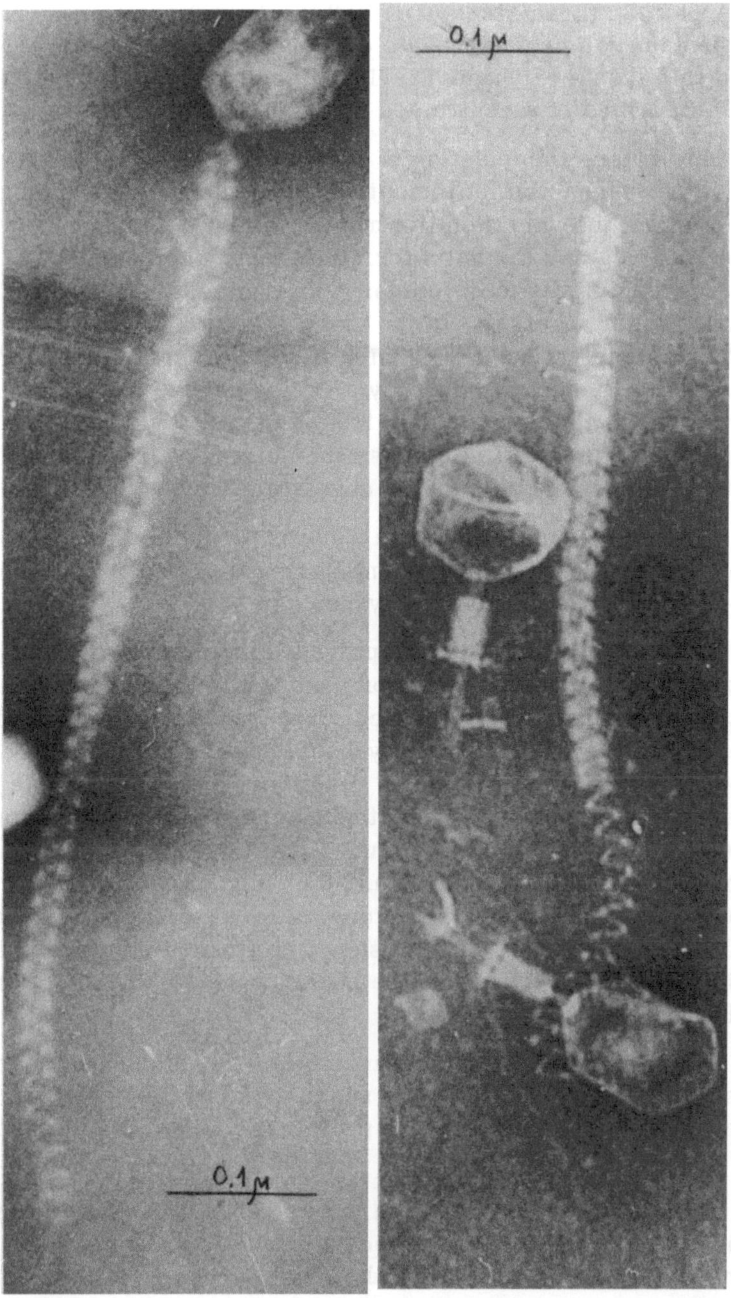

Fig. 120. Polysheaths of phage T2 with greatly stretched helix. PTA. 200,000 ×.

What can these structures be? In their diameter and fine structure, the compact aggregate corresponds precisely to the contracted tail sheath of phage T2. In all probability they are the continuous structure of a contracted tail sheath.

This raises the question of the cause of the structural variation and the mechanism of formation of the discovered aggregate. In my opinion, the variation in structure is due to the fact that in different aggregates the helix forming them is compressed to a different degree. In the more compact aggregates the turns of the helix are closer together. In the more uncoiled helices, it can be seen more clearly that they consist of a single strand. The intermediate state is characterized by a varied degree of compactness or stretching of the helix. Some fragments are evidently formed of two or three turns. In this case the helix appears coarser and the impression is created that it consists of several strands.

Kellenberger and Boy de la Tour [234] showed that a suspension of phage T4 also contains long aggregates of contracted sheaths, which they also described as polysheaths.

Just as with phage T2, the polysheaths of phage T4 vary in structure. Some appear more compact, and were described as smooth, while others have a helical appearance. Kellenberger and Boy de la Tour conclude that polysheaths are formed by two or three strands coiled into a helix. However, they were unable to see any helices so strongly unwound that a single strand was clearly visible. On this basis they concluded that the strands composing the turns of the helix are labile and they suggested that the helix of the polysheath is distinguishable only after association of several strands. In my opinion, the polysheath is formed by one strand. This is proved by the appearance of the outstretched end of the polysheath helix (Fig. 120).

The reason for the appearance of polysheaths in a phage suspension is not yet clear. All the suggestions which have been made are based on the ability of phage proteins to undergo aggregation [32].

Kellenberger and Boy de la Tour [234] put forward a number of hypothetical claims for the mechanism of formation of polysheaths which seem to me to be the most probable. These claims are based mainly on Caspar's theory [122] of the ability of virus proteins to organize themselves from separate protein subunits, provided that the thermodynamic and ionic state of the medium is suitable. They assume that protein subunits themselves carry all the necessary information for building the typical structure. The fact that compact polysheaths are similar in structure to contracted tail sheaths leads naturally to the conclusion that they are formed from subunits which have undergone conformational changes.

It must be pointed out that stretched sheaths have never yet been observed in an isolated state. From this, Kellenberger and Boy de la Tour [234] conclude that an additional morphopoietic factor must be present which influences each subunit in such a way that they aggregate to form a stretched sheath. In their opinion, this factor may be carried either by the tail rod or by a chemical agent, or by both together. In fact, the stretched and contracted sheaths differ from each other in their fine structure. The turn of the helix in the stretched sheath lies at an angle of 60°, compared with 30° in the contracted sheath. During contraction, changes are also observed in the shape of the separate subunits composing the sheath, which become longer.

The change of the subunits from one shape to another during contraction of the sheath is most likely to be the cause and not the effect of the contraction. Kellenberger and Boy de la Tour [234] suggest that changes in shape of the subunits may be produced by the presence or absence of the "allosteric effector." This view is based on investigations by Monod and co-workers [284], who concluded from their observations on the activity and structure of enzyme proteins that interaction between an allosteric effector and individual segments of the protein molecule may give rise to conformational and structural changes in the molecule. These changes may liberate or may conceal active areas of the protein. The role of allosteric effector for phage is possibly played by ATP, which was discovered by Kozlov and Lute [253] in the normal tail of phage T2, whereas in the phage particle with a contracted sheath most of the ATP has disappeared.

For the reasons given above it may be supposed that polysheaths, on the one hand, can be formed from subunits which have undergone conformational changes. Disintegrated sheath structures may provide a stock of such subunits. On the other hand, sheath subunits synthesized in excess in the bacterial cell infected by the

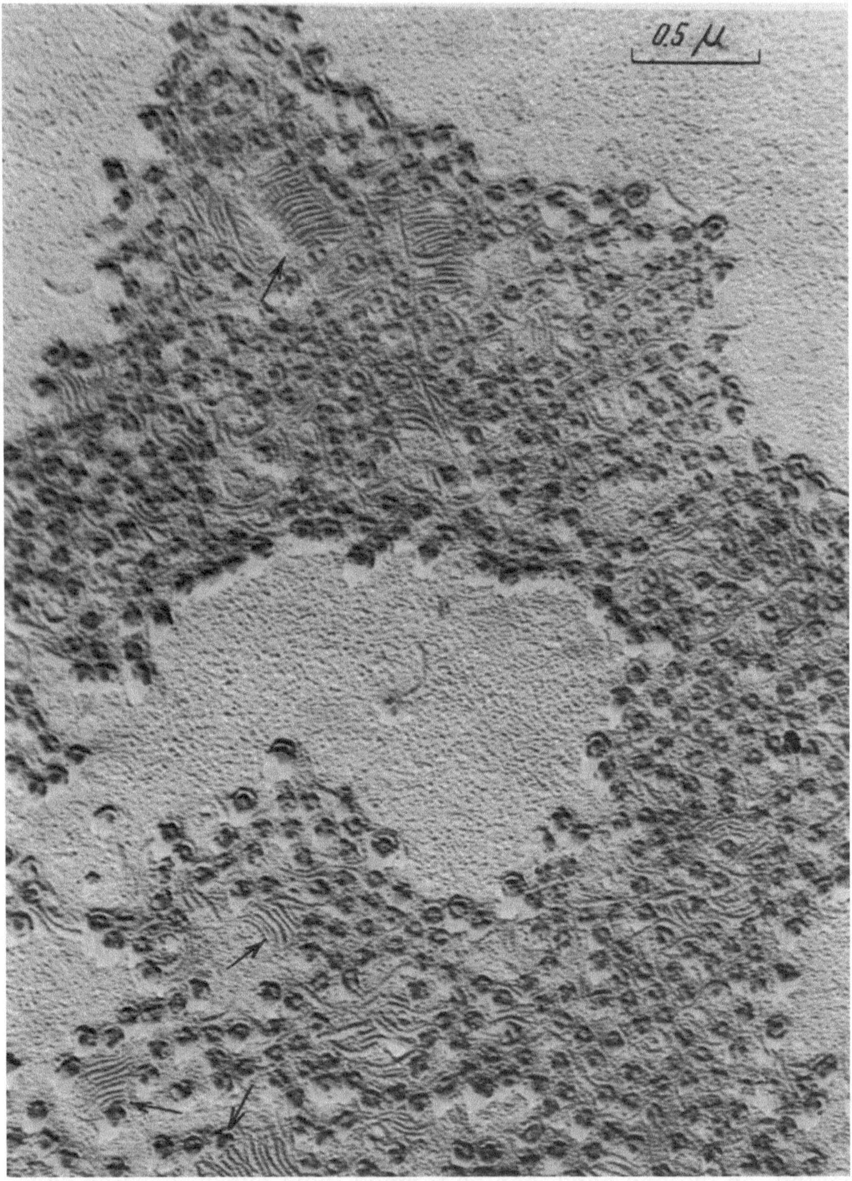

Fig. 121. Lysis of cells of *Bacillus mycoides* by phage No. 1 on a support film. Groups of phage tails are indicated by arrows. Shadowed with chromium. 35,000 ×.

phage particle may subsequently organize themselves uncontrollably into polysheaths.

The probability also is not ruled out that isolated contracted sheaths or their fragments, which are always present in a certain amount in a phage suspension, may act as centers of crystallization for the formation of polysheaths.

The ability of sheath subunits to organize themselves has been confirmed directly by the experiments of Poglazov and co-workers [31], who reconstructed the tail sheaths of phage T2 after lysis under alkaline conditions. It is, admittedly, somewhat surprising that the length of the reconstructed sheaths does not exceed the length of the normal contracted rod.

When studying lysis of cells of *B. mycoides* by phage No. 1 by the method described by Pokotinskii and co-workers [34], which enables lysis to be observed actually on the supporting film without disturbing the spatial relationships of the object examined, I found that in addition to phage particles, large clusters of tails without heads also are formed in place of the lysed cell (Fig. 121). I consider that these clusters are evidence of excessive protein synthesis in the infected cell, and that the surplus proteins are organized into incomplete phage particles, in this particular case, into tails. Stefanov and Smirnova [39] calculated the ratio between the number of complete particles and separate structural elements of phage No. 1 of *B. mycoides* and found an excess of isolated phage tails in the lysates. These results also suggest possible synthesis of an excess of some phage proteins in the infected cell.

As Kellenberger [229] suggests, the possibility also is not ruled out that aberrant phage structures may be formed in infected cells through mutation of hypothetical genes responsible for morphopoiesis of the phage particle as a whole. As a result of disturbance of the work of these genes, polysheaths, polyheads, and atypical phage particles with two or three tails [39, 98, 285, 347] or heads of modified shape [229] may appear.

A tendency toward polysheath formation also was found when I treated phage No. 1 of *B. mycoides* by various procedures causing destruction of the tail (Figs. 106 and 108). However, they were much shorter than the polyheads of phage T2. I also found a few comparatively short polysheaths in a suspension of phage No. 1 in

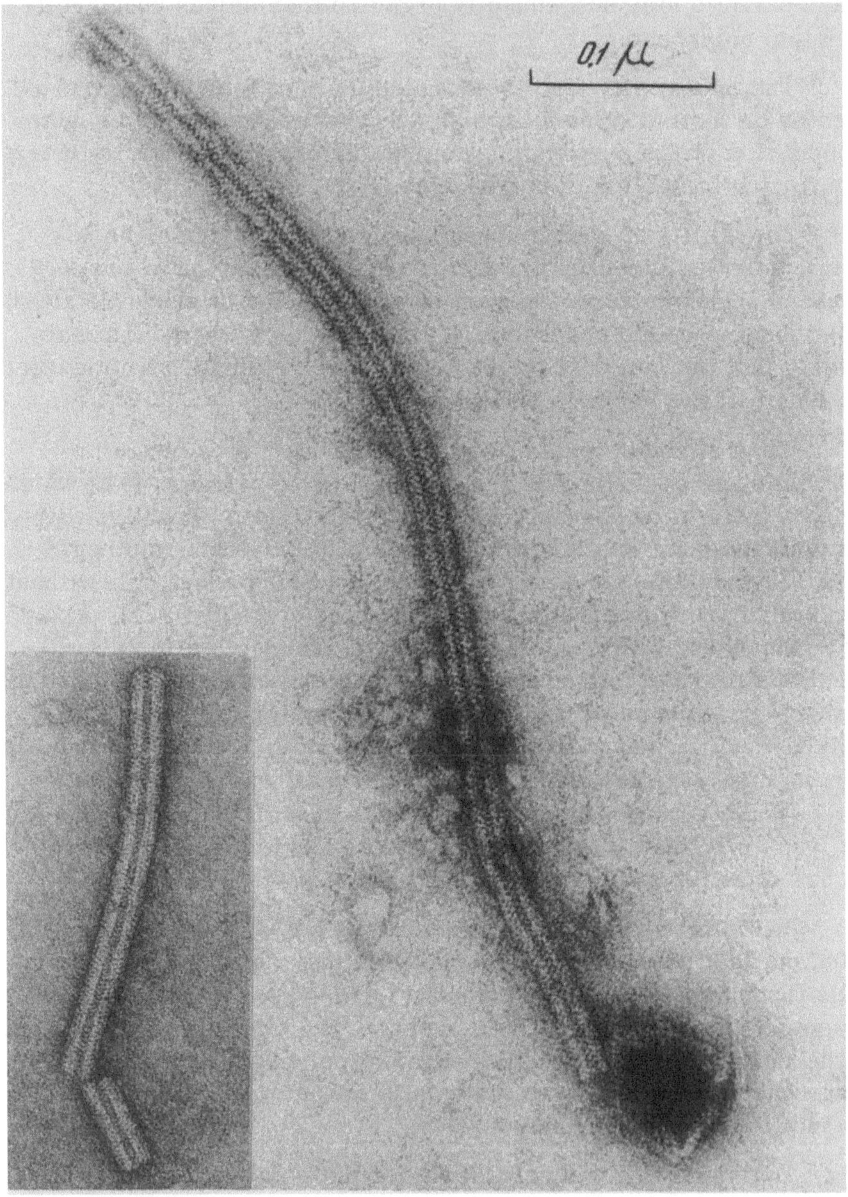

Fig. 122 Fig. 123

Fig. 122. Polysheaths appearing in a suspension of phage No. 1 of *Bacillus mycoides* in physiological saline after keeping for 1 year. Uranyl acetate. 240,000×.

Fig. 123 . Polysheaths of phage No. 1 of *Bacillus mycoides* after dialysis of phage suspension in physiological saline kept for 1 year. 240,000×.

physiological saline kept for a long time in a refrigerator (Fig. 122). As the electron-microscopic study of such phage preparations showed, prolonged refrigeration leads to destruction of the great majority of phage particles. In such preparations mainly empty heads with a tail rod and separate contracted sheaths or fragments of them are mainly found. Destruction of the sheath is evidently accompanied by its disintegration into separate morphological subunits.

I found polysheaths which attained a considerable length [48] after dialysis of a suspension of phage No. 1 containing fragmented particles against distilled water (Fig. 123). In all probability, more favorable conditions for aggregation or self-organization of the fragmented sheaths and of their component subunits into structures of polysheath type were thereby created.

Polysheaths of phage No. 1 always had a compact structure similar to that characteristic of the normal contracted sheath. The tail sheath of phage No. 1 has not yet been found in the form of a stretched helix.

The view is held that the bonds holding the sheath helix of phage T2 in a compact state are weaker than the bonds between the separate subunits forming the strand of the sheath helix, and, because of this, uncoiling of the helix of phage T2 can be observed.

The bonds between individual morphological subunits and between the turns of the helix in phage No. 1 are evidently equally strong, so that when they are broken the tail sheath of this phage either breaks up into separate fragments or into its component subunits.

POLYRODS

As was mentioned above, it was not only the tail sheaths that are built from morphological subunits. The structure of the capsid and tail rod is also formed of homogeneous subunits. Therefore, it must be expected that the tail rods must also possess powers of aggregation, although so far no reports of crystallization of the phage rods have appeared in the literature.

Long aggregates of rod-like structures (polyrods) were obtained in my experiments [51, 364] in which phages No. 1 and N19

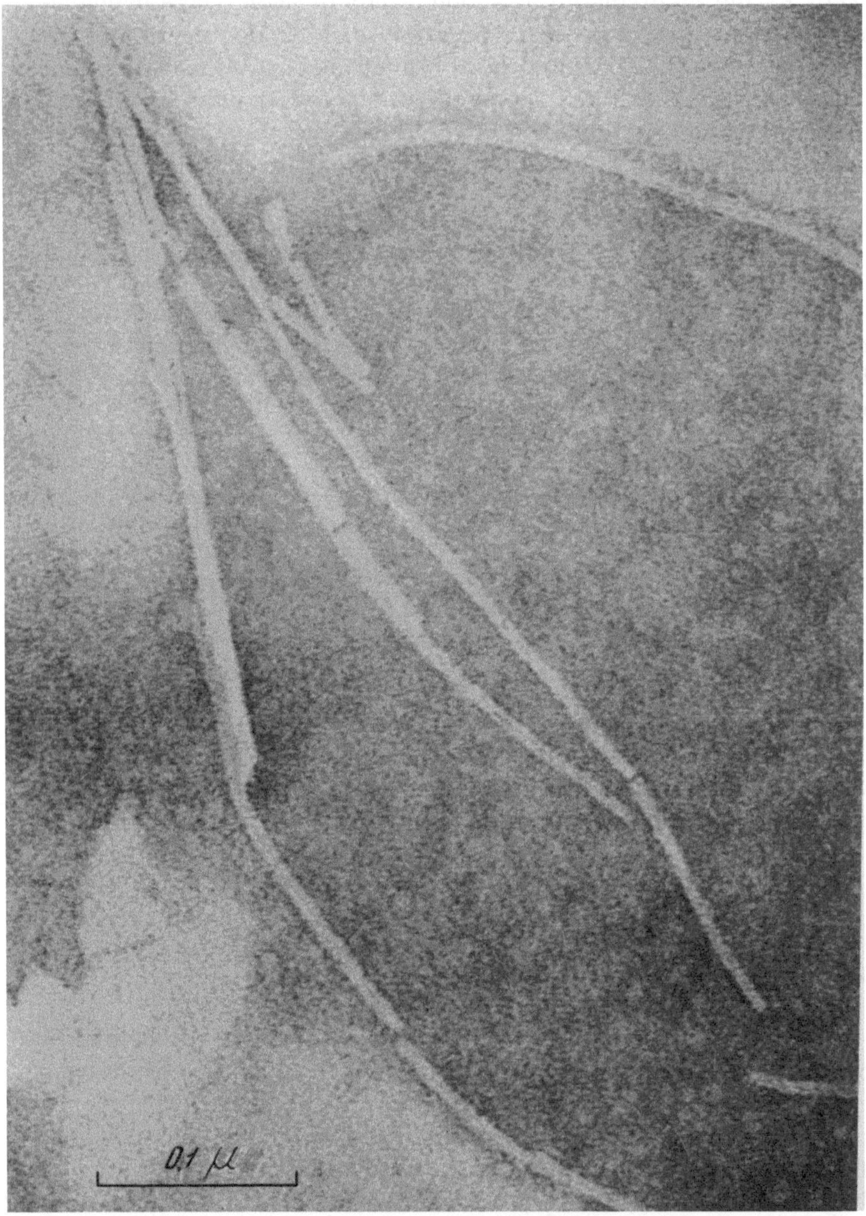

Fig. 124. Polyrods of phage T2 after treatment with acetic acid (pH 2) followed by dialysis against distilled water. PTA. 260,000×.

of *B. mycoides* were treated with different physical agents, including freezing and thawing (Fig. 108) and heating to 90-100°C. Particularly long polyrod structures are formed during exposure to heat (Figs. 112 and 113). These were fully described and their fine structure examined in Chapter 8.

I first observed this ability of the tail rods to undergo aggregation only in phages No. 1 and N19 of *B. mycoides*. Recently, however, by choosing the proper conditions, I obtained the formation of polyrods of phage T2 of *E. coli* [52].

A study of changes in the structure of phage T2 particles during treatment with 1 N acetic acid to different pH values, followed by dialysis against distilled water, showed that acidification of a suspension of phage T2 to pH 2.25-1.75 completely destroys all structural components of the phage, except the rod. However, in the course of this treatment, the tail rods undergo profound changes. Hollow rigid rod-like structures, corresponding in diameter and morphology to the tail rod, yet much greater in length, appear in dialyzed preparations obtained from these suspensions. Some polyrods may attain a length of several microns, and in addition they show a tendency to aggregate side-to-side, to form bundles (Fig. 124).

However, after stronger acidification of a suspension of phage T2 to pH 1.0, no long polyrods are formed. Only rod-like structures of about the same length as normal phage rods can be seen in such specimens.

During treatment of phage T2 with acetic acid, the rod structure probably disintegrates into smaller fragments or even into individual subunits. Dialysis restores the neutral pH of the medium, and, under these conditions, rod-like structures composed of small fragments and subunits evidently organize themselves into larger aggregates. In a phage suspension similarly treated, but not dialyzed, structures analogous to polyrods are absent.

In specimens obtained from phage suspensions fixed with formaldehyde for 2 h immediately after treatment with acetic acid, and then dialyzed, no polyrods likewise are formed.

The formation of long rod-like structures (polyrods) by phages No. 1 and N19 of *B. mycoides* and phage T2 is evidence that both the protein forming the sheath and also the tail rod protein possess powers of aggregation.

POLYHEADS

The proteins forming the phage capsid may also possess aggregating properties. As long ago as 1950, Herčik [195] and Wyckoff [393] directed attention to unusual filamentous structures appearing in lysates of *E. coli* B after infection with T-even phages. These filamentous structures, sometimes of considerable length, are flat bands or collapsed tubes, corresponding in width to the width of the phage head. The low resolving power of electron microscopes at that time and the less advanced staining technology did not allow the fine structure of these filaments to be studied. These workers postulated that the filamentous structures were directly related to phage and represented a stage in the process of its formation in the cell. This suggestion was confirmed by the fact that large numbers of filamentous structures appeared when phagolysis took place, not at the optimal temperature, but at low temperature [393].

A group of workers headed by Professor Kellenberger [161, 163, 164, 235] found that in *E. coli* B cells infected by the amber mutant of phage T4 an unusual development of phage particles takes place. Instead of normal phage particles, long flat bands appear in the cells. They vary considerably in length, individual bands reaching 10 μ. The width of these bands is 900 Å, corresponding to the width of the head of normal phage T4. The name polyheads was given to these structures. The study of their fine structure showed that they consist of individual morphological subunits shaped like short hollow cylinders, with an external diameter of 70-80 Å and an internal diameter of 20-40 Å. However, Kellenberger and his collaborators point out that no such subunits can be distinguished in the heads of normal phage T4 [235].

In my electron-microscopic study of phage No. 1 [47], I sometimes found among normal phage particles distinctive flat bands of different lengths, but always strictly of the same width. The fine structure of these bands resembles the structure of the head capsid of phage No. 1. The bands consist of morphological subunits of the same diameter (50 ± 10 Å) as the capsomeres of the phage capsid and they possess the same structure of short, hollow, hexagonal tubes. The width of the band is equal to the diameter of the head of a normal phage No. 1 particle. However, they are much longer than the normal head.

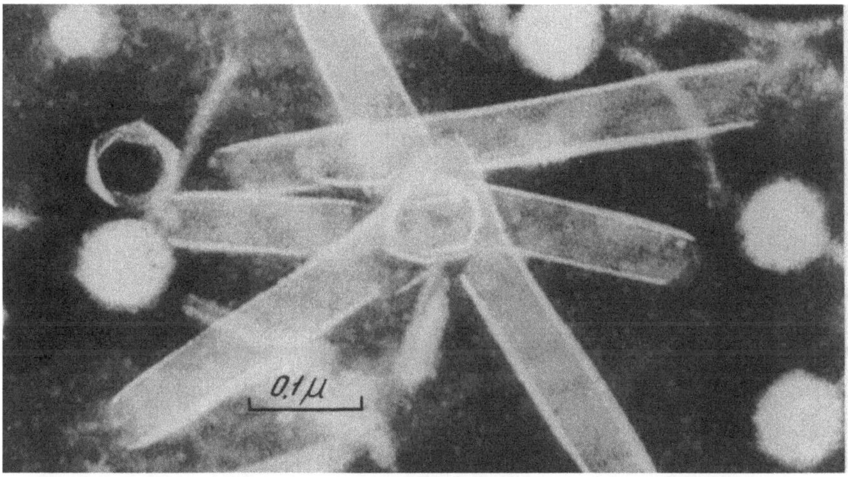

Fig. 125. Formation of polyheads after lysis of *Bacillus mycoides* cells at 10-12°C. PTA. 150,000×.

Allowing for the considerable lability of particles of phage No. 1, I originally suggested that the flat bands appear in phage preparations as the result of aggregation of fragmented head envelopes. However, a further study of the causes leading to the appearance of flat bands in specimens of phage No. 1 compelled me to change my mind. If lysis of a culture of *B. mycoides* by phage No. 1 takes place at low temperatures of 10-12°C, the number of flat bands in the lysate is increased. Under these conditions, they are found in almost every field of vision of the microscope and sometimes form small groups (Fig. 125).

The detailed study of these structures showed that they are not bands but collapsed tubes. Proof of this is given in Fig. 126, showing that when the upper surface of the tube is ruptured its lower surface is exposed. Both surfaces of the tube are composed of subunits. By analogy with the structures found in phage T4, these hollow tubes are in all probability polyheads of phage No. 1.

The atypical strain No. 1 of *B. mycoides*, on which phage No. 1 is cultivated, has a very narrow temperature optimum of growth (27-30°C). It does not grow at low temperatures (+4°C). Even a culture which has completed its growth dies if kept in a refrigerator for one month. At 37°C, this strain gives very weak growth.

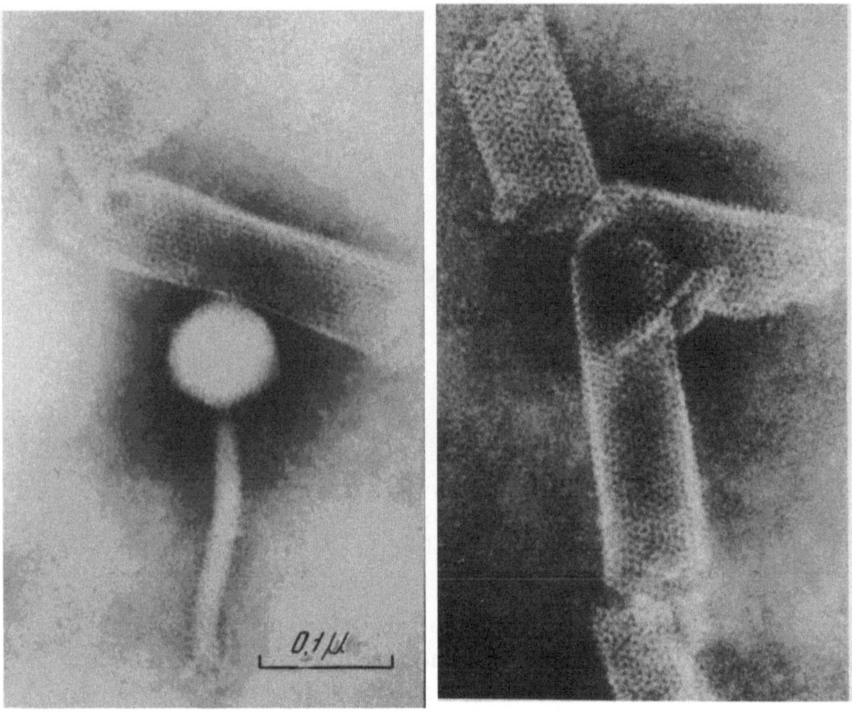

Fig. 126. Polyheads of phage No. 1 of *Bacillus mycoides* consisting of hollow cylinders with clearly distinguishable capsomeres. PTA. 180,000 ×.

In view of the special features of this strain, I consider that slight variations in the temperature of cultivation may lead to defective development of part of the phage progeny, as a result of which not only normal phage particles, but also polyheads appear in the cell.

Development of phage at low temperatures (10–12°C) promotes defective phage development, leading to accumulation of polyheads in the lysates.

The polyheads found in phage No. 1 of *B. mycoides* are similar in structure to the polyheads appearing in *E. coli* B cells when infected with the amber mutant of phage T4. However, in their fine structure, the latter differ from the structure of normal phage T4 capsids, because they are built of readily distinguishable capsomeres [117, 161, 163, 164, 235], whereas the individual capsomeres of the normal capsid of the phage T4 head are distinguishable with difficulty.

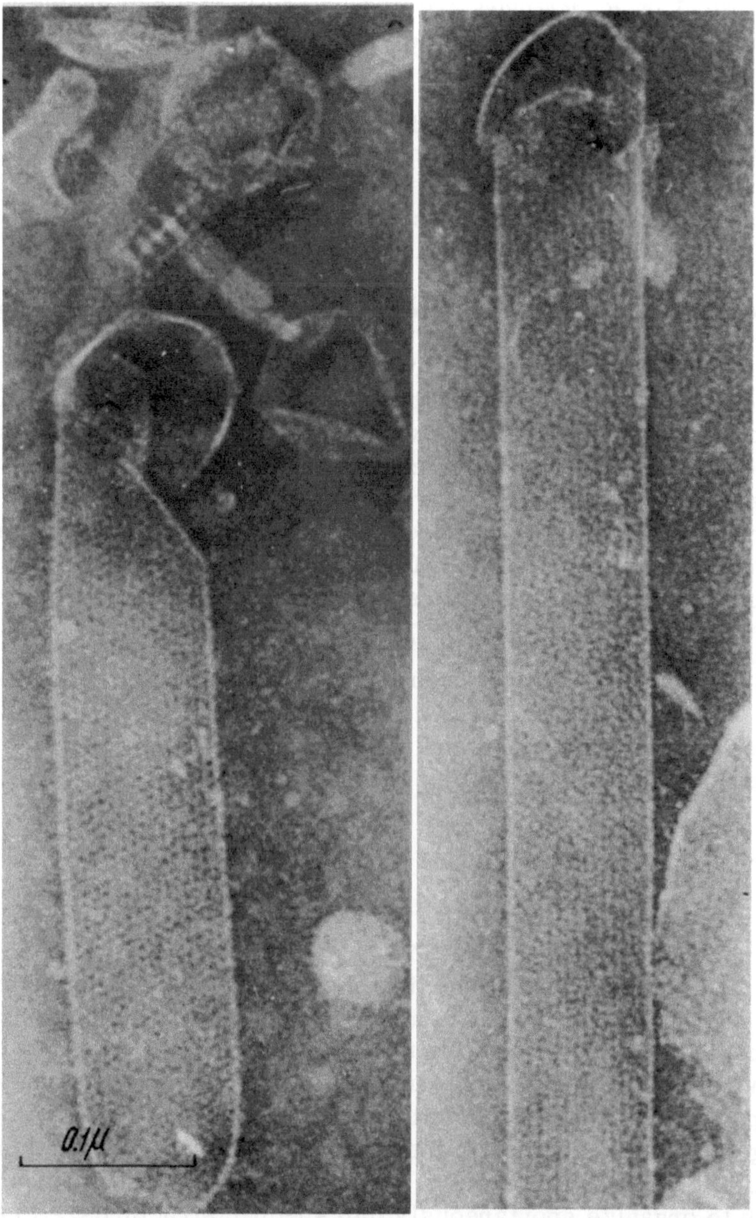

Fig. 127. Polyheads of phage AR1 of *Bacillus subtilis* . PTA. 230,000×.

In contrast to phage T4, capsomeres of the normal capsid of phage No. 1 of *B. mycoides* are just as easily distinguishable as the individual capsomeres on the polyheads and are similar to them in their fine structure.

In all probability it is impossible to form a capsid of the normal shape for phage No. 1, namely an octahedron, from long hollow tubes. In my opinion, therefore, these structures cannot be "blanks" of head capsids. They are most probably the result of abnormal assembly of capsomeres into a continuous, cylindrical tube.

In contrast to the amber mutant of T4, in which abnormal morphogenesis is associated with genetic disturbances [164], in the case of phage No. 1, these disturbances become manifest only in part of the phage progeny, so that the normal stages of formation of the phage particle occur as well as defective morphogenesis of the head capsid. In the latter case it can be postulated that all that happens is some degree of abnormal working of the normal gene which determines morphogentic processes in the phage head. This abnormality is perhaps due to unfavorable conditions for the gene to exhibit its function, leading to spontaneous organization of capsomeres into polyheads.

Polyheads have also been found among particles of phages AR1, AR2, and AR3 of *B. subtilis* [3]. They resemble polyheads of phage No. 1 of *B. mycoides* and are formed from capsomeres with the appearance of short hollow tubes (Fig. 127).

It will be noted that long tubular structures resembling phage polyheads are frequently found in a number of animal viruses [168, 245].

* * *

The study of the properties of the various phage proteins has thus shown they all possess the ability to aggregate. Proteins of the capsid and proteins of the tail sheath and rod are all capable of increasing in length uninterruptedly. The study of the aggregating properties of phage proteins suggests that the formation of phage protein structures in the cell may be based on a single principle, the expression of which is the ability of protein macromolecules to organize spontaneously into specific structures. A particular sort of protein macromolecule can recognize only those similar to it and can aggregate with them. This spontaneous organization evidently depends on the presence of a medium of appropriate thermodynamic and ionic state [122].

The ability of the various phage protein subunits to undergo spontaneous organization *in vitro* is most probably reflected also *in vivo* , except that, in the latter case, this self-assembly is presumably under genetic control also, and determines the shape and size of the corresponding phage components.

Chapter 10

Phosphatase Activity of Phages and Some Properties of the Contractile Phage Protein

An important function of the contractile proteins is their ability to transform chemical energy directly into mechanical work. This phenomenon has been called the mechanicochemical effect. Many structures in the living organism possess mechanicochemical activity. This is seen in its most perfect form in the muscles of higher animals. Mechanicochemical activity has also been found on many occasions in the structures of much simpler organisms, such as plants with motor responses, cilia of *Paramoecium*, flagella of bacteria, and even in cell organelles, such as mitochondria [29]. The most remarkable discovery has been that of contractile properties in the smallest of all biological structures – bacteriophages. As mentioned above, these properties are exhibited by the tail sheath of certain phages.

Engel'gardt and Lyubimova [72] showed for the first time that the isolated contractile muscle protein actomyosin can perform mechanical work if adenosinetriphosphate (ATP), a universal carrier of chemical energy in biological systems, is added. The same workers showed [159] that the contractile protein possesses ATPase activity. Besides its contractile properties, this protein also possesses the function of an enzyme. It is obvious that actomyosin-like proteins are widely distributed in nature and play an important role in the living organism.

To study the properties of the contractile protein of phages by analogy with muscle proteins, its ATPase activity has been investigated. Dukes and Kozloff [155] demonstrated the phosphatase activity of phages T2, T4, and T5 of *E. coli* B. Kozloff and Lute [253] obtained evidence to show that proteins with actomyosin-like properties are present in phage tails.

Tikhonenko and Poglazov [60] have studied phosphatase activity in phages differing in their morphology [60]. Phages No. 1 of *B. mycoides* and T2 of *E. coli* B, with a contractile tail sheath, phage T1 of *E. coli* B, with a noncontracting tail, and phage s_d of *E. coli* SK, with a very short tail, were used for this purpose. Experiments were carried out on concentrated, purified phage suspension in 0.9% NaCl solution. The purified phage preparations contained about 10^{12} phage particles/ml.

Phosphatase activity was determined from the ability of the phage particles to hydrolyze ATP. The reaction mixture used consisted of 0.3 ml borate buffer, pH 8.0; 0.3 ml 0.008 M ATP; 0.1 ml 0.005 M $CaCl_2$ or $MgCl_2$; and 0.3 ml of phage suspension. Preparations of intact phage and also of phage broken up by freezing and rapid thawing were used in the experiment. Samples were incubated at 37°C for 3 h. The enzyme reaction was stopped by addition of 5% trichloroacetic acid. The quantity of phosphorus hydrolyzed was determined by the method of Fiske and Subbarow [171]. The end result was expressed as the number of micrograms of phosphorus split from ATP by a phage suspension containing 1 mg protein/ml in the course of 1 h.

The investigation began with determination of the ATPase activity of phage No. 1.

When phage No. 1 of wild type was seeded on a plate culture of *B. mycoides*, besides plaques of the usual type, plaques differing considerably from the original in size also appeared. The diameter of the central zone of complete lysis of plaques of wild type is 5–7 mm, whereas the mutant gives plaques with a central zone of lysis measuring 1–3 mm. Both types of plaques are surrounded by an extensive halo of incomplete lysis. The plaque attains its largest size after 72 h. By isolation of single plaques of different types and after repeated subcultures, phage No. 1 of wild type (Fig. 128a) and its mutant, described as phage No. 1a (Fig. 128b) were obtained in a pure form.

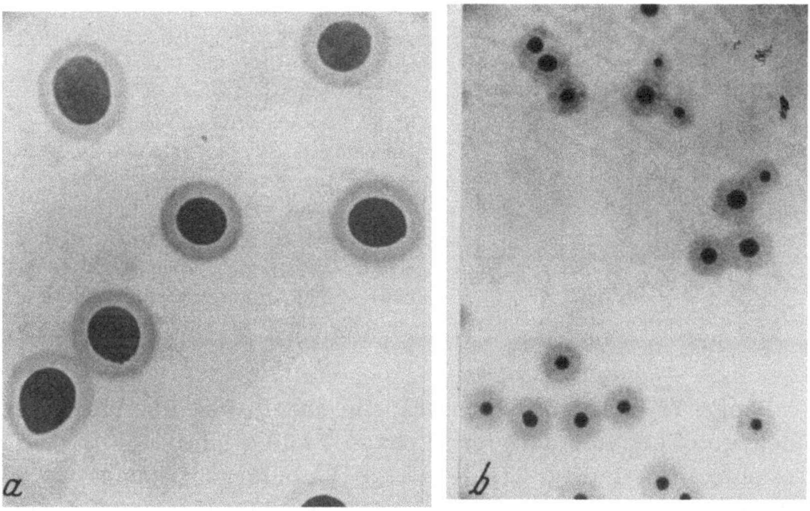

Fig. 128. Plaques of phages of *Bacillus mycoides*. a) phage No. 1; b) phage No. 1A.

The electron-microscopic study of phages Nos. 1 and 1A showed that phage particles of wild type and of its mutant are morphologically absolutely identical.

The complete identity of phages Nos. 1 and 1A in their structure and in the ability of their tail sheath to contract, combined with their ability to form different plaques, made it imperative to study the cause of this difference. It was necessary to determine whether differences in the degree of phosphatase activity are present in phage No. 1 and its mutant.

Experiments showed that phage No. 1 possesses high phosphatase activity, several times higher than the activity of phage No. 1A (Fig. 129a). I consider that this fact shows that the mutant possesses defective phosphatase. A unique type of "enzyme disease" arises, leading to the appearance of a biochemical mutant, and is expressed outwardly by plaques of reduced size.

Since the first investigations of phosphatase properties of phages were carried out on the T-series of coli phages, I also investigated the phosphatase activity of phages T1 and T2 of *E. coli* B for comparison.

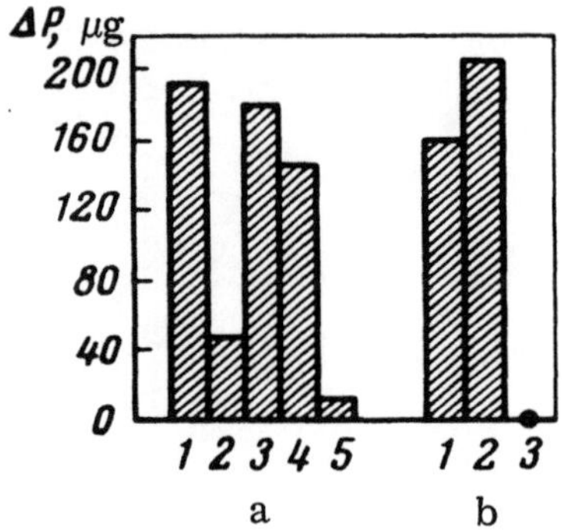

Fig. 129. Phsophatase activity of different phages. A: 1) Phage No. 1 *Escherichia coli* 2) phage No. 1A of *Bacillus mycoides*; 3) phage T2 of *Escherichia coli* B; 4) phage T1 of *Escherichia coli* B; 5) phage s_d of *Escherichia coli* SK. b: Action of Ca^{++} and Mg^{++} ions on phosphatase of phage No. 1 of *Bacillus mycoides*. 1) In the presence of 0.005 M $CaCl_2$; 2) in the presence of 0.005 M $MgCl_2$; 3) in the presence of 0.001 M EDTA. Activity expressed in μg phosphorus split per hour by 1 mg protein.

Phage T2 possesses a contractile sheath just like phage No. 1. The degree of enzyme activity of phage T2 is slightly lower than that of phage No. 1 (Fig. 129a). Phage T1 belongs to the group of phages with noncontracting tails. Nevertheless, it possesses fairly high phosphatase activity (Fig. 129a), of approximately the same order as phages No. 1 and T2. The presence of phosphatase activity suggests that contractile acts of a different type may take place in phage T1. It must be remembered that phosphatase activity also was found by Dukes and Kozloff [155] in phage T5, belonging to the same morphological group as phage T1.

Phage s_d of *E. coli* SK, which I studied, differs morphologically from all the other phages described above. It has a very short tail. Because of the morphology of this phage, it might be assumed that it would contain a relatively smaller amount of protein possessing phosphatase properties than the other phages studied. This hypothesis was confirmed experimentally. As is clear from Fig. 129a, the phosphatase activity of phage s_d, although measurable, was extremely low.

To obtain a more complete picture of the properties of the phosphatase discovered in phage No. 1, and to compare it with myosin, some properties of this enzyme were studied. Investigation of the effect of pH on the action of the phage phosphatase showed that its activity is lower in the acid zone, reaches a maximum at pH 8, and thereafter changes very little with further alkalification.

A very clear relationship was established between the phosphatase activity of phage No. 1 and Ca^{++} and Mg^{++} ions (Fig. 129b).

Ca^{++} ions, and to an even greater degree Mg^{++} ions, activate the phage phosphatase. The optimal concentration of these ions was 0.005 M. Addition of ethylenediaminetetraacetate (EDTA), binding these ions, leads to complete inactivation of the enzyme. This relationship is similar to the action of these ions on actomyosin ATPase. In the case of actomyosin, Ca^{++} and Mg^{++} ions also have an activating effect, activity in the presence of Mg^{++} being higher than in the presence of Ca^{++}.

Thiol groups play an important role in manifestation of the ATPase activity of myosin. Addition of SH-reagents to myosin in comparatively low concentrations inhibits the activity of the enzyme. The study of the action of p-chloromercuribenzoate (PCMB) on phage phosphatase revealed a similar relationship. In a concentration of 10^{-5} M, PCMB activated the enzyme by 40% and abolished enzyme activity in higher concentrations.

These results demonstrate the similarity between phosphatase of phage and the actomyosin-like enzyme of muscle. It may be supposed that the presence of this protein in phage is responsible for the contractile movements taking place in the phage particle on contact with the bacterial cell.

All phages thus possess phosphatase activity. The only difference lies in the amount, which correlates to some degree with the size of the tail on different phage particles, and evidently reflects individual features of the mechanism of interaction between the phage particle and bacterial cell.

In this connection, special interest is attached to the sharp difference in phosphatase activity of phage No. 1 of *B. mycoides* and of its mutant, phage No. 1A, with tails of absolutely identical size and structure. The deficiency of enzyme activity in phage No. 1A is apparently expressed functionally as loss of its ability to produce extensive lysis of the culture.

The comparative study of phosphatase activity in phages of different tail morphology suggests that it is mainly connected with tail structure.

The object of my later investigations was to determine more precisely with which protein structures of the phage particle phosphatase activity is connected.

LOCALIZATION OF PHOSPHATASE ACTIVITY IN STRUCTURAL ELEMENTS OF PHAGE T2

To determine the localization of phosphatase activity in the phage particle, it was first necessary to find a method of separating the phage particle into its structural components and yet at the same time preserve the native properties of the protein to the greatest degree, avoiding the introduction of proteolytic enzymes and additional strongly active compounds into the system, as was done in the investigations of Brenner and co-workers [111]. For this purpose, a method of alkalification of the phage suspension was developed by the author and Poglazov [61] which has proved effective whenever it has been necessary to dissolve or separate protein aggregates.

Successive disintegration of phage T2 was carried out with KOH, the pH of the phage suspension being adjusted to various values from 10.0 to 12.5.

Untreated and treated phage suspensions were precipitated by high-speed centrifugation at 100,000 g for 1 h. The residue was suspended in physiological saline and used for electron microscopy and for determination of phosphatase activity. Electron-microscopic observations of the process of disintegration of phage T2 particles at different pH values were fully described in Chapter 8. Here, it will be recalled that at pH 10.0–10.8 rupture of the head envelope takes place, accompanied by liberation of DNA. In the pH range from 10.8 to 11.5 the head envelope is separated from the tail (Fig. 92) and begins to break up gradually until it disappears completely as a morphological structure. At pH 11.5 only contracted sheaths with their rods remain in the specimen (Fig. 94); at pH 11.8–12.0, the sheaths and rod are separated (Fig. 95) and this is accompanied by fragmentation of the rod. At pH 12.0–12.5 only contracted tail sheaths remain in the preparation (Fig. 96).

When a phage suspension treated with alkali at pH 12.0 or above was centrifuged, only tail sheaths passed into the residue. Rod protein, like head protein, remained principally in the supernatant.

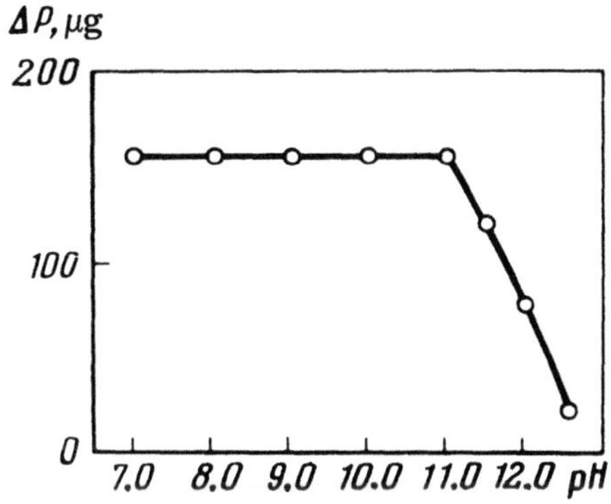

Fig. 130. Effect of pH on phosphatase activity of phage T2.

Phosphatase activity was determined by the method described above and also by electrophoretic fractionation on paper of the products of enzymic hydrolysis of ATP, followed by their elution in 0.2 M HCl and determination of the ratio between nucleotides on a type SF-4 spectrophotometer. The final results were expressed as the number of micrograms of phosphorus split from ATP by a suspension containing 1 mg protein/ml in 1 h. Electrophoretic fractionation was carried out at a voltage of 1000 V in CCl_4. A chromatographically pure ATP preparation containing 92% triphosphate was used in the experiments. Protein was determined by the biuret reaction.

Before investigating the phosphatase activity of the phage fractions, the total phosphatase activity of the preparation as a whole was studied to discover whether the phosphatase had survived alkalification. To do this, samples were taken from a phage suspension which had been gradually alkalified, neutralized, and the total phosphatase activity determined. The phosphatase activity remained constant up to pH 11.0 (Fig. 130). Further alkalification reduces activity of the enzyme. The results of these experiments demonstrate that alkalification to pH 11.5-11.8 causes comparatively slight damage to enzyme protein. Preparations treated in this way can be used for investigation of their enzymic properties. Under more alkaline conditions, marked denaturation changes take place, making it impossible to carry out the enzyme experiments.

Table 10

Fraction	pH at which fraction was obtained	ΔP
Tail sheath with rods (residue)	11.8	77
Dissolved head envelopes (supernatant)	11.8	9
Tail sheaths (residue)	12.4	20
Supernatant obtained after sedimentation of sheath	12.4	3

Next, the phosphatase activity of the phage fractions was determined. Results showing the relative proportion of the total phosphatase activity contained in the various structural components of the phage T2 particle are given in Table 10 (activity expressed in micrograms phosphorus split by 1 mg phage protein per hour).

These results show that the relative activity of the fraction consisting of contracted sheaths with rods is much higher (in this case more than 8 times) than the activity of the head fraction. It can be concluded from the results of these experiments that protein possessing phosphatase properties is concentrated mainly in the phage tail. Later experiments showed that this protein is contained in the tail sheath, because the specific phosphatase activity of this fraction is much higher than that of the other elements of the phage particle. As a result of strong alkalification to pH 12.0-12.5, which is required to cause complete separation of sheaths from rods and destruction of the rods, the phosphatase activity in the complete preparations is reduced, so that it cannot be compared in absolute units with the activity of the fraction containing contracted sheaths with rods obtained at lower pH values. However, the specific phosphatase activity of the tail sheaths was 7 times higher than the activity of the supernatant remaining after sedimentation of the sheaths.

Phosphatase activity is thus mainly concentrated in the tail sheath.

The localization of protein possessing phosphatase properties in the tail sheath enables the sheath to contract. This is evidently necessary for penetration of the bacterial cell wall.

The presence of some degree of phosphatase activity in the head fraction can be explained either by the presence of small traces of sheath as an impurity in this fraction or by the presence of a small quantity of contractile protein in the composition of the phage head also.

This latter suggestion is confirmed by the fact that phosphatase activity is also found in phages with a very short tail.

The presence of contractile protein in the phage head may perhaps enable changes to take place in the shape of the capsid under certain conditions, thereby increasing the pressure within the head and causing liberation of the DNA contained in it.

PHYSICOCHEMICAL PROPERTIES OF THE CONTRACTILE PROTEIN OF PHAGE T2

The nature of the reaction causing contraction of the tail sheath has not been adequately explained. Kozloff and his collaborators suggested that contraction of the sheath is similar to muscular contraction and the proteins composing the sheath are of actomyosin type [253]. These workers found that the tail of phage T2 contains about 115 ATP molecules, hydrolyzed to ADP and inorganic phosphates during contraction. They also state that sodium salts and EDTA, which prevent contraction of muscle actomyosin, also prevent contraction of the tail sheath. Brenner and co-workers [111] claim that the sheath protein does not resemble actomyosin in its chemical composition and structure.

To study the nature and physicochemical properties of the protein composing the tail sheath of phage T2, Poglazov and I [32] investigated a pure fraction of tail sheath obtained after treatment of a concentrated phage suspension with alkali at pH 11.9. To purify the sheath fraction from contamination with DNA and to render the sheath protein soluble, Fraenkel-Conrat's method [174] was used. This method was developed for the purification of tobacco mosaic virus protein, and it was subsequently used by Brenner and co-workers [111] to purify the tail sheaths of phage T2. The procedure was as follows. To one volume of a suspension of tail sheaths two volumes of glacial acetic acid cooled to a temperature close to the freezing point was added. The sheaths thereupon dissolved and the DNA present in the solution was precipitated. The DNA thus thrown down was separated from the dissolved sheaths by low-speed centrifugation and the pure supernatant was dialyzed against borate buffer, pH 5.5. During dialysis the dissolved sheath protein is precipitated as a sparingly soluble residue. Brenner and co-workers [111] were able to prevent this precipitation to some extent by carrying out the dialysis against 8 M urea.

However, dialysis against 8 M urea makes investigation of the physicochemical properties of the protein difficult. The precipitated (during dialysis against borate buffer) phage sheath protein does not pass into solution again, even as a result of treatment with alkali, powerful reducing agents (Na_2SO_3, ascorbic acid), urea, and p-chloromercuribenzoate. To stabilize the protein dissolved in acetic acid until it begins to be precipitated, I used reducing agents. To the solution of sheath protein, 40 μg/ml cysteine and the same amount of neutralized ascorbic acid were added, after which dialysis was carried out against borate buffer, pH 5.5, containing cysteine and ascorbic acid in the same concentrations. The protein precipitate formed during dialysis under these conditions is readily soluble at pH 7.0-8.0. These experiments demonstrate that aggregation of phage sheath protein molecules in the absence of reducing agents takes place with the participation of thiol groups and is accompanied by formation of stable bonds which determine the rigid tertiary structure of the tail sheath. If conditions are created which prevent the formation of these bonds, looser and more readily dissociated aggregates appear. The solution of tail sheath protein of phage T2 thus obtained was used for investigation of the Tyndall effect, optical activity, and for viscosimetry.

Since the protein preparation thus obtained is only sparingly soluble in the absence of reducing agents and tends to form a solid residue, the ability of this protein to polymerize and form aggregates was tested. By analogy with the contractile muscle protein actin, which can undergo polymerization in the presence of Mg^{++} ions, I investigated the action of Mg^{++} and Ca^{++} ions on phage sheath protein. Addition of $MgCl_2$ or $CaCl_2$ to the protein solution increases its viscosity, Ca^{++} ions having a stronger effect than

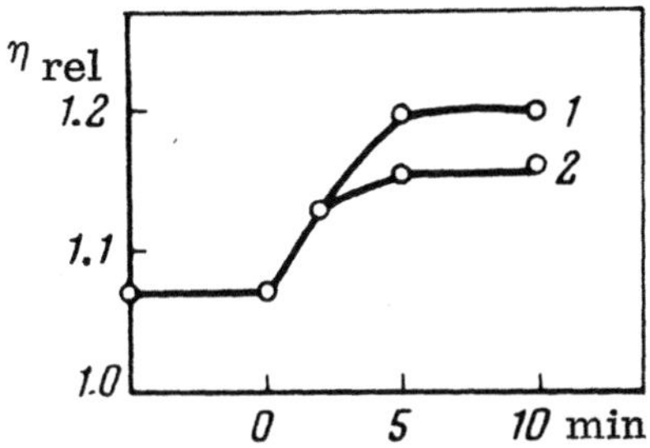

Fig. 131. Action of Ca^{++} and Mg^{++} ions on viscosity of a solution of sheath protein of phage T2; an aqueous solution of protein containing 0.14 mg/ml at pH 8.0 was used for the determination: 1) after addition of 0.01 M $CaCl_2$; 2) after addition of 0.01 M $MgCl_2$. Abscissa, time in min after addition of salt.

Mg^{++} (Fig. 131). Addition of an excess of the salt or exposure for a longer time to it causes the formation of a sparingly soluble residue. The increase in viscosity is small, but it is accompanied by a marked increase in the Tyndall effect. As is evident from Fig. 132, Ca^{++} also has a much stronger action on the increase in absorption of the protein solution at 400 mμ, doubling the turbidity in this case. If Ca^{++} is added after Mg^{++}, a further increase in absorption of the solution is observed, but the final absorption in this case is still less than if only Ca^{++} ions are added to the protein preparation. These results indicate the presence of competitive relationships between Mg^{++} and Ca^{++} ions.

If Ca^{++} ions are added first, and after absorption of the solution has reached its maximum, Mg^{++} ions are added, only a very slight decrease in turbidity takes place as a result of their competitive action. The fact that Ca^{++} ions considerably strengthen the action of Mg^{++} ions, while Mg^{++} ions have almost no effect on the action of Ca^{++}, suggests that calcium has a greater affinity for sheath protein and is bound more firmly to it than magnesium. As curve 3 shows, in Fig. 132 addition of EDTA slightly reduces the absorption of the solution, but does not return it to its initial value. This may be evidence that a certain number of Ca^{++} ions are bound comparatively weakly to protein, but most calcium ions are so firmly bound with the protein that they do not react with EDTA and the protein retains its property of aggregation. The results strongly suggest that the tail sheath protein has the property of aggregation under the influence of Ca^{++} and Mg^{++} ions.

To verify the hypothesis that phage sheath protein is similar to actin, I investigated its interaction with myosin obtained from rabbit muscle by Bailey's method as modified by Poglazov and co-

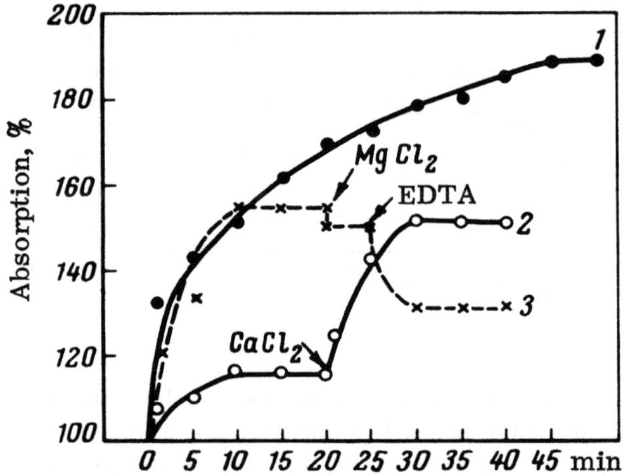

Fig. 132. Action of Ca^{++} and Mg^{++} ions on absorption of a solution of sheath protein of phage T2 at 400 mμ: 1) after addition of 0.01 M $CaCl_2$; 2) after addition of 0.01 M $MgCl_2$ followed by 0.01 M $CaCl_2$; 3) successive action of 0.01 M $CaCl_2$, 0.01 M $MgCl_2$, and 0.002 M EDTA.

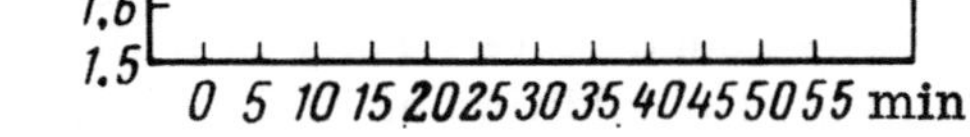

Fig. 133. Changes in total viscosity on addition of sheath protein of phage T2 to a solution of myosin and its dependence on addition of ATP. To 3.5 ml of myosin solution containing 3.1 mg protein/ml, 1 ml of a solution of polymerized sheath protein containing 0.2 mg protein/ml was added. After reaching a steady level of viscosity, 10^{-3} M ATP was added (marked by an arrow). Additive viscosity of the mixture of proteins was taken as the initial value.

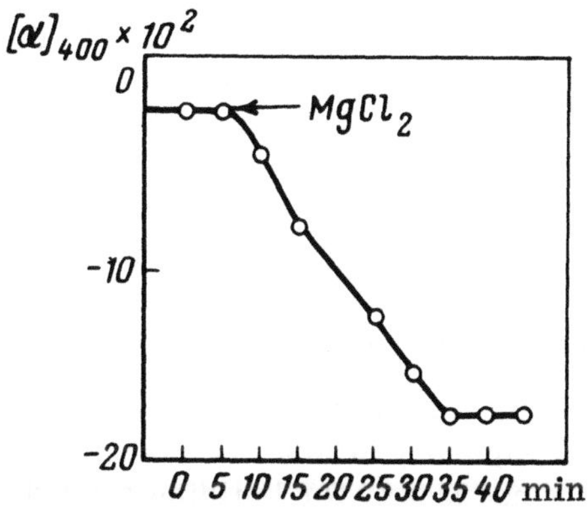

Fig. 134. Changes in optical rotation of a solution of sheath protein of phage T2 in the course of aggregation. Protein concentration 0.0073%, length of cuvette 0.3 cm. Aggregation carried out with 5 times 10^{-3} M $MgCl_2$ solution; measurements made at 400 mμ.

workers [30]. The most characteristic feature of actomyosin formation is the fact that the viscosity of the complex is higher than the simple arithmetic sum of the viscosities of its components. This interaction may be disturbed by the addition of ATP, which causes dissociation of the complex and a corresponding decrease in the viscosity of its solution. In my experiments the addition of a solution of phage tail sheath protein, polymerized with the aid of Ca^{++}, to myosin led to a small increase in viscosity, the value of which was greater than the sum of the viscosities of these proteins separately (Fig. 133). The increase in viscosity ended 10 min after mixing the solutions. Addition of ATP in a concentration of 10^{-3} M causes a decrease in viscosity, just as with actomyosin. These results suggest that some similarity exists between the phage tail sheath protein and muscle actin.

However, differences between the properties of tail sheath protein and muscle actin must be emphasized. Polymerization of phage sheath protein is accompanied by a marked increase in the turbidity of the solution, the formation of insoluble aggregates, and by a comparatively small increase in viscosity, whereas the most characteristic feature of actin polymerization is a considerable increase in viscosity and only a slight increase in opalescence of the solution. Polymerization of actin, in contrast to that of sheath protein, takes place more strongly by the action of Mg^{++} ions than of Ca^{++} ions. Interaction between phage sheath protein and myosin is not so marked as in the case of muscle actin. These findings, and many others, make it impossible to identify phage sheath protein with actin, but when these proteins are studied from the standpoint of their contractile functions, the existence of common properties is of greater interest.

As was shown above, the tail sheath is a helix. Uncoiled tail sheath helices frequently attain a considerable length, many times longer than is necessary for building a single sheath. The formation of long helices is evidently due to the fact that during stretching of the tightly compressed sheath structure, the bonds responsible for aggregation are liberated. Compact tail sheaths also possess a tendency to undergo aggregation. This property of sheaths to form long structures is evidently a reflection of the ability of sheath protein to undergo polymerization, which is observed by the action of Ca^{++} and Mg^{++} ions.

The helix of the tail sheath is in a comparatively stretched state in the intact phage particle and it shortens as the tail sheath contracts. This change in the state of the quaternary structure of the sheath is naturally closely connected with changes in the configuration of the polypeptide chain.

On the assumption that shortening of the helix may take place as a result of the action of aggregating forces with the participation of Ca^{++} or Mg^{++} ions, I investigated changes in the secondary structure of sheath protein taking place during its polymerization under the influence of these ions [32]. The method used was to study the optical activity of sheath protein solution during its aggregation.

The protein preparation obtained had strongly negative rotation. The main measurements of optical activity were made at 400 mμ. If the measurements were made at a shorter wavelength, a strong absorption effect was superimposed, and in some cases it prevented the measurements from being made. The initial specific rotation of the unpolymerized protein at 400 mμ was $-140°$ (Fig. 134). On the addition of the polymerizing agent, in this case $MgCl_2$, the optical rotation begins to increase in a negative direction, reaching a maximum of $-1730°$ after incubation for 35 min.

The increase in negative rotation during aggregation of the protein is evidence of changes taking place in the secondary structure of the polypeptide chains, causing a change from the α-configuration to the β-configuration.

According to Brenner and co-workers [111], the molecular weight of the sheath protein of phage T2 is about 54,000, and the weight of the whole sheath is $7.8 \cdot 10^6$ [377]. From these results, the claim has been made [377] that the sheath of phage T2 consists of 144 ± 20 protein subunits.

Sarkar and co-workers [328] also studied the properties of isolated contracted tail sheaths of phage T2 using methods of sedimentation analysis, diffusion of light, electrophoresis, amino acid analysis, and electron microscopy. They showed that sheath protein contains numerous amino acids and also a certain amount of hexosamine. No other carbohydrates were found in it. The molecular weight of the sheath, determined by the light diffusion method, was $8.0 \cdot 10^6$. On the basis of a minimal number of 144 histidine residues per sheath, these workers conclude that sheath protein contains 144 subunits, each with a molecular weight of 55,500.

These calculations are in agreement with the morphological findings. In the contracted sheath lying on its end, 12 morphological subunits can be counted in each turn of the helix (Fig. 54) and the contracted sheath consists of 12 turns. Consequently, the total number of morphological subunits in the sheath is about 144.

As Sarkar and co-workers [328] point out, the sedimentation coefficient of sheaths in a neutral buffer is 118S. On the addition of various substances, especially nucleotides, these workers observed transformation of the sheaths into a form in which they are sedimented more slowly. After removal of the nucleotides by dialysis the sedimentation rate returned to its original level. A 0.02 M solution of ATP is most effective for this purpose. Sarkar and co-workers consider that in the subunits of the sheath histidine residues are bound with ATP, and because of this the sheath as a whole acquires a more extended structure. The sedimentation coefficient of such sheaths is reduced by 18%.

Kozloff and co-workers [253] found that the tail sheath of phage T2 contains 142 ± 25 molecules of nucleoside triphosphates and 160 ± 30 calcium ions. It can thus be deduced that for each protein subunit there is one molecule of nucleoside triphosphate and 1 Ca^{++} ion. The same workers showed that interaction between the phage particle and bacterial cell, during which the sheath contracts, is accompanied by splitting of inorganic phosphate from nucleoside triphosphates. The role of nucleoside triphosphates, including ATP and desoxy-ATP, in this process thus consists essentially of maintaining the quaternary structure of the sheath in the relaxed state [377], while Ca^{++} ions participate in activation of their enzymic hydrolysis [254].

Poglazov and I [32] showed that Mg^{++} ions, and to a greater extent Ca^{++} ions, cause aggregation of the sheath protein. Some Ca^{++} ions are so firmly bound with protein that it cannot be removed by means of EDTA. These results agree with the concept of Kozloff and Lute [254] that some (about 40) Ca^{++} ions are more firmly bound with the tail sheath.

This discovery of the ability of tail protein to undergo polymerization under the influence of Ca^{++} and Mg^{++} ions, and more especially the ability of this protein to interact with muscle myosin, justified the conclusion that it bears some resemblance to actin. The molecular weight of the sheath protein is the same as that established for actin, namely 54,000 [257]. If this conclusion is correct, the act of splitting of ATP during contraction of the tail sheath as the phage interacts with the bacterial cell is evidently analogous to the splitting of ATP during polymerization of actin, and the spontaneous contraction of the sheath is a process of aggregation similar to the process of actin polymerization. Calcium ions, a component of the contractile structure, thus participate in the process of contraction of the tail sheath. At the same time, it must be remembered that phage sheath protein is a special type of protein possessing unique individual properties. Its amino acid composition [111, 328] differs from the composition of actin and myosin and in its resistance to various harmful agents it has a stronger resemblance to keratin.

To study the change in the secondary structure of the tail protein molecules during its aggregation, a polarimetric method was used [32]. The changes in the quaternary and tertiary structure during contraction are closely connected with changes in the configuration of the polypeptide chains of the protein. Astbury [87] first postulated that shortening of contractile muscle proteins is accompanied by replacement of the α-configuration by the cross (x)β-configuration of polypeptide chains. The work of Robertson and Bott [314] and of other investigators has shown that the increase in specific rotation of the polypeptide chains correlates precisely with the change from the α- to the β-configuration.

My own investigation [32] showed that aggregation of the phage sheath protein is accompanied by a marked increase in levorotation, reflecting an $\alpha \rightarrow \beta$ conversion. The decrease in the number of hydrogen bonds within the chains themselves, which accompanied such conversions, must lead to the appearance of new bonds between the chains and, consequently, to a change in the tertiary and quaternary protein structure, such as is observed during contraction of the tail sheath, which under these circumstances becomes shorter and wider. Such a change in quaternary structure is probable in the presence of conversion of the α-configuration into the transverse (x)β-configuration.

Standaert and Laki [349], using a polarimetric method, also showed that the $\alpha \rightarrow$ (x)β configurational change takes place during polymerization of actin obtained from animal muscles. The quaternary structure of filaments of polymerized actin, the precise nature of which was discovered by Hanson and Lowy [192], resembles the structure of the stretched helix of the tail sheaths of phage T2 (Fig. 120).

Another interesting point is that the structure of the flagella of bacteria is very similar to the structure of the contractile phage sheath [264, 265]. These observations are evidence of the existence of elements of similarity both in the structure and in the behavior of the protein of phage sheath, actin, and bacterial flagella. It would be too much to expect complete identity of the contractile proteins in different members of the organic world, so widely different in their levels of development, but nevertheless it appears that the elementary physicochemical reaction which leads to contraction is the same in all of them.

Chapter 11

Organization of Phage DNA During Its Replication in the Bacterial Cell

As Thomas [68] points out, DNA molecules can assume a contracted, compact configuration. This property is characteristic of the DNA of chromosomes, spores, heads of spermatozoa, and so on, and also for the compact arrangement of the DNA within the phage head. The study of the organization of DNA within the phage capsid may shed light on the causes and the requirements determining the manner of this organization.

One possible approach to the study of organization of phage DNA is by investigating the stages of its formation within an infected cell.

The process of phage-formation in the bacterial cell begins from the moment of adsorption of the phage particle on the host cell. This is clear from Fig. 139, showing that adsorbed particles of phage No. 1, with empty heads, are attached to the cell wall by their tail.

Hershey and Chase [200, 201] showed that phage DNA, together with a small quantity of internal protein, play the role of infective principle after penetration into the cell. Phage ghosts, consisting of external protein, remain on the surface of the cell.

The time from entry of the phage DNA into the bacterial cell until full maturation of phage particles in it is called the latent period. Every bacterium – phage system has its own latent period,

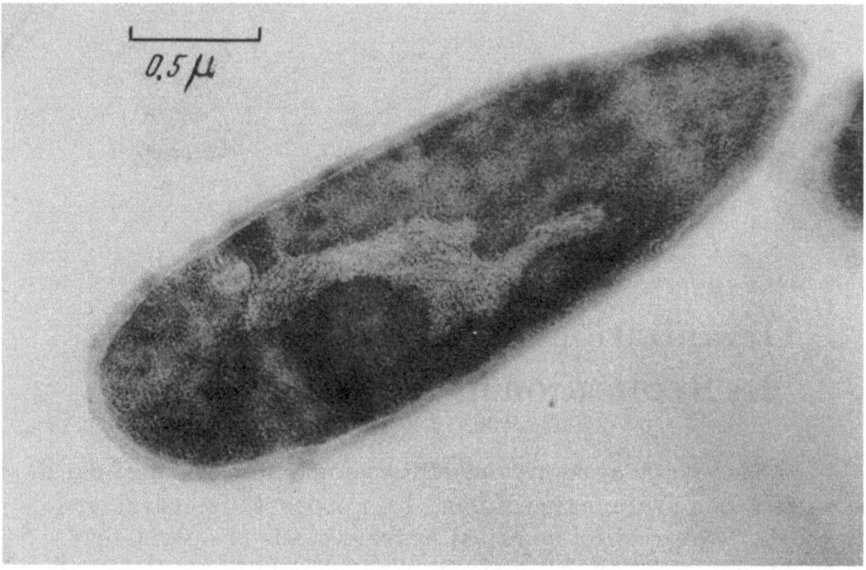

Fig. 135. Section through *Bacillus mycoides* cell (control). 35,000 ×.

during which biochemical changes concerned with the synthesis of new material, foreign to the host cell, takes place. From this material phage particles will subsequently be formed. The biochemical processes taking place in this period must be accompanied by morphological changes in the bacterial cell, leading to the appearance of new structures which are gradually transformed into phage particles. However, the study of the morphology of intracellular development of the phage particle is attended by considerable difficulties which have now been partly overcome as the result of improvements in the techniques of cutting ultrathin sections and the use of new methods of fixation of bacteria, enabling the internal structure both of the bacterial cell and of the phage particles developing in it to be preserved in the sections.

Kellenberger and co-workers [236, 239, 322] have given the clearest picture of changes taking place in cells of *E. coli* B after infection with phage T2. They found that immediately after introduction of phage DNA into the cell, the nuclear material of the cell is destroyed and this is accompanied by biochemical changes leading to the formation and accumulation of a stock of phage DNA.

Subsequent processes taking place in the bacterial cell, as Kellenberger [228] suggests, follow the line of condensation of phage DNA. Discrete, labile structures are formed and subsequently undergo condensation accompanied by dehydration. However, these early stages of phage formation were not identified morphologically by these workers.

Tikhonenko and Bespalova [361] carried out a morphological study of the stages of phage formation in a different bacterium–phage system with a longer latent period than that of *E. coli* cells infected with phage T2. The longer latent period allowed a more detailed study to be made of changes in the bacterial cell in the early stages of phage infection and the stages of formation of the phage particle in the cell to be examined consecutively.

A culture of atypical strain No. 1 of *B. mycoides*, grown in nutrient broth for 4h at 27°C until the cell concentration was $5 \cdot 10^7$/ml, was used for this purpose. This culture was infected by phage No. 1, the multiplicity of infection being 10 phage particles per bacterial cell.

Experiments to study changes in the optical density of the broth culture of bacteria after infection with phage showed that the turbidity of the culture begins to diminish toward the end of the second hour and completely disappears between the sixth and seventh hour. Samples were taken after 30 min, 60 min, 90 min, and 2, 3, 4, 5, and 6 h. The latent period of this phage, determined by studying a single replication cycle, is 60–70 min.

To prepare ultrathin sections, the suspension of bacterial cells, both uninfected and infected with phage, was fixed, dehydrated, and embedded in a mixture of butyl and methyl-methylmethacrylates by the method of the author and Bespalova [54, 361] described in Chapter 1.

Electron-microscopic study of sections of cells from a 4-h culture of *B. mycoides*, uninfected with phage, showed that they possess a fairly thick, amorphous cell wall, separated from the cytoplasmic membrane by a narrow layer transparent to electrons. The cytoplasmic membrane of *B. mycoides* cells consists of two layers. The cell cytoplasm is finely granular and appears dense to electrons. In the center of the section through the cell there is a more electron-transparent area filled with tightly packed, reticu-

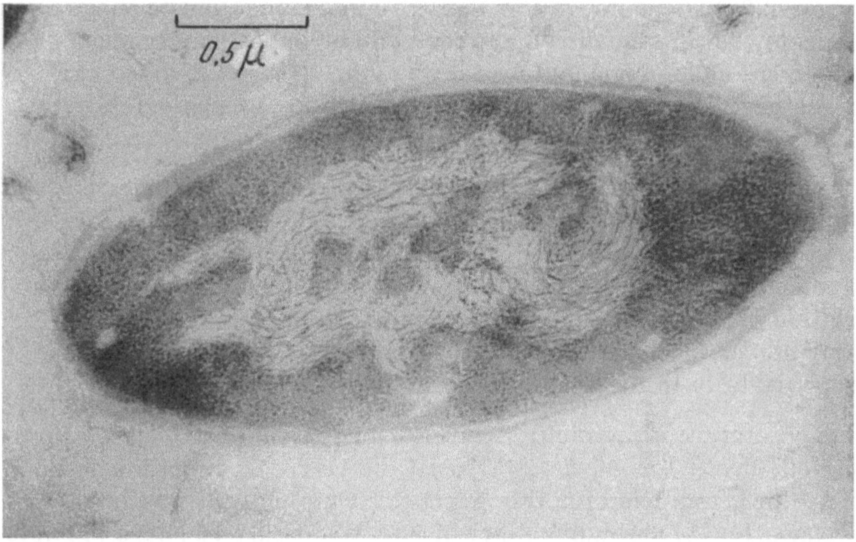

Fig. 136 . Section through *Bacillus mycoides* cell 1.5 h after infection with phage No. 1. 35,000×.

lar material, consisting of the nucleoid. As a rule, it stretches along the long axis of the cell and is irregular in shape, occupying a comparatively small area of the cell in section (Fig. 135).

Infection of bacterial cells leads in the early stages (between 30 min and 2 h) to intense hypertrophy of the nucleoid, which comes to occupy a larger part of the cell, displacing the cytoplasm to the periphery. It is noteworthy that in the early stages of infection the reticular material occupying the region of the nucleoid is more loosely arranged than in the nucleoid of the normal cell. This is presumably associated with intensive hydration of the nucleoplasm. Individual filaments become more clearly distinguishable and when these invade the cytoplasm they make the border between nucleoid and cytoplasm less sharp (Fig. 136). Similar hypertrophy of the nucleoid was observed by Kellenberger and co-workers [236, 239] in *E. coli* B cells soon after infection by phage T2.

In all probability these changes in the structure and shape of the nucleoid are associated with intensive synthesis of phage DNA taking place in the nucleoid under the influence of infection.

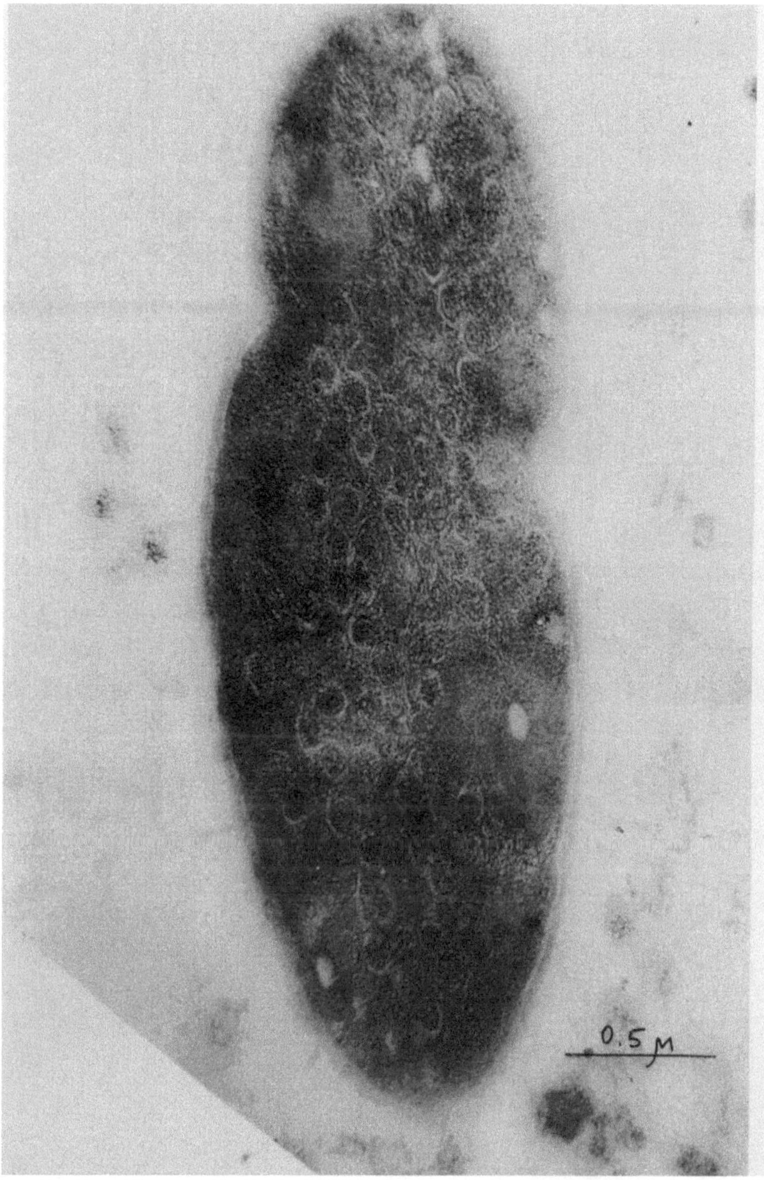

Fig. 137. Section through *Bacillus mycoides* cell 3 h after infection with phage No. 1. Loose balls of varied diameter can be seen. 40,000 ×.

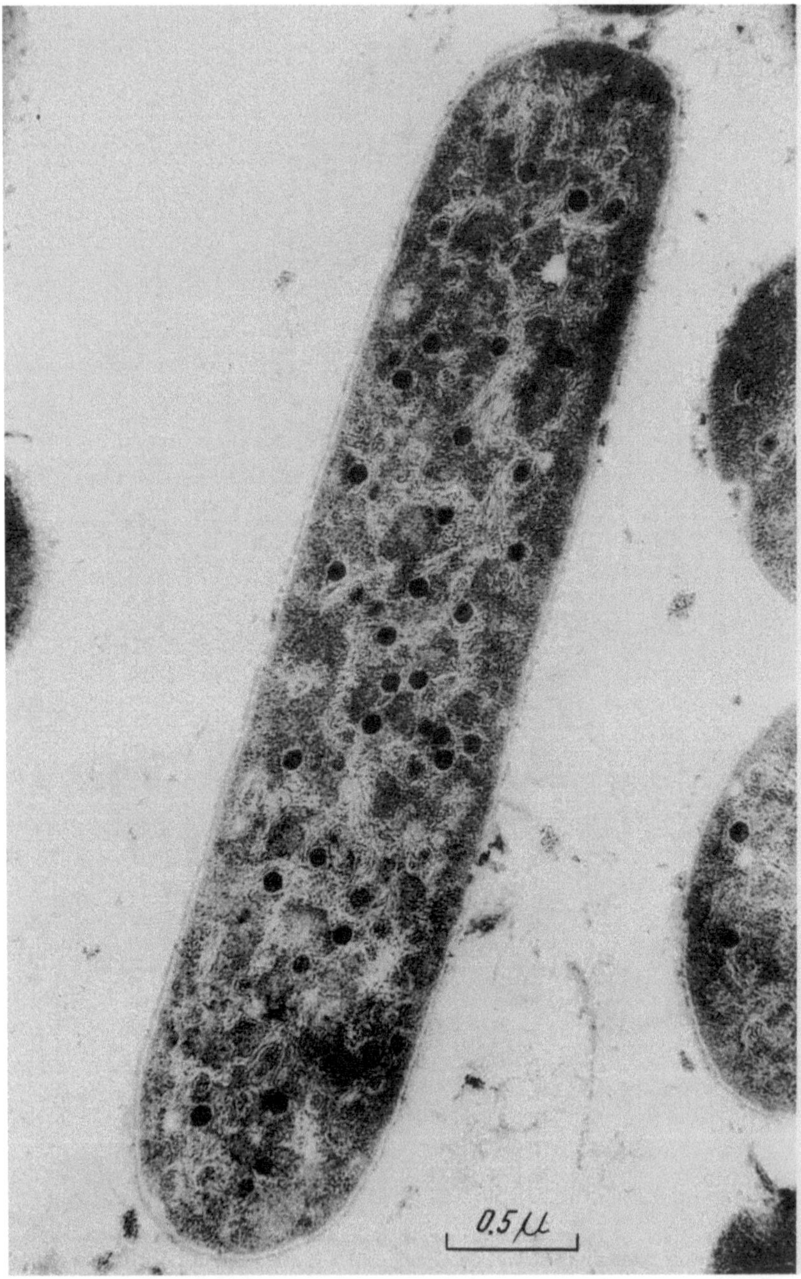

Fig. 138. Section through *Bacillus mycoides* cell 4 h after infection with phage No. 1. Electron-dense phage particles, circular and hexagonal in shape, have appeared. 35,000×.

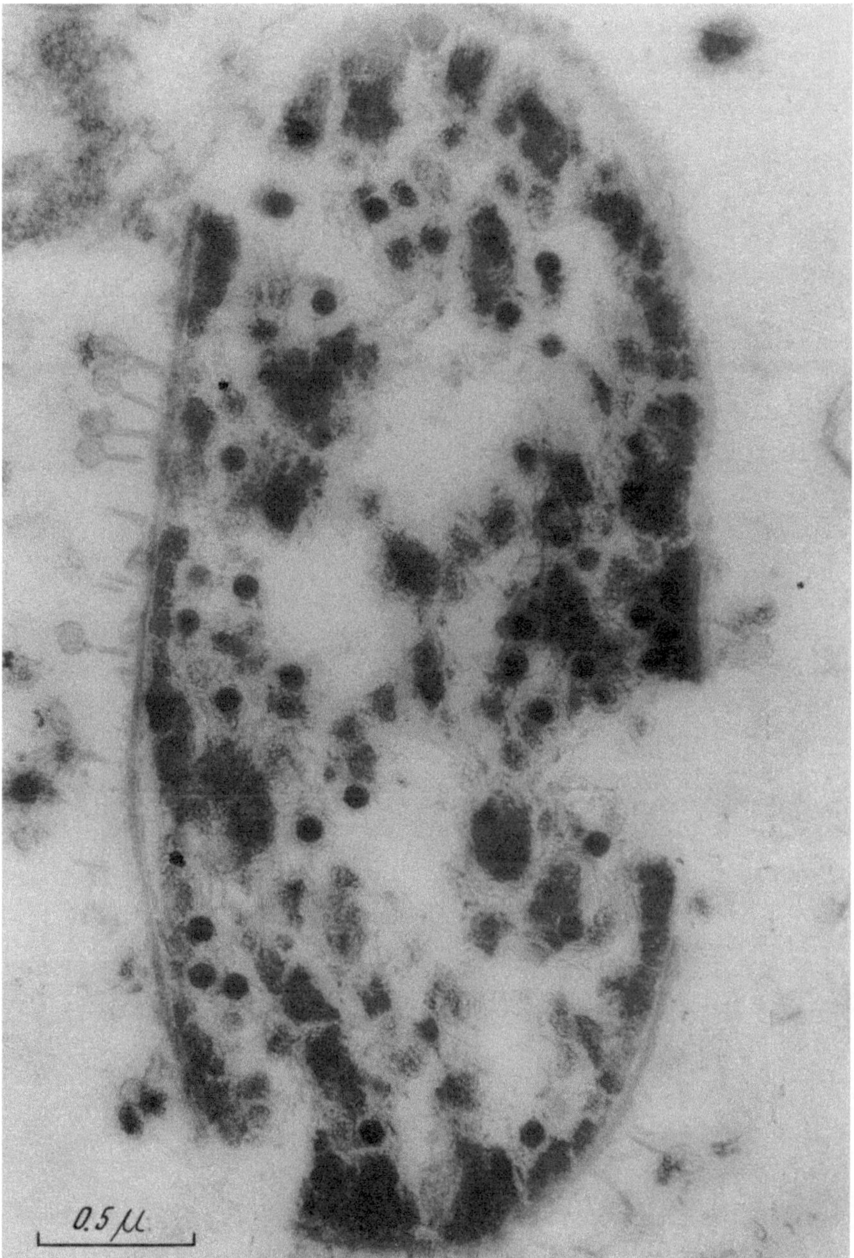

Fig. 139. Section through *Bacillus mycoides* cell 6 h after infection with phage No. 1. Hexagonal phage particles can be seen inside the half-destroyed cell, and adsorbed phage particles with empty heads are visible outside. 42,000 ×.

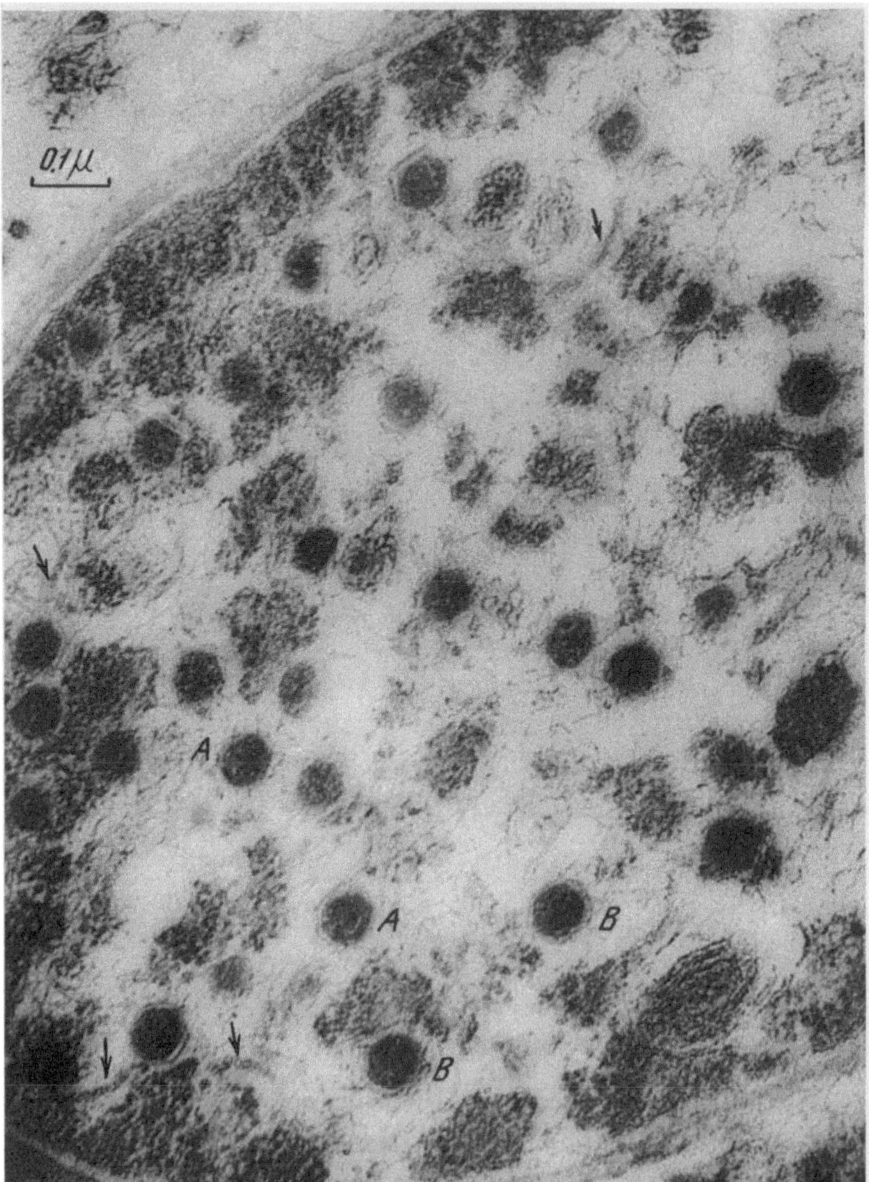

Fig. 140. Fragment of section through a *Bacillus mycoides* cell 6 h after infection with phage No. 1. A) Helical arrangement of DNA within the phage head (cut longitudinally); B) arrangement of DNA in the form of dots (cut transversely). Arrows indicate phage tails. 100,000×.

Toward 3 h after infection the structure of the cell becomes profoundly modified, acquiring completely new morphological features, specific of phage infection. By this time, loosely arranged circular structures, resembling balls of wool, appear in the diffusely outlined, greatly hypertrophied nucleoid. They are probably formed by coiling of strands of phage DNA and they act as centers of formation of phage particles.

The diameters of these balls differ, some of them being about 1500 Å, whereas the diameter of the mature phage head is 800 Å. Variations in size are evidently attributable to differences in the stages of coiling of the strands during formation of the DNA of the phage particle (Fig. 137).

I consider that these loose ball-like structures appearing in the process of phage infection reproduce the stages of DNA "condensation" whose existence in the early stages of phage formation was postulated by Kellenberger [228]. These centers of condensation are, in all probability, precursors of future phage particles, i.e., to use Kellenberger's terminology, they are particles of the first type.

Toward 4 h after infection, besides these loose balls, electron-dense bodies of circular and hexagonal shape begin to appear in the cell. In size these bodies correspond to heads of particles of phage No. 1 of *B. mycoides*. At this stage of maturation of the phage particle, it is not yet possible to distinguish the envelope surrounding the head clearly. However, the possibility cannot be ruled out that it has begun to form in some particles, because it is only through the formation of a rigid structure of some sort on the surface of the phage head that transformation of the circular shape of the head into hexagonal can be explained (Fig. 138).

At a later stage (5-6 h) after infection, the bacterial cell appears half fragmented. Only certain areas of cytoplasm and fragments of reticular material remain in it. Highly electron-dense bodies, consisting of mature hexagonal phage particles, are present in the devastated cell (Fig. 139).

Even in the late stages of phage formation, however, a few of the loose ball-like structures still remain in the cell (Figs. 138 and 139).

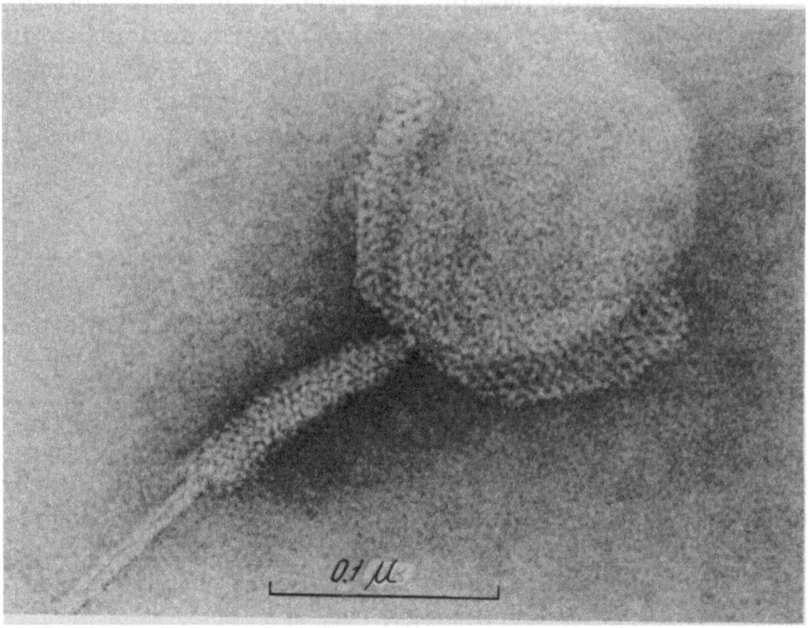

Fig. 141. Discharge of a solid block of DNA from the ruptured capsid of phage No. 1. of *Bacillus mycoides*. Hollow hexagonal capsomeres are clearly distinguishable. PTA. 300,000×.

The simultaneous presence of particles of different morphology in a section through the cell (loose or dense oval, dense hexagonal particles) suggests that maturation of phage particles takes place asynchronously in the cell. In all probability, some phage particles never attain a state of complete maturation.

Unfortunately, the phage tail can rarely be distinguished in the sections because of the very slight chance that the section passes through the plane of this slender structure. However, in some cases the phage tail structure is clearly distinguishable (Fig. 140). The head envelope, or capsid, can also be seen on this same photomicrograph. It is also apparent that the DNA filling the phage head is very tightly packed there and has a definite structure, visible in the sections in different projections either as dots (transverse section A) or as compactly coiled strands (longitudinal section B). Tightly packed DNA forming the contents of the phage head is surrounded by a clearly distinguishable envelope or capsid (Fig. 140).

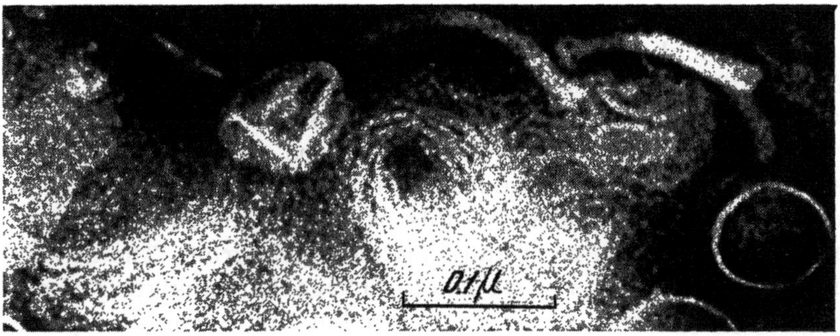

Fig. 142. Loose ball of DNA strands liberated from the head of phage No. 1 of *Bacillus mycoides* after treatment with ATP. PTA. 190,000×.

The study of intracellular phage by the negative staining method sometimes revealed particles with a ruptured head envelope from which the internal contents (DNA) have escaped. It is also noteworthy that, at the moment when it is discharged from the ruptured capsid, the DNA has the appearance of a very tightly wrapped ball, usually irregular in shape, in which the separate strands can no longer be distinguished (Fig. 141). At the moment of discharge of the DNA, it is still evidently in an extremely condensed state, characteristic of its arrangement within the phage head. Later, these balls become looser, acquiring a structure in which the separate strands are readily distinguishable (Fig. 142).

The organization of phage DNA during its replication in the bacterial cell thus takes place as follows. In the early stages, strands of phage DNA begin to coil into discrete, loose balls of different sizes. In the process of maturation they become compact and are turned into circular structures of the same size, and when completely mature they are hexagonal in shape. The process of phage formation in the cell thus takes place through condensation of phage DNA, accompanied, in all probability, by dehydration, leading to a very compact arrangement of the DNA in the mature particle. Protein subunits forming the capsid and tail of the phage particle are subsequently formed on this compactly arranged DNA. However, the precise character of arrangement of the DNA strands cannot be determined in these sections. The possibility cannot be ruled out that the arrangement of the reticular material during formation of the head determines its shape. Hence, it can be postulated that in phage No. 1 the DNA is coiled into a compact ball of spherical shape, on which protein subunits are subsequently formed to give the head its regular polyhedral shape. In the case of phage T2, the long DNA molecule is packed into an oval structure, the strands of which lie along one of the axes, as various investigators have suggested [184, 240]. The formation of protein subunits on DNA packed in this oval arrangement gives the phage particle the shape of an elongated polyhedron. The appearance of aberrant forms of the head in phage T2, consisting of an isometric polyhedron, is evidently attributable to defective packing of the DNA in the process of intracellular phage formation, and associated, as Kellenberger [229] suggests, with a disturbance of morphopoiesis.

The facts described above indicate that DNA strands, under certain conditions, can change from a loose to a more compact arrangement, and vice versa. This property of DNA is probably utilized in the mechanism of infection of the bacterial cell by the phage particle.

Conclusion

Despite the great morphological variation existing among the bacterial viruses, they nevertheless possess common features in their structural organization. A common feature of all phages, as well as of viruses of plants and animals, is that they consist of nucleic acid, of a single type (either DNA or RNA), and a protein envelope formed from morphological subunits which are identical in particular structural components. The strict arrangement of the morphological subunits is responsible for the regular shape of the virion.

The head of different phage particles can be either regular or elongated in shape. In my opinion, this depends on the character of arrangement of the nucleic acid: spherical packing creates conditions for the formation of protein subunits on it which fit together perfectly to form a regular polyhedron; the elongated arrangement of the nucleic acid creates conditions for the formation of an elongated polyhedral head.

In contrast to viruses of plants and animals, nearly all bacteriophages (except the filamentous type) possess a characteristic structure in the form of a tail. Phages can be distinguished by the shape, structure, and size of their tail. In some phages (the RNA-phages, phages of type ϕX 174) this structure shows only very slight differentiation and is merely a short projection. In other phages, despite their small size, signs of structural differentiation of the tail can be found (phages of type s_d). Phages with a well-defined, long tail also show great structural variety and are distinguished primarily by the ability of their tail to contract.

Increased complexity of structural organization among phages is in all probability, associated with their nucleic acid content. Virulent phages of complex organization contain a nucleic acid with higher molecular weight.

The tail of most phage particles terminates in an end plate, the structure of which varies among different phages. Most frequently the end plate is pentagonal or hexagonal in shape, with projections from which thin fibers emerge. In all probability, the end plate is the structure in which the proteolytic enzymes of the phage particle, destroying the bacterial cell wall, are concentrated. In phages with a contractile tail sheath the end plate evidently has another function, namely, that of keeping the sheath in a stretched state. While the end plate produces hydrolysis of the bacterial cell wall, it is partially destroyed itself, and this leads to contraction of the tail sheath. This hypothesis is confirmed by comparing the structure of the end plate in particles with an uncontracted and contracted tail sheath. The end plate on uncontracted tails has pro-projections with circular outlines.

On the contracted sheath the projections of the end plate become longer and pointed in shape, as if liberated from the structures constraining them.

My study of the fine structure of different phages showed that some of them have a tail of intermediate morphological type. These include phage VI of *Proteus mirabilis* (Fig. 25a, b, c), possessing a short, conical tail, resembling that of phages T3 and T7. However, an end plate is formed in the phage VI particle, but not in phages of types T3 and T7, although a well-developed end plate is possessed by phage s_d of *E. coli* SK, which also has a short tail.

An additional structural component is found in the head of many phage particles, consisting of a compact membrane situated at the point of attachment of the tail to the head. The functional role of this structure is not yet clear; it may perhaps participate in the process of transmission of nucleic acid from the head into the tail canal.

Phage Plonus I of *Mycobacterium tuberculosis* , in which differentiation of the tail into an outer sheath and inner rod is observed (Fig. 35a, b, c), is an example of a tail of intermediate structure between noncontracting and contracting.

Infection of animal and plant tissue by viruses can take place either through a wound surface, by phagocytosis, pinocytosis [8], or insects [42]. In bacteria, because of their very small size, these pathways of infection are impossible.

Bacteria, being unicellular organisms, are securely protected against external environmental influences by a comparatively strong outer membrane. In order for bacterial cells to be infected by viruses, a special adaptation is necessary to overcome this obstacle. The tail or its analogous part of the phage particles may serve as this adaptive device. In fact, if the obstruction of the bacterial membrane is removed, the process of phage reproduction can take place by the bare phage nucleic acid along (development of phage in protoplasts and sheroplasts).

However, the question arises why this great variation in tail structure is found among the bacteriophages. It is difficult at present to find an answer. It would seem that the main reason for the existence of phages varying in the degree of complexity of the structural organization of their tail is connected with the structure of the bacterial cell wall.

Electron-microscopic investigations have shown that the outer membrane of bacterial cells is a mosaic consisting of heterogeneous areas [95, 97, 325].

Fractionation of the bacterial membrane has revealed the presence of definite structures specifically reacting with phage [149, 221, 258, 315, 382, 383, 384].

These structures have been called receptors of the cell wall. Although the chemical nature of the cell receptors for many phages has not been discovered, it must be considered to be highly varied. The specificity of the reaction between the cell receptor and a particular species of phage is evidently based on this variety. Some receptors evidently require a less complex structural organization of the phage particle tail, others a more complex orgainzation. From this point of view, it is an interesting fact that certain phages (filamentous, RNA-containing) are specifically adsorbed on the fimbriae of male types of bacterial cell. Information has also been obtained to show that receptor areas for certain phages are localized on bacterial flagella [178, 223, 282].

As Stent [37] points out, the structure of receptor areas can be modified by genetic changes in the bacterial cell, after which specific interaction between a given receptor and the homologous phage particle becomes impossible. It is therefore logical to suppose that the tail is the specialized organ which must be actively modified, depending on changes in the fine structure of the cell membrane, and, conversely, changes in the tail structure of the phage particle compel the cell to evolve new protective adaptation.

Variation in tail structure observed among the bacteriophages can thus, in my opinion, arise in response to changes in the receptor apparatus of the cell membrane. The specific structure of the cell receptor and its localization, in all probability, lead to the development of specific structural adaptations in the phage particle embodied in its definitive shape. In the process of evolution, changes in structure of the receptor apparatus of the cell from simpler to more complex have evidently led to variety and increasing complexity of the structural organization and functions of the phage tail. Phages with complex tail organization, with a contractile sheath, have evidently appeared in response to increasingly complex conditions of interaction between phage particle and bacterial cell.

The discovery, in the future, of still finer structural details of the structure both of the phage particle and of the cell receptors will undoubtedly help to elucidate this problem.

It can thus be concluded that the role of the protein structures of bacteriophages is not simply one of protecting the nucleic acid which is the infective principle. The various structural proteins of the phage particle undoubtedly play a complex role in the process of infection of the bacterial cell.

Literature Cited

1. Adams, M., Bacteriophages. Interscience, New York (1959).
2. Azizbekyan, R. R., and Kriviskii, A. S., The system phage – *Bacillus subtilis* cell as an object for the study of genetics of microorganisms. Genetika, No. 5, p. 111 (1966).
3. Azizbekyan, R. R., Belyaeva, N. N., Kriviskii, A. S., and Tikhonenko, A. S., Structure of the phages of *Bacillus subtilis* and lysogeny of host cells. Mikrobiologiya, 35:279 (1966).
4. Belykh, R. A., and Kriviskii, A. S., Lysogeny of strains of *Escherichia coli* 600 and SK, host bacteria for phage s_d. Mikrobiologiya, 34:819 (1965).
5. Belyaeva, N. N., The unique morphology of phage AR9 of *Bacillus subtilis*. Abstracts of Proceedings of the 6th All-Union Conference on Electron Microscopy, Novosibirsk (1967).
6. Belyaeva, N. N., and Azizbekyan, R. R., A new phage of *Bacillus subtilis* of unusual morphology. Mikrobiologiya, 36:1054 (1967).
7. Biryuzova, V. I., Borovyagin, V. L., Gilev, V. P., Kiselev, N. A., Tikhonenko, A. S., and Chentsov, Yu. S., Electron-Microscopic Methods of Investigation of Biological Objects. Moscow, Izd. AN SSSR (1963).
8. Bykovskii, A. F., Ontogenesis of some viruses of man and animals, in: Virology and Immunobiology. Moscow, Nauka Press (1964).
9. Vainshtein, B. K., and Kiselev, N. A., The structure of viruses, in: Virology and Immunobiology. Moscow, Nauka Press (1964).
10. Velikodvorskaya, G. A., Chikova, T. S., and Lysenko, A. M., Identification of lipids in the phage s_d corpuscle. Acta Virologica, 9:558 (1965).
11. Gol'dfarb, D. M., Bacteriophagy. Moscow, Medgiz (1961).
12. Gol'dfarb, D. M., Avdeeva, A. V., and Borisova, N. B., Spheroplasts of *Escherichia coli* obtained by means of phage ghosts. Mikrobiologiya, 31:869 (1962).
13. Zavil'gel'skii, G. B., Il'yashenko, B. N., Minyat, É. E., and Rudchenko, O. N., Protective action of acridine orange on infective DNA of bacteriophage 1φ7 with ultraviolet radiation. Dokl. Akad. Nauk SSSR, 155:937 (1964).
14. Ivanovskii, D. I., On two diseases of tobacco: Tobacco rattle; Mosaic disease. Sel'skoe Khozyaistvo i Lesovodstvo, No. 3, p. 1 (1892).

15. Il'yashenko, V. N., Infection of lysozyme spheroplasts of isolated DNA of phage φX174. Vopr. Virusol., No. 6, p. 667 (1963).

16. Il'yashenko, V. N., Infectivity of DNA of phage φX174, in: Genetics of Microorganisms, Moscow, Medgiz (1963).

17. Il'yahsenko, V. N., and Rudchenko, O. N., Single-stranded infectious DNA of a small enteric bacteriophage. Dokl. Akad. Nauk SSSR, 157:198 (1964).

18. Il'yashenko, B. N., Tikhonenko, A. S. Dityatkin, S. Ya , and Rudchenko, O. N., Biological properties of small enteric phages containing DNA. Mikrobiologiya, 34:814 (1965).

19. Kiselev, N. A., Electronmicroscopy of Biological Macromolecules, Moscow, Nauka Press (1965).

20. Kiselev, N. A., and Poglazov, B. F., The molecular organization of the tail sheath of phage T2. Dokl. Akad. Nauk SSSR, 155:442 (1964).

21. Kiselev, N. A., Tikhonenko, T. I., Kaftanova, A. S., and Kiselev, F. L., Investigation of phage s_d and its nucleic acid by the method of electron microscopy. Biokhimiya, 28:1065 (1963).

22. Crick, F., and Watson, J., General principles of the structure of viruses. The Nature of Viruses [Russian translation], Moscow, IL (1958).

23. Kriss, A. E., Biryuzova, V. I., and Zolkover, A.M., Drop analysis, a method of preparation of biological specimens for electronmicroscopy. Mikrobiologiya, 17:484 (1948).

24. Kriss, A. E., and Tikhonenko, A. S., Uncoiling of the helix formed by the bacteriophage head under the influence of high pressures. Dokl. Akad. Nauk SSSR, 93:353 (1953).

25. Kriss, A. E., and Tikhonenko, A. S., Action of high pressures on the particles of various phages. Mikrobiologiya, 24:677 (1955).

26. Marikhin, V. A., and Romankova, L. P., Preparation of microgrids for the electron microscope. Zavodskaya Lab., 29:975 (1963).

27. Nikitin, L. I., and Vasil'eva, L. V., The fimbriae of soil microorganisms. Izv. Akad. Nauk SSSR, Seriya Biol., No. 3, p. 400 (1965).

28. Peshkov, M. A., Tikhonenko, A. S., and Marek, B. I., A virulent phage against the multicellular bacterium *Caryophanon tenue* Peshkoff. Mikrobiologiya, 35:684 (1966).

29. Poglazov, B. F., Structure and Function of Contractile Protein, Moscow, Nauka Press (1965).

30. Poglazov, B. F., Bilushi, V., and Baev, A. A., Sulfhydryl groups of myosin adenophosphatase. Biokhimiya, 23:269 (1958).

31. Poglazov, B. F., Borkhsenius, S. N., and Belavtseva, E. M., Reconstruction and crystallization of tail sheaths of phage T2. Biokhimiya, 29:1143 (1964).

32. Poglazov, B. F., and Tikhonenko, A. S., A study of the properties of the contractile protein of phage T2. Biokhimiya, 28:888 (1963).

33. Poglazov, B. F., Tikhonenko, A. S., and Engel'gardt, V. A., The action of ATP on the liberation of DNA from bacteriophage. Dokl. Akad. Nauk SSSR, 145:450 (1962).

34. Pokotinskii, I. S., Kriviskii, A. S., and Luzyanina, T. Ya., A new method of studying the development of microorganisms and bacterial viruses in the electron microscope. Zh. Mikrobiol., Epidemiol. Immunobiol., No. 5, p. 19 (1961).

35. Rautenshtein, Ya. I., Stefanov, S. B., Smirnova, E. I., and Khadzhi-Murat, L.° N., Defective lysogeny of a culture of *Act. streptomycini* Kras., a streptomycin producer. Mikrobiologiya, 35:860 (1966).
36. Rautenshtein, Ya. I., Tikhonenko, A. S., and Retinskaya, V. I., Electron-microscopic study of actinophages of a lysogenic strain of *Act. erythreus* Mikrobiologiya, 31:49 (1962).
37. Stent, G. S., Molecular Biology of Bacterial Viruses, San Francisco, Freeman (1963).
38. Stefanov, S. B., and Graf, I. A., Collodion microgrids for high-resolution electron microscopy. Biofizika, 7:357 (1962).
39. Stefanov, S. B., and Smirnova, E. I., A surplus of free tails in suspensions of bacteriophage No. 1 of *Bac. mycoides*. Mikrobiologiya, 32:819 (1963).
40. Stefanov, S. B., and Smirnova, E. I., Bacteriophage particles with two tails. Mikrobiologiya, 33:643 (1964).
41. Stefanov, S. B., Rautenshtein, Ya. I., and Khachaturyan, L. S., Structures of some bacteriophages of strains of the group *Bac. cereus-thuringiensis*. Mikrobiologiya, 35:1064 (1966).
42. Sukhov, K. S., General Virology, Moscow, Nauka Press (1959).
43. Tikhonenko, A. S., Comparative study of the morphology of phage particles by means of shadowing and negative staining in phosphotungstic acid. Biofizika, 6:372 (1961).
44. Tikhonenko, A. S., The fine structure of phage of *Bacillus mycoides*. Dokl. Akad. Nauk SSSR, 138:1449 (1961).
45. Tikhonenko, A. S., Structural elements of the phage corpuscle. Biofizika, 2:247 (1962).
46. Tikhonenko, A. S., Effect of contrasting substances on biological objects. Thematic Collection on Current Problems in Electron Microscopy [in Russian], No. 1, p. 59 (1966).
47. Tikhonenko, A. S., Distorted morphogenesis of the head envelope of phage No. 1 of *Bacillus mycoides*. Mikrobiologiya, 35:118 (1966).
48. Tikhonenko, A. S., Structure of the head capsomeres and polysheaths of phages T2 of *E. coli* and No. 1 of *Bacillus mycoides*. Abstracts of Proceedings of the 9th International Congress on Microbiology [in Russian] (1966), p. 476.
49. Tikhonenko, A. S., The Ultrastructure of Bacterial Viruses (phages). Doctoral dissertation (1966).
50. Tikhonenko, A. S., and Belyaeva, N. N., The morphology of new phages of *Bacillus mycoides* Report of Paper given at the 5th All-Union Conference on Electron Microscopy [in Russian], Sumy (1965), p. 41.
51. Tikhonenko, A. S., and Belyaeva, N. N., Changes in the Protein structure of phages No. 1 and N19 of *Bacillus mycoides* during heating. Mikrobiologiya, 36:475 (1967).
52. Tikhonenko, A. S., and Belyaeva, N. N., Polymerization of the rod protein of the phage T2 tail.. Report of a Paper given at the 6th All-Union Conference on Electron Microscopy, Novosibirsk (1967).
53. Tikhonenko, A. S., and Bespalova, I. A., On two forms of phage of *Bacillus mycoides*. Mikrobiologiya, 30:867 (1961).

54. Tikhonenko, A. S., and Bespalova, I. A., A method of preserving the fine structure of bacteria infected with phage in ultrathin sections. Mikrobiologiya, 33:353 (1964).

55. Tikhonenko, A. S., and Bespalova, I. A., Development of two forms of phage in one cell of *Bacillus mycoides*. Abstracts of Proceedings of the 5th All-Union Conference on Electron Microscopy [in Russian], Sumy (1965), p. 42.

56. Tikhonenko, A. S., Bespalova, I. A., and Kriviskii, A. S., Electron-microscopic study of RNA-containing phage MS2 and its reproduction in the bacterial cell. Dokl. Akad. Nauk SSSR, 160:704 (1965).

57. Tikhonenko, A. S., Velikodvorskaya, G. A., and Belykh, R. A., The action of various agents on phage s_d. Mikrobiologiya, 33:824 (1964).

58. Tikhonenko, A. S., and Zavarzina, N. B., Morphology of a lytic agent of *Chlorella pyrenoidosa*. Mikrobiologiya, 35:856 (1966).

59. Tikhonenko, A. S., and Kuimova, T. F., Effect of fixation on morphology of the bacteriophage of *Bacillus mycoides*. Mikrobiologiya, 29:395 (1960).

60. Tikhonenko, A. S., and Poglazov, B. F., Adenosinetriphosphatase activity of various phages. Dokl. Akad. Nauk SSSR, 145:218 (1962).

61. Tikhonenko, A. S., and Poglazov, B. F., Localization of adenosinetriphosphatase activity in the structural elements of bacteriophage T2. Biokhimiya, 28:340 (1963).

62. Tikhonenko, A. S., and Él'piner, I. E., Electron-microscopic study of a phagolysate of *Bacillus mycoides* irradiated by ultrasonic waves. Biofizika, 7:610 (1959).

63. Tikhonenko, T. I., Vinetskii, Yu., and Zemtsova, É., A method of obtaining phagelysate of *Escherichia coli* s_d with high initial titers. Mikrobiologiya, 30:1020 (1961).

64. Tikhonenko, T. I., Velikodvorskaya, G. A., and Zemtsova, É., Chemical and biological properties of bacteriophage s_d. Biokhimiya, 27:726 (1962).

65. Tikhonenko, T. I., and Zak, V. I., The molecular weight of the DNA of phage s_d of *E. coli* SK. Biokhimiya, 31:33 (1966).

66. Tikhonenko, T. I., and Solov'eva, N. Ya., Concentration and purification of phage s_d of *Escherichia coli* strain SK. Biokhimiya, 26:794 (1961).

67. Thomas, J., Biological reproduction of macromolecules [Russian translation], Moscow, IL (1960).

68. Thomas, C. A., Molecular Genetics [Russian translation], Moscow, IL (1964).

69. Ulanov, B. P., Il'yashenko, B. N., and Tashpulatov, R. Yu., Electron-microscopic investigation of DNA of bacteriophage 1ϕ7. Dokl. Akad. Nauk SSSR, 169:965 (1966).

70. Khavina, É. S., and Rautenshtein, Ya. I., Bacteriophage for strains of bacteria from the genus *Caulobacter*. Dokl. Akad. Nauk SSSR, 153:197 (1963).

71. Khachaturyan, L. S., and Rautenshtein, Ya. I., Comparative study of some bacteriophages of strains of the group *Bac. cereus-thuringiensis*. Mikrobiologiya, 32:813 (1963).

72. Engel'gardt, V. A., and Lyubimova, M. N., The mechanicochemistry of muscles. Biokhimiya, 7:205 (1942).

73. Adams, M., Stability of bacterial viruses in solutions of salts. J. Gen. Physiol., 32:579 (1949).

74. Aiello, I., Frontali, C., and Tangucci, F., Descrizione di un fago temperato del *Bacillus megaterium*. Ann. Inst. Super. Sanita (ex. Rend. Ist Super. Sanita), 1:119 (1965).

75. Almeda, J., A classification of virus particles based on morphology. Can. Med. Assoc. J., 89:787 (1963).

76. Amako, K., and Takeya, K., Electron microscopy of colicin 15. J. Electron Microscopy, 14:149 (1965).

77. Ames, B., and Dubin, D., The role of polyamines in the neutralization of bacteriophage deoxyribonucleic acid. J. Biol. Chem., 235:769 (1960).

78. Anderson, T., The reactions of bacterial viruses with their host cells. Bot. Rev., 15:464 (1949).

79. Anderson, T., Destruction of bacterial viruses by osmotic shock. J. Appl. Phys., 21:70 (1950).

80. Anderson, T., The morphology and osmotic properties of bacteriophage systems. Cold Spring Harbor Sympos. Quant. Biol., 18:197 (1953).

81. Anderson, T., On the fine structure of the temperate bacteriophages P1, P2, and P22. Proc. European Region Conf. on Electron Microscopy, 2:10008 (1960).

82. Anderson, T., and Krimm, S., Diffraction of light from electron micrographs of helical structures in bacteriophage tail sheaths. Proc. VI Congr. Electron Microscopy, Kyoto, Japan 2:145 (1966).

83. Anderson, T., Rappaport, C., and Muscatine, A., On the structure and osmotic properties of phage particles. Ann. Inst. Pasteur, 84:5 (1953).

84. Anderson, T., and Stephens, R., Decomposition of T6 bacteriophage in alkaline solutions. Virology, 23:113 (1964).

85. Anderson, D., Hickman, D., and Reilly, B., Structure of *Bacillus subtilis* bacteriophage ϕ29 and the length of ϕ29 deoxyribonucleic acid. J. Bacteriol., 91:2081 (1966).

86. Arber, W., and Kellenberger, E., Untersuchungen der Feinstrukture eines Bakteriophagen mit Hilfe von Oxydativen Abbau. Schweiz. Z. Pathol., 18:1118 (1955).

87. Astbury, W., On the structure of biological fibres and the problem of muscle. Proc. Roy. Soc., 134:303 (1947).

88. Bacq, V., and Dierickx, Z., Purification de l'actinophage ϕ17. Biochem. Biophys. Acta, 61:19 (1962).

89. Bacq, C., and Horne, R., Morphology of actinophage ϕ17. J. Gen. Microbiol., 32:131 (1963).

90. Baigent, I., De Vey, J., and Starr, M., Bacteriophages of *Pseudomonas syringae* N. Z. J. Sci., 6:75 (1963).

91. Barrington, L., Kozloff, L., Action of bacteriophage on isolated host cell walls. J. Biol. Chem., 223:615 (1956).

92. Bendet, J., Schachter, E., and Lauffer, M., The size of T3 DNA. J. Mol. Biol., 5:76 (1962).

93. Bendich, A., and Rosenkranz, H., Some thoughts on the double-stranded model of deoxyribonucleic acid, in: Progress in Nucleic Acid Research, Vol. 1, New York, Academic Press (1963), p. 219.

94. Bespalova, I., and Tikhonenko, A., The membrane structure of bacterial cells. Proc. 3rd European Region. Conf. on Electron Microscopy, Prague, 2:523 (1964).

95. de Boer, W., and Spit, B., A new type of bacterial cell wall structure revealed by replica technique. Antonie van Leeuwenhock. J. Microbiol. Serol., 30:239 (1964).

96. Bonifas, V., and Kellenberger, E., Etude de l'action des membranes du bacteriophages T2 sur *Escherichia coli*. Biochim. Biophys. Acta, 16:330 (1955).

97. Boy de la Tour, E., Bolle, A., and Kellenberger, E., Nouvelles observations concernant l'action du laurylsulfate de sodium sur la paroi et la membrane d'*E. coli*. Pathol. Microbiol. (Suisse), 28:229 (1965).

98. Boy de la Tour, E., and Kellenberger, E., Aberrant forms of the T-even phage head. Virology, 27:222 (1965).

99. Bradley, D., Negative staining of bacteriophage ϕR. Virology, 15:203 (1961).

100. Bradley, D., Some new small bacteriophages (ϕX174 type). Nature, 195:622 (1962).

101. Bradley, D., The structure of coliphages. J. Gen. Microbiol., 31:435 (1963).

102. Bradley, D., The structure of some *Staphylococcus* and *Pseudomonas* phages. J. Ultrastruct. Res., 8:552 (1963).

103. Bradley, D., The structure of some bacteriophages associated with male strains of *Escherichia coli*. J. Gen. Microbiol., 35:471 (1964).

104. Bradley, D., The morphology and physiology of bacteriophages as revealed by the electron microscope. J. Roy. Microscop. Soc., 84:257 (1965).

105. Bradley, D., The isolation and morphology of some new bacteriophages specific for *Bacillus* and *Acetobacter* species. J. Gen. Microbiol., 41:233 (1965).

106. Bradley, D., The morphology of some bacteriophages specific to *Serratia marcescens*. J. Appl. Bacteriol., 28:271 (1965).

107. Bradley, D., The structure of protein particles released from *Pseudomonas aeruginosa* by mitomycin C. Proc. VI Congr. Electron Microscopy, Kyoto, Japan, 2:115 (1966).

108. Bradley, D., and Kay, D., The fine structure of bacteriophages. J. Gen. Microbiol., 23:553 (1960).

109. Brenner, S., and Horne, R., A negative staining method for high resolution electron microscopy of viruses. Biochim. Biophys. Acta, 34:103 (1959).

110. Brenner, S., and Horne, R., The structure of bacteriophage. Times Sci. Rev. 33:10 (1959).

111. Brenner, E., Streisinger, G., Horne, R., Champe, S., Barnett, L., Benzer, S., and Rees, M. Structural components of bacteriophage. J. Mol. Biol., 1:281 (1959).

112. Brinley-Morgan, W., Kay, D., and Bradley, D., *Brucella* bacteriophage. Nature, 188:74 (1960).

113. Brown, D., and Kozloff, L., Morphological localization of the bacteriophage tail enzyme. J. Biol. Chem., 225:1 (1957).

114. Burchard, R., and Dworkin, M., A bacteriophage for *Myxococcus xanthus*: isolation, characterization, and relation of infectivity to host morphogenesis. J. Bacteriol., 91:1305 (1966).

115. Burgi, E., and Hershey, A., A relative molecular weight series derived from the nucleic acid of bacteriophage T2. J. Mol. Biol., 3:458 (1961).
116. Burnet, F., The relationship between heat-stable agglutinogens and sensitivity to bacteriophage in the *Salmonella* group. Brit. J. Exper. Pathol., 8:121 (1927).
117. Burnet, F., Classification of dysentery — coli bacteriophages. III. Correlation of the serological classification with certain biochemical tests. J. Pathol. Bacteriol., 37:179 (1933).
118. Cairns, J., An estimate of length of the DNA molecule of T2 bacteriophage by autoradiography. J. Mol. Biol., 3:756 (1961).
119. Calderone, J., and Pickett, M., Characterization of brucellaphages. J. Gen. Microbiol., 39:1 (1965).
120. Caro, L., The molecular weight of Lambda DNA. Virology, 25:226 (1965).
121. Caro, L., and Schnos, M., The attachment of the male-specific bacteriophage f1 to sensitive strains of *Escherichia coli*. Proc. Nat. Acad. Sci. USA, 56:126 (1966).
122. Caspar, D., Assembly and stability of the tobacco mosaic virus particle. Advances in Protein Chem., 18:37 (1963).
123. Caspar, D., Design principles in organized biological structures, in: Principles of Biomolecular Organization, Ciba Foundation Sympos. (1966), p. 7.
124. Caspar, D., and Klug, A., Physical principles in the construction of regular viruses. Cold Spring Harbor Sympos. Quant. Biol., 27:1 (1962).
125. Caspar, D., Dulbecco, R., Klug, A., Lwoff, A., Stocker, M., Tournier, P., and Wildy, P., Proposals. Cold Spring Harbor Sympos. Quant. Biol., 27:49 (1962).
126. Caulfield, J., Effects of varying the vehicle for OsO_4 in tissue fixation. J. Biophys. Biochem. Cytol., 3:827 (1957).
127. Chapman, H., and Norris, J., Four new bacteriophages of *Bacillus thuringiensis* J. Appl. Bacteriol., 29:529 (1966).
128. Chiozzoto, A., Coppo, A., Donini, P., and Grazioci, F., The icosahedral form of a temperate phage of *Bacillus megaterium*. Proc. European Reg. Conf. Electron Microscopy, Delft, 2:1012 (1960).
129. Coetzee, J. N., Smit, J. A., and Prozesky, O. W., Properties of providence and *Proteus morganii* transducing phages. J. Gen. Microbiol., 44(2):167 (1966).
130. Cohen, S., The synthesis of bacterial viruses in infection cells. Cold Spring Harbor Sympos. Quant. Biol., 12:35 (1947).
131. Cooper, S., and Zinder, N., The growth of RNA bacteriophage: the role of DNA synthesis. Virology, 18:405 (1962).
132. Cota-Robles, E., and Coffman, M., Fine structure of the bacteriophage attachment process. J. Bacteriol., 86:266 (1963).
133. Crawford, E., and Gesteland, R., The absorption of bacteriophage R17. Virology, 22:165 (1964).
134. Crick, F., and Watson, J., Structure of small viruses. Nature, 177:473 (1956).
135. Cummings, D., Subunit basis of head configurational changes in T2 bacteriophage. Biochim. Biophys. Acta, 68:472 (1963).
136. Cummings, D., and Kozloff, L., Biophysical properties of bacteriophage T2. Biochim. Biophys. Acta, 44:445 (1960).
137. Cummings, D., and Kozloff, L., Various properties of the head protein of T2 bacteriophage. J. Mol. Biol., 5:50 (1962).

138. Daems, W., A preliminary report on the fine structure of a bacteriophage of *Arthrobacter polychromogenes*. Schippers, Lammertse, Muysers, et Klatser-Oedekerk. Antonie van Leeuwenhoek. J. Microbiol. and Serol., 29:16 (1963).
139. Daems, W., van de Pol, J., and Cohen, J., Some remarks on the morphology ot bacteriophage T4B. J. Mol. Biol., 3:225 (1961).
140. Daems, W., Eigner, J., Sluys, J., and Cohen, J., The fine structure of the 114-S and 70-S components of bacteriophage ϕX174 as revealed by negative and positive staining methods. Biochim. Biophys. Acta, 55:801 (1962).
141. Dalton, A., A chrome — osmium fixative for electron microscopy. Anat. Rec. 121:281 (1955).
142. Davis, J., Strauss, J., Sinsheimer, R., Bacteriophage MS2: another RNA phage. Science, 134:1427 (1961).
143. Davison, P., The structure of bacteriophage SP8. Virology, 21:146 (1963).
144. Davison, P., and Freifelder, D., The physical properties of T7 bacteriophage. J. Mol. Biol., 5:635 (1962).
145. Davison, P., and Freifelder, D., Physical properties of the deoxyribonucleic acid from T7 bacteriophage. J. Mol. Biol., 5:643 (1962).
146. Davison, P., Freifelder, D., Hede, R., and Levinthal, C., The structural unity of DNA of T2 bacteriophage. Proc. Nat. Acad. Sci. USA, 47:1123 (1961).
147. Dawson, J., Smillie, E., and Norris, J., The morphology of *Bacillus cereus* bacteriophage. J. Gen. Microbiol., 28:517 (1962).
148. Day, L., Protein conformation in fd bacteriophage as investigated by optical rotatory dispersion. J. Mol. Biol., 15(1):395 (1966).
149. Demeurisse, G., and Sanabria, J., Recepteurs de phages coli-dysenteriques chez *Pseudomonas aeruginosa*. Ann. Inst. Pasteur, 106:449 (1964).
150. Dettori, R., and Neri, M. G., Batteriofago filamentoso specifico per cellule Hfr ed F^+ di *E. coli* K 12. Giorn. Microbiol., 13:111 (1965).
151. Doi, R. H., and Spiegelman, S., Homology test between the nucleic acid of an RNA virus and the DNA in the host cell. Science, 138:1270 (1962).
152. Doi, R. H., Spiegelman, S., Conservation of viral RNA genome during replication and translation. Proc. Nat. Acad. Sci. USA, 49:353 (1963).
153. Drummond, D. G., The practice of electron microscopy. J. Roy. Microsc. Soc., 70:1 (1950).
154. Dugid, J., Smith, W., et al., Non-flagellar filamentous appendages ("fimbriae") and haemagglutinating activity in *Bacterium coli*. J. Pathol. Bacteriol., 70:335 (1955).
155. Dukes, P., and Kozloff, L., Phosphatases in bacteriophages T2, T4, and T5. J. Biol. Chem., 234:534 (1959).
156. Eiserling, F., The structure of *Bacillus subtilis* bacteriophage PBS1. J. Ultrastruct. Res., 17:342 (1967).
157. Eiserling, F., and Boy de la Tour, E., Capsomeres and structure observed on some bacteriophages. Pathol. Microbiol. (Suisse), 28:175 (1965).
158. Eiserling, F., and Romig, W., Studies of *Bacillus subtilis* bacteriophages. Structural characterization by electron microscopy. J. Ultrastruct. Res., 6:540 (1962).
159. Engel'gardt, V. A., and Lyubimova, M. N., Myosin and adenosintriphosphatase. Nature, 144:663 (1939).

160. Enger, M., Stubbs, E., Mitra, S., and Kaesberg, P., Biophysical characteristics of the RNA-containing bacterial virus R17. Proc. Nat. Acad. Sci. USA, 49: 857 (1963).

161. Epstein, R., Bolle, A., Steinberg, C., Kellenberger, E., Boy de la Tour, E., and Chevalley, R., Physiological studies of conditional lethal mutants of bacteriophage T4D. Cold Spring Harbor Sympos. Quant. Biol., 28:375 (1963).

162. Farrant, J., An electron microscopic study of ferritin. Biochim. Biophys. Acta, 13:569 (1954).

163. Favre, E., Boy de la Tour, E., Kellenberger, E., and Sechaud, J., Morphogenese de la tete du bacteriophage T4: Observations sur les polytetes. Proc. 3rd European Reg. Conf. on Electron Microscopy, Prague, 2:541 (1964).

164. Favre, R., Boy de la Tour, E., Segre, N., and Kellenberger, E., Studies on the morphopoiesis of the head of phage T-even. I. Morphological immunological and genetic characterization of polyheads. J. Ultrastruct. Res., 13:318 (1965).

165. Feary, R., Fisher, E., and Fisher, T., A small RNA containing *Pseudomonas aeruginosa* bacteriophage. Biochim. Biophys. Acta Res. Commun., 10:359 (1963)

166. Feary, T., Fisher, E., and Fisher, T., Isolation and preliminary characteristics of three bacteriophages associated with a lysogenic strain of *Pseudomonas aeruginosa*. J. Bacteriol., 87:196 (1964).

167. Fernandez-Moran, H., New approaches in the study of biological ultrastructure by high-resolution electron microscopy. Sympos. Internat. Soc. Cell. Biol., 1:411 (1962).

168. Finch, J., and Klug, A., The structure of viruses of the papilloma-polyoma type III. Structure of rabbit papilloma virus with an appendix on the topography of contrast in negative staining for electron microscopy. J. Mol. Biol., 13:1 (1965).

169. Finch, J., Klug, A., and Stretton, A. O. W., The structure of the "polyheads" of T4 bacteriophage. J. Mol. Biol., 10:570 (1964).

170. Fischbach, F., Harrison, P., and Anderson, J., An X-ray scattering study of the bacterial virus R17. J. Mol. Biol., 13(3):638 (1965).

171. Fiske, C., and Subbarow, J., The colorimetric determination of phosphorus. J. Biol. Chem., 66:375 (1925).

172. Földes, J., and Trautner, T., Infectious DNA from a newly isolated *B. subtilis* phage. Z. Vererbungslehie, 95:57 (1964).

173. Fraenkel-Conrat, H., The role of the nucleic acid in the reconstitution of active tobacco mosaic virus. J. Am. Chem. Soc., 78:882 (1956).

174. Fraenkel-Conrat, H., Degradation of tobacco mosaic virus with acetic acid. Virology, 4:1 (1957).

175. Fraenkel-Conrat, H., and Williams, R., Reconstitution of active tobacco virus from its inactive protein and nucleic acid components. Proc. Nat. Acad. Sci. USA, 41:690 (1955).

176. Frampton, E., and Brinkley, B., Evidence of lysogeny in derivatives of *Escherichia coli*. J. Bacteriol., 90(2):446 (1965).

177. Frank, H., Zarnitz, M., and Weidel, W., Über die Rezeptorsubstanz für den Phagen T5. VII Mitt. Electronenoptische Darstellung und Längenbestimmung der aus T5/R5-Komplexen freigesetzen DNA. Z. Naturforsch., 18b:281 (1963).

178. Frankel, R., and Joys, T., Adsorption specificity of bacteriophage PBS1. J. Bacteriol., 92:388 (1966).
179. Franklin, R., and Granboulan, N., Ultrastructure of *Escherichia coli* cells infected with bacteriophage R-17. J. Bacteriol., 91:834 (1966).
180. Fraser, D., Mahler, H., Shug, A., and Thomas, C., The infection of subcellular *Escherichia coli* strain B, with a DNA preparation from T2 bacteriophage. Proc. Nat. Acad. Sci. USA, 43:939 (1957).
181. Fraser, D., and Williams, R., Electron microscopy of nucleic acid released from individual bacteriophage particles. Proc. Nat. Acad. Sci. USA, 39:750 (1953).
182. Freifelder, D., Kleinschmidt, A. K., and Sinsheimer, R. L., Electron microscopy of single-stranded DNA: circularity of DNA of bacteriophage φX174. Science, 146:254 (1964).
183. French, R., and Siminovitch, L., The action of T2 bacteriophage ghosts on *Escherichia coli* B. Can. J. Microbiol., 1:757 (1955).
184. Gellert, M., Davies, D., Organization of DNA in bacteriophage T4. J. Mol. Biol., 8:341 (1964).
185. Goebel, W., and Jesaitis, M., Chemical and antiviral properties of the somatic antigens of phage II *Shigella sonnei* and of a phage-resistant variant. Ann. Inst. Pasteur, 84:66 (1953).
186. Granboulan, N., and Franklin, R., High-resolution autoradiography of *Escherichia coli* cells infected with bacteriophage R17. J. Bacteriol., 91:849 (1966).
187. Gratia, A., Le phénomène du halo et la synergie des bacteriophages. Compt. Rend. Soc. Biol., 126:418 (1937).
188. Gratia, A., De l'action antogoniste du calcium contre la toxicité exercée par le potassium sur un bactèriophage du *Bacillus megaterium*. Compt. Rend. Soc. Biol., 133:1253 (1940).
189. Guthrie, D., and Sinsheimer, R., Infection of protoplasts of *Escherichia coli* by subviral particles of bacteriophage φX174. J. Mol. Biol., 2:297 (1960).
190. Hall, C., Electron densitometry of stained virus particles. J. Biophys. Biochem. Cytol., 1:1 (1955).
191. Hall, C., Maclean, E., and Tessman, I., Structure and dimensions of bacteriophage φX174 from electron microscopy. J. Mol. Biol., 1:192 (1959).
192. Hanson, J., and Lowy, J., The structure of F-actin and actin filaments isolated from muscle. J. Mol. Biol., 6:46 (1963).
193. Harrington, W., and Schachaman, H., Studies on the alkaline degradation of tobacco mosaic virus. I. Ultracentrifugal analysis. Arch. Biochem. Biophys. 65:278 (1956).
194. Harris, W. J., Holey films for electron microscopy. Nature, 196:499 (1962).
195. Herčik, F., Some observations about the morphology of bacteriophage. Experientia, 6:64 (1950).
196. d'Herelle, F., The bacteriophage and its behavior. Baltimore, Williams and Wilkins (1962).
197. Herriott, R., and Barlow, J., Preparation, purification, and properties of *E. coli* virus T2. J. Gen. Physiol., 36:17 (1952).

198. Herriott, R., and Barlow, J., Protein coats or "ghosts" of coliphage T2.2. Biological functions. J. Gen. Physiol., 41:307 (1957).

199. Hershey, A., An upper limit to the protein content of the germinal substance of bacteriophage T2. Virology, 1:108 (1955).

200. Hershey, A., Some minor components of bacteriophage T2 particles. Virology, 4:237 (1957).

201. Hershey, A., and Chase, M., Independent function of viral protein and nucleic acid in growth of bacteriophage. J. Gen. Physiol., 36:39 (1952).

202. Hillier, J., and Baker, R., The mounting of bacteria for electron microscope examination. J. Bacteriol., 52:411 (1946).

203. Hoffmann-Berling, H., Marvin, D., and Pürwald, H., Ein fädiger DNS Phäge (fd) und ein sphärischer RNS-Phage (fr), wirtspezifisch für männliche Stämme von *E. coli* I. Praparation und chemische Eigenschaften von fd und fr. Z. Naturforsch., 18b:876 (1963).

204. Hoffmann-Berling, H., Dürwald, H., and Beulke, I., Ein fadiger DNS-phage (fd) und ein sphärischer RNS-Phage (fr) wirtspezifisch für männliche Stämme von *E. coli*. III. Biologisches Verhalten von fd und fr. Z. Naturforsch., 18b:893 (1963).

205. Hoffmann-Berling, H., and Maze, R., Release of male-specific bacteriophages from surviving host bacteria. Virology, 22:305 (1964).

206. Hofschneider, P., Über ein infektiöses Desoxyribonucleinsäure Agens aus dem ϕX174. Z. Naturforsch., 15b:441 (1960).

207. Hofschneider, P., Untersuchungen über "Kleine" *E. coli* K-12 Bakteriophagen 1, 2 Mitt. Z. Naturforsch., 18b:203 (1963).

208. Hofschneider, P., and Müller-Jensen, K., Über infektiöse Substrukturen aus *E. coli* — Bakteriophagen. 3. Mitt. Nachweis und Eigenschaften der "HT2" Partikel. Z. Naturforsch., 18b:922 (1963).

209. Hofschneider, P., and Preuss, A., M13 bacteriophage liberation from intact bacteria as revealed by electron microscopy. J. Mol. Biol., 7:450 (1963).

210. Holmes, F., The Filtrable Viruses. Baltimore, Williams and Wilkins (1948).

211. Horne, R., Russell, G., and Trim, A., High resolution electron microscopy of beet yellows virus filaments. J. Mol. Biol., 1:234 (1959).

212. Horne, R., and Wildy, P., Symmetry in virus architecture. Virology, 15:248 (1961).

213. Horne, R., and Wildy, P., Recent studies on the fine structure of viruses by electron microscopy using negative staining techniques. Brit. Med. Bull., 18:199 (1962).

214. Huet, M., and Thouvenot, H., Etude d'un bactériophage actif sur une bactérie anaérobie: *Sphaerophorus varius*. Ann. Inst. Pasteur, 106:867 (1964).

215. Huxley, H., Some observations on the structure of tobacco mosaic virus. Proc. European Reg. Conf. on Electron Microscopy. Stockholm (1956), p. 260.

216. Huxley, H., Electron microscopy studies on the structure of natural and synthetic protein filaments from striated muscle. J. Mol. Biol., 7:281 (1963).

217. Huxley, H., and Zubay, G., Electron microscopy observations on the structure of microsomal particles from *Escherichia coli*. J. Mol. Biol., 2:10 (1960).

218. Huxley, H., and Zubay, G., Preferential staining of nucleic acid-containing structures for electron microscopy. J. Biophys. Biochem. Cytol., 11:273 (1961).

219. Ionesco, H., Ryter, A., and Schaeffer, P., Sur un bactériophage hébergé par la souche Marburg de *Bacillus subtilis*. Ann. Inst. Pasteur, 107 : 764 (1964).
220. Ishii, S., Nishi, Y., and Egami, F., The fine structure of a pyocin. J. Mol. Biol., 13 : 428 (1965).
221. Jesaitis, M., and Goebel, W., Lysis of T4 phage by the specific lipocarbohydrate of phage I1 *Shigella sonnei*. J. Exper. Med., 102 : 733 (1955).
222. Jesaitis, M., and Hutton, J., Properties of a bacteriophage derived from *Escherichia coli* K 235. J. Exper. Med., 117 : 285 (1963).
223. Joys, T. M., Correlation between susceptibility to bacteriophage PBS1 and motility in *Bacillus subtilis*. J. Bacteriol., 90(6) : 1575 (1965).
224. Junasz, S., and Bonicke, R., Possible classification of rapidly growing mycobacteria on the basis of their phage susceptibility. Can. J. Microbiol., 11 : 235 (1965).
225. Kanner, L., and Kozloff, L., The reaction of indole and T2 bacteriophage. Biochemistry, 3 : 215 (1964).
226. Kay, D., The nucleic acid composition of bacteriophage ϕR. J. Gen. Microbiol., 27 : 201 (1962).
227. Kay, D., and Bradley, D., The structure of bacteriophage ϕR. J. Gen. Microbiol., 27 : 195 (1962).
228. Kellenberger, E., Vegetative bacteriophage and the maturation of virus particles. Advances Virus Res., 8 : 1 (1961).
229. Kellenberger, E., Control mechanisms in bacteriophage morphopoiesis, in: Principles of Biomolecular Organization. Ciba Foundation Sympos. (1966). p. 192.
230. Kellenberger, E., The genetic control of the shape of a virus. Scient. Am., 215 : 32 (1966).
231. Kellenberger, E., and Arber, W., Die Structur des Schwanzes der Phagen T2 und T4 und der Mechanismus der irreversiblen Adsorption. Z. Naturforsch., 10b : 698 (1955).
232. Kellenberger, E., and Arber, W., Electron microscopical studies of phage multiplication. I. A method for quantative analysis of particle suspensions. Virology, 3 : 245 (1957).
233. Kellenberger, E., Bolle, A., Boy de la Tour, E., Eptstein, R., Franklin, N., Jerne, N., Reale-Scafati, A., Séchaud, Y., Bendet, I., Goldstein, D., and Lauffer, M., Functions and properties related to the tail fibers of bacteriophage T4. Virology, 26 : 419 (1965).
234. Kellenberger, E., and Boy de la Tour, E., On the fine structure of normal and "polymerized" tail sheath of phage T4. J. Ultrastruct. Res., 11 : 545 (1964).
235. Kellenberger, E., and Boy de la Tour, E., Studies on the morphopoieses of the head of phage T-even. II. Observations on the fine structure of polyheads. J. Ultrastruct. Res., 13 : 343 (1965).
236. Kellenberger, E., Ryter, A., and Sechaud, J., Electron microscope study of DNA-containing plasms. II. Vegetative and mature nucleoids in different physiological states. J. Biophys. Biochem. Cytol., 4 : 671 (1958).
237. Kellenberger, E., and Sechaud, J., Electron microscopical studies of phage multiplication. II. Production of phage-related structures during multiplication of phages T2 and T4. Virology, 3 : 256 (1957).

238. Kellenberger, G., and Kellenberger, E., Electron microscopical studies of phage multiplication. III. Observation of single cell bursts. Virology, 3: 275 (1957).

239. Kellenberger, E., Sechaud, J., and Ryter, A., Electron microscopical studies of phage multiplication. IV. The establishment of the DNA pool of vegetative phage and the maturation of phage particles. Virology, 8:478 (1959).

240. Kilkson, R., and Maestre, M., Structure of T2 bacteriophage. Nature, 195:494 (1962).

241. Klein, M., Kalter, S., and Mudd, S., The action of synthetic detergents upon certain strains of bacteriophage and virus. J. Immunol., 51:389 (1945).

242. Kleinschmidt, A., Lang, D., Jacherts, S., and Zahn, R., Darstellung und Längenmessungen der gesamten Desoxyribonucleinsäure-Inhaltes von T2-Bakteriophagen. Biochim. Biophys. Acta, 61:857 (1962).

243. Klerk, H., and Coetzee, J., The fine structure of lactobacillus bacteriophages. J. Gen. Microbiol., 38:35 (1965).

244. Klug, A., and Caspar, D., The structure of small viruses. Advances Virus Res., 7:225 (1960).

245. Klug, A., Finch, J., Leberman, R., and Longley, W., Design and structure of regular virus particles, in: Principles of Biomolecular Organization. Ciba Foundation Sympos. (1966), p. 158.

246. Knapp, W., and Zwillenberg, L., Morphological differences between *Pasteurella* bacteriophages. Arch. Ges. Virusforsch., 14:563 (1964).

247. Koch, G., and Weidel, W., Abspaltung chemischer Komponenten der Coli-Membran durch daran absorbierte Phagen. I. Mitt: Allgemeine Charakterisierung des Effekts und partial Analyse einer des abgespaltenen Komponenten. Z. Naturforsch., 11b:345 (1956).

248. Kolstad, R., and Bradley, S., Purification of *Streptomyces venezuelae* phage. J. Bacteriol., 87:1157 (1964).

249. Kozloff, L., Mechanism of viral invasion, in: Sympos. on Mol. Biol. (1959), p. 178.

250. Kozloff, L., and Henderson, K., Action of complexes of zinc group metals on the tail protein of bacteriophage T2r^{+}. Nature, 176:1169 (1955).

251. Kozloff, L., and Lute, M., Viral invasion. II. The role of zinc in bacteriophage invasion. J. Biol. Chem., 228:529 (1957).

252. Kozloff, L., and Lute, M., Viral invasion. III. The release of viral nucleic acid from its protein covering. J. Biol. Chem., 228:537 (1958).

253. Kozloff, L., and Lute, M., A contractile protein in the tail of bacteriophage T2. J. Biol. Chem., 234:239 (1959).

254. Kozloff, L., and Lute, M., Calcium content of bacteriophage T2. Biochim. Biophys. Acta, 37:420 (1960).

255. Kozloff, L., Lute, M., and Henderson, K., Viral invasion. I. Rupture of thiol ester bonds in the bacteriophage tail. J. Biol. Chem., 228:511 (1957).

256. Krueger, A., The heat inactivation of antistaphylococcus bacteriophage. J. Gen. Physiol., 15:363 (1932).

257. Laki, K., and Standaert, J., The minimal molecular weight of actin estimated with the use of carboxypeptidase. Arch. Biochem. Biophys., 86:16 (1960).

258. Lantos, J., and Ivanovics, G., The phage receptors of *Bacillus anthracis* Acta Microbiol. Hung., 8:379 (1961).
259. Lapchine, L., and Engalbert, L., Étude morphologique de quelques phages staphylococciques. J. Microscopie, 4:33 (1965).
260. Lark, K., and Adams, M., The stability of phages as a function of the ionic environment. Cold Spring Harbor Symps. Quant. Biol., 18:171 (1953).
261. Lewin, R., Crothers, D., Correll, D., and Reimann, B., A phage infecting *Saprospira grandis*. Can. J. Microbiol., 10:75 (1964).
262. Loeb, T., The isolation of a bacteriophage specific for the F^+ and Hfr mating types of *Escherichia coli* K-12. Science, 131:932 (1960).
263. Loeb, T., and Zinder, N., A bacteriophage containing RNA. Proc. Nat. Acad. Sci. USA, 47:282 (1961).
264. Lowy, J., and Hanson, J., Structure of bacterial flagella. Nature, 202:538 (1964).
265. Lowy, J., and Hanson, J., Electron microscope studies of bacterial flagella. J. Mol. Biol., 11:293 (1965).
266. Luft, J. H., Permanganate – a new fixative for electron microscopy. J. Biophys. Biochem. Cytol., 2:799-801 (1956).
267. Lwoff, A., Anderson, T., and Jacob, F., Remarques sur les characteristiques de la particule virale infectieuse. Ann. Inst. Pasteur, 97:281 (1959).
268. Mach, F., Fortsatzstrukturen bei Actinophagen. Electron Microscopy, 2:10 (1962).
269. MacHattie, L., and Thomas, C., DNA from bacteriophage lambda: molecular length and conformation. Science, 144:1142 (1964).
270. Maclean, E., and Hall, C., Studies on bacteriophage ϕX174 and its DNA by electron microscopy. J. Mol. Biol., 4:173 (1962).
271. Mayers, V., and Spizizen, J., The isolation of desoxyribonucleic acid from bacteriophages by an improved method. J. Biol. Chem., 210:877 (1954).
272. Mare, I. J., Klerk, H. C., and Prozesky, O. W., The morphology of *Alcaligenes faecalis* bacteriophages. J. Gen. Microbiol., 44(1):23 (1966).
273. Marvin, D., and Hoffmann-Berling, H., Physical and chemical properties of two new small bacteriophages. Nature, 197:517 (1963).
274. Marvin, D., and Hoffmann-Berling, H., A fibrous DNA phage (fd) and spherical RNA phage (fr) specific for male strains of *E. coli*. II. Physical characteristics. Z. Naturforsch., 18b:884 (1963).
275. Marvin, D., X-ray diffraction and electron microscope studies on the structure of the small filamentous bacteriophage fd., J. Mol. Biol., 15(1):8 (1966).
276. Marvin, D., and Schaller, H., The topology of DNA from the small filamentous bacteriophage fd., J. Mol. Biol., 15:1 (1966).
277. Matthews, M., and Bradley, D., Preliminary observations on two bacteriophages from *Pseudomonas* and *Serratia*. Proc. 3rd European Reg. Conf. on Electron Microscopy, Prague, 2:543 (1964).
278. Matthews, M., Miller, P., and Pappenheimer, A., Morphological observations on some diphtherial phages., Virology, 29:402 (1966).
279. Maxted, W., The active agent in nascent phage lysis of Streptococci. J. Gen. Microbiol., 16:584 (1957).

280. McDuff, C., Jones, L., and Wilson, H., Characteristics of brucellaphage., J. Bacteriol., 83:324 (1962).
281. Mennigmann H. D., Electron microscopy of the antibacterial agent produced by *Escherichia coli* 15., J. Gen. Microbiol., 41:151 (1965).
282. Meynell, E., A phage ϕX, which attacks motile bacteria., J. Gen. Microbiol., 25:253 (1961).
283. Mohelska, H., Morphological study of mycobacterial phage MyF_3P/59a., Proc. 3rd European Reg. Conf. on Electron Microscopy, Prague, 2:551 (1964).
284. Monod, J., Changeux, J., and Jacob, F., Allosteric proteins and cellular control systems., J. Mol. Biol., 6:306 (1964).
285. Moody, M. F., The shape of the T-even bacteriophage head., Virology, 26:567 (1965).
286. Müller-Jensen, R., and Hofschneider, P., Infectious substructures of *E. coli* bacteriophages. IV. The nature of infectious urea T2 particles., Biochim. Biophys. Acta, 80:422 (1964).
287. Murphy, J., An agent derived from *B. megaterium* phage G which dissolves the bacterial cell wall., Virology, 11:510 (1960).
288. Murray, R., Gillen, D., and Heagy, F., Cytological changes in *Escherichia coli* produced by infection with phage T2. J. Bacteriol., 59:603 (1950).
289. Nanavutty, S., The thermal death rate of bacteriophage., J. Path. Bacteriol., 33:203 (1930).
290. Nathaus, D., Notani, G., Schwartz, J., and Zinder, N., Biosynthesis of the coat protein of coliphage f2 by *E. coli* extracts., Proc. Nat. Acad. Sci. USA, 48:1424 (1962).
291. Nishi, Y., Ishii, S., and Egami, F., The fine structure of a pyocin., J. Electron Microscopy, 14:158 (1965).
292. Nixon, H., and Harrison, B., Electron microscopic evidence on the structure of the particles of tobacco rattle virus., J. Gen. Microbiol., 21:582 (1959).
293. Painter, B., and Bradley, S., Electron microscopic observations on actinophages for *Streptomyces venezuelae*., J. Bacteriol., 89:240 (1965).
294. Palade, G., A study of fixation for electron microscopy., J. Exper. Med., 95:285 (1952).
295. Panter, R. A., and Symons, R. H., Isolation and properties of a DNA containing rod-shaped bacteriophage., Austral. J. Biol. Sci., Vol. 19, No. 565 (1966).
296. Paranchych, W., Stages in phage R-17 infection: the role of divalent cations., Virology, 28(1):90 (1966).
297. Paranchych, W., and Graham, A., Isolation and properties of RNA-containing bacteriophage., J. Cell. Comp. Physiol., 60:199 (1962).
298. Parnas, J., and Bradley, D., Characteristics of *Brucella* phages: negative colonies and morphology., Bull. Acad. Polon. Sci. Ser. Biol., 12:13 (1964).
299. Parnas, J., and Chiozzotto, A., Further studies on *Brucella* phage morphology., Bull. Acad. Polon. Sci. Ser. Biol., 10:135 (1962).
300. Parnas, J., and Sarnecka-Szunke, B., Weitere Charakteristik der Brucellaphagen., Arch. Exper. Veterinärmed., 19:497 (1965).
301. de Petris, S., and Nava, G., Osservazioni sul fago μ_2., Atti IV Congr. microscopia electronica (1963), p. 123.

302. dePetris, S., and Nava, G., Sex specific bacteriophages of *E. coli* K-12. II. Electron microscope observation on bacteriophage μ_2., Giorn. Microbiol., 11:1 (1963).

303. de Petris, S., and Nava, G., Infection of *E. coli* K-12 by the RNA phage μ_2., Proc. 3rd European Reg. Conf. on Electron Microscopy, Prague, 2:547 (1964).

304. Pohjanpelto, P., and Nyholm, M., Fine structure of subilis phage SP-50., Arch. Ges. Virusforsch., 17:481 (1965).

305. Pollard, E., and Reaume, M., Thermal inactivation of bacterial viruses., Arch. Biochem. Biophys., 32:278 (1951).

306. Pottinger, M., and Bachofer, C., Protection of bacteriophage T1 against x-rays and heat., Arch. Biochem. Biophys., 70:499 (1957).

307. Prozesky, O., Klerk, H., and Coetzee, J., The morphology of *Proteus* bacteriophages., J. Gen. Microbiol., 41:29 (1965).

308. Puck, T., A reversible transformation of T1 bacteriophage., J. Bacteriol., 57:647 (1949).

309. Putnam, F., Miller, D., Palm, L., and Evans, E., Biochemical studies of Bacteriophage reproduction. X. Precursors of bacteriophage T7., J. Biol., Chem., 199:177 (1952).

310. Putnam, F., Kozloff, L., and Neil, J., Biochemical studies of virus reproduction. I. Purification and properties of *E. coli* bacteriophage T6., J. Biol. Chem., 179:303 (1949).

311. Ralston, D., Liebermann, M., Baer, B., and Krueger, A., Staphylococcal virolysin, a phage-induced lysin. Its differentiation from the autolysin of normal cells., J. Gen. Physiol., 40: 791 (1957).

312. Ray, D., Preuss, A., and Hofschneider, P., Replication of the single-stranded DNA of the male-specific bacteriophage M13. Circular forms of the replicative DNA., J. Mol. Biol., 21:485 (1966).

313. Ris, H., and Chandler, B., The ultrastructure of genetic systems in prokaryotes and eukaryotes., Cold Spring Harbor Sympos. Quant. Biol., 28:1 (1963).

314. Robertson, C., and Bott, M., Optical rotation and chain folding in synthetic polypeptides and gelatin., Nature, 168:325 (1951).

315. Rosato, R., and Cameron, J., The bacteriophage receptor sites of *Staphylococcus aureus*. Biochem. Biophys. Acta, 83:1737 (1964).

316. Rosenblum, E., and Tyrone, S., Serology, density, and morphology of staphylococcal phages., J. Bacteriol., 88:1737 (1964).

317. Roslycky, E., Allan, O., and McCoy, E., Physicochemical properties of phages for *Agrobacterium radiobacter*., Can. J. Microbiol., 9:199 (1963).

318. Roth, Th. F., and Hayashi, M., Allomorphic forms of bacteriophage ϕX174 replicative DNA., Science, 154:658 (1966).

319. Rubenstein, I., Thomas, C., and Hershey, A., The molecular weights of T2 bacteriophage and its first and second breakage product., Proc. Nat. Acad. Sci. USA, 47:1113 (1961).

320. Ruska, H., Über ein neues der Bakteriophagen Lyse auftretendes Formelement., Naturwissenschaften, 29:363 (1941).

321. Ruska, E., Zur Entstehung der Säume um übermicroskopisch abgebildete Partikel und über ihre Veränderung mit der optischen Einstellung., Kolloid. Z., 105:43 (1943).

322. Ryter, A., Kellenberger, E., Birch-Anderson, A., and Maaleφe, O., Étude au microscope électronique de plasmas contenant de l'acide desoxyribonucléique., Z. Naturforsch., 13b: 597 (1958).
323. Sacata, S., J. Electron Microscopy, 6: 75 (1958).
324. Salivar, V., Tzagiloff, H., and Pratt, D., Some physicalchemical and biological properties of the rod-shaped coliphage M13., Virology, 24: 359 (1964).
325. Salton, M., Bacterial cell walls, in: Bacterial Anatomy. Sixth Sympos. Soc. Gen. Microbiol., Cambridge (1956).
326. Sandoval, H., Reilly, C., and Tandler, B., Colicin 15: possibly a defective bacteriophage., Nature, 205: 522 (1965).
327. Sanyal, A., Ganguly, P., and Das Cupta, M., Interaction of phosphotungstate with haemoglobin., J. Mol. Biol., 8: 325 (1964).
328. Sarkar, M., Sarkar, S., and Kozloff, L., Tail components of T2 bacteriophage. I. Properties of the isolated contractile tail sheath., Biochemistry, 3: 511 (1964).
329. Sarkar, S., Sarkar, M., and Kozloff, L., Tail components of T2 bacteriophage. II. Properties of isolated tail cores., Biochemistry, 3: 517 (1964).
330. Sato, G., Activation of bacteriophage by urea., Science, 123: 891 (1956).
331. Schmidt, J., and Stanier, R., Isolation and characterization of bacteriophages active against stalked bacteria., J. Gen. Microbiol., 39: 95 (1965).
332. Schramm, G., Über die Spaltung des Tabakmosaikvirus in niedermolecularen Proteine und die Rückbildungen hochmolecularen Protein aus dem Spaltstüken., Naturwissenschaften, 31: 94 (1943).
332. Schramm, G., Über die Spaltung der Tabak-Mosaik-Virus und die Wiedervereinigung der Spaltstücke zu höhermolecularen Proteinen. I. Die Spaltungst-Reaktion., Z. Naturforsch., 2b: 112 (1947).
334. Schramm, G., and Zillig, W., Über die Struktur des Tabakmosaikvirus. IV. Mitt: Die Reaggregation des nucleinsäure-freien Proteins., Z. Naturforsch., 10b: 493 (1955).
335. Schwartz, F., and Zinder, N., Crystalline aggregates in bacterial cells infected with the RNA bacteriophage f2., Virology, 21: 276 (1965).
336. Seaman, E., Tarmy, E., and Marmur, J., Inducible phages of *Bacillus subtilis* Biochemistry, 3: 607 (1964).
337. Sekiguchi, M., Taketo, A., and Takagi, Y., An infective deoxyribonucleic acid from bacteriophage φX174, Biochim. Biophys. Acta, 45: 199 (1960).
338. Sertic, V., Origine de la lysine d'une race du bactériophage., Compt. Rend. Soc. Biol., 100: 477 (1929).
339. Sertic, V., and Boulgakov, N., Classification et identification des typhiphages., Compt. Rend. Soc. Biol., 119: 1270 (1935).
340. Setlow, R., and Boyce, R., The ultraviolet light inactivation of φX174 bacteriophage at different wavelengths and pH's., Biophys. J., 1: 29 (1960).
341. Siefert-Gertchman, H., and Lippert, W., Elektronenmikroskopische Untersuchung zweier temperieter Phagen von *Serratia marcescens* . Z. Allg. Mikrobiol., 1: 87 (1960).
342. Sinsheimer, R., Purification and properties of bacteriophage φX174., J. Mol. Biol., 1: 37 (1959).

343. Sjöstrand, F., The ultrastructure of the outer segments of rods and cones of the eye as revealed by the electron microscope., J. Cell. Comp. Physiol., 42:15 (1953).
344. Sjöstrand, F., An improved method to prepare formvar nets for mounting thin sections for electron microscopy., Proc. First European Reg. Conf. on Electron Microscopy, Stockholm (1956), p. 120.
345. Slayter, H., Holloway, B., and Hall, C., The structure of *Pseudomonas aeruginosa* phages B3, E79, and F116., J. Ultrastruct. Res., 11:274 (1964).
346. Smith, K., Brown, R., and Walne, P., Electron microscopy of the infection process of the blue-green alga virus., Virology, 30:182 (1966).
347. Smith, K., and Troousdale, M., Multiple-tailed T4 bacteriophage., J. Bacteriol., 90:796 (1965).
348. Staehelin, M., Reaction of TMV nucleic acid with formaldehyde. Biochim. Biophys. Acta, 29:410 (1958).
349. Standaert, J., and Laki, K., Conformation of the peptide chain in actin molecules., Biochim. Biophys. Acta, 60:641 (1962).
350. Stickler, D., Tucker, R., and Kay, D., Bacteriophage-like particles released from *Bacillus subtilis* after induction with hydrogen peroxide., Virology, 26:142 (1965).
351. Strauss, J., and Sinsheimer, R., Purification and properties of bacteriophage MS2 and of its rubonucleic acid., Mol. Biol., 7:43 (1963).
352. Swanstrom, M., and Adams, M., Agar layer method for production of high titer phage stocks., Proc. Soc. Exper. Biol. Med., 78:372 (1951).
353. Takahashi, J., Genetic transduction in *Bacillus subtilis*. Biochem. Biophys. Res. Commun., 5:171 (1961).
354. Takeya, K., and Amako, H., The structure of mycobacteriophages., Virology., 24:461 (1964).
355. Takeya, K., and Amako, K., A rod-shaped *Pseudomonas* phage., Virology, 28(1):163 (1966).
356. Takeya, K., Mori, R., Ueda, S., and Toda, T., Bacteriophage of *Pseudomonas aeruginosa* with unfamiliar head morphology., J. Bacteriol., 78:332 (1959).
357. Takeya, K., Minamishima, Y., and Amako, K., Electron microscopy of a pseudomonas-phage and a pyocin., Proc. VI Congr. Electron Microscopy Kyoto, Japan, 2:135 (1966).
358. Taubeneck, U., Über die Produktion biologische aktiver Phagen-Schwanze durch einen defekt lysogenen *Proteus mirabilis* -stamm., Z. Naturforsch., 18b:898 (1963).
359. Taubeneck, U., and Zickler, F., Inaktivierung inkompletter Proteus-Phagen durch eine Rezeptorsubstanz im zellfreien Kulturfiltrat der Indikatorbakterien., Z. Allg. Mikrobiol., 5:78 (1965).
360. Tessman, I., Some unusual properties of the nucleic acid in bacteriophage S13 and φX174., Virology, 7:263 (1959).
361. Tikhonenko, A., and Bespalova, I., Phage maturation in *Bacillus mycoides* cells., Virology, 23:259 (1964).
362. Tikhonenko, A., Bespalova, I., and Krivisky, A., Electron microscopy studies of RNA phage MS2 and its reproduction in bacterial cells., Proc. 3rd European Reg. Conf. on Electron Microscopy, Prague, 2:545 (1964).

363. Tikhonenko, A., and Bespalova, I., Development of two phage forms in a cell of *Bacillus mycoides*. Proc. VI Congr. Electron Microscopy, Kyoto, Japan, 2:141 (1966).

364. Tikhonenko, A., and Belyaeva, N., Contraction process of tail sheath and "polymerization" of some proteins of phage N1 *Bacillus mycoides* on heating., Proc. VI Congr. Electron Microscopy, Kyoto, Japan, 2:143 (1966).

365. Tokunaga, T., Mizuguchi, Y., and Murohashi, T., Deoxyribonucleic acid base composition of mycobacteriophage., J. Bacteriol., 86:608 (1963).

366. Tromans, W., and Horne, R., The Structure of bacteriophage ϕX174., Virology, 15:1 (1961).

367. Tzagaloff, H., and Pratt, D., The initial steps in infection with coliphage M13. Virology, 24:372 (1964).

368. Valentine, A., Chen, P., Colwell, R., and Chapman, G., Structure of a marine bacteriophage as revealed by the negative-staining technique., J. Bacteriol., 91:819 (1966).

369. Valentine, R., and Strand, M., Complexes of F-pili and RNA bacteriophage., Science, 148:511 (1965).

370. Valentine, R., Wedel, H., and Ippen, K., F-pili-requirements for RNA bacteriophage adsorption., Biochim. Biophys. Acta, 21:277 (1965).

371. Van Vunakis, H., Baker, W., and Brown, R., Structural studies on the proteins of bacteriophages. I. Alkaline dissociation of the protein coat "ghosts" of bacteriophage T2 r^+., Virology, 5:327 (1958).

372. Van Vunakis, H., and Herriott, R., Inactivation of the T-even coliphages by pyrophosphate., J. Bacteriol., 83:590 (1962).

373. Viev; J., Croissant, O., and Dauguet, C., Sur La morphologie du bacteriophage Twort au microscope electronique., Compt. Rend. Acad. Sci., 257:553 (1963).

374. Viev, J., Croissant, O., and Dauguet, C., Ultrastructure du bactériophage Staphylococcique Twort., J. Microscopie, 3:403 (1964).

375. Viev, J., Croissant, O., and Dauguet, C., Structure des Bactériophages responsables des phenomenes de conversion chez des *Salmonella*. Ann. Inst. Pasteur, 108:160 (1965).

376. Viev, J., Guelin, A., and Dauguet, C., Morphologie du bactériophage 80 de *Welchia perfringens* Ann. Inst. Pasteur, 109:157 (1965).

377. Wahl, R., and Kozloff, L., The nucleoside triphosphate content of various bacteriophages., J. Biol. Chem., 237:1953 (1962).

378. Watanabe, K., Studies on the bacteriophage and desoxyribonuclease of a *B. subtilis* strain producing amylase (Part 4). The electron micrograph of a bacteriophage active against *B. subtilis* var. *amyloliquefaciens* Fukumoto K49., Sci. Bull. Fac. Agric. Kyushu Univ., 18:147 (1960).

379. Watanabe, K., and Yamafuji, K., Studies on the bacteriophage and desoxyribonuclease of a *B. subtilis* strain., Enzymologia, 23:353 (1961).

380. Webb, J., and Levy, J., A sensitive method for the determination of deoxyribonucleic acid in tissues and microorganisms., J. Biol. Chem., 213:107 (1955).

381. Weidel, W., Further studies on the membrane of *E. coli* B., Ann. Inst. Pasteur, 84:61 (1953).

382. Weidel, W., Frank, H., and Martin, H., The rigid layer of the cell wall of *Escherichia coli* strain B., J. Gen. Microbiol., 22:158 (1960).
383. Weidel, W., and Kellenberger, E., The *E. coli* B receptor for the phage T5. II. Electron microscopic studies., Biochim. Biophys. Acta, 17:1 (1955).
384. Weidel, W., Koch, G., and Bobosch, K., Über die Rezeptorsubstanz für den Phagen T5. I. Reindarstellung aus *E. coli* B. Physikalische, chemische und funktionelle Charakterisierung., Z. Naturforsch., 9b:573 (1954).
385. Weissmann, C., and Borst, D., Double-stranded ribonucleic acid formation in vitro by MS2 phage-induces RNA synthetase., Science, 142:1188 (1963).
386. Weissmann, C., Borst, D., Simon, L., and Ochoa, S., Induction by an RNA phage of an enzyme catalyzing incorporation of ribonucleotides into ribonucleic acid., Proc. Nat. Acad. Sci. USA, 49:407 (1963).
387. Welker, N., and Campbell, L., Induction and properties of temperate bacteriophage from *Bacillus stearothermophilus*., J. Bacteriol., 89:175 (1965).
388. White, R., Georgi, C., and Militzer, W., The heat studies on a thermophylic bacteriophage., Proc. Soc. Exp. Biol. Med., 85:137 (1954).
389. Williams, R., and Fraser, D., Morphology of the seven T-bacteriophages., J. Bacteriol., 66:458 (1953).
390. Williams, R., and Fraser, D., Structural and functional differentiation in T2 bacteriophage., Virology, 2:289 (1956).
391. Williams, R., and Wyckoff, R., Applications of metallic shadow-casting to microscopy., J. Appl. Phys., 17:23 (1946).
392. Winkler, U., Johns, H., and Kellenberger, E., Comparative study of some properties of bacteriophage T4D irradiated with monochromatic ultraviolet light., Virology, 18:343 (1962).
393. Wyckoff, R., Filaments in cultures of bacteriophage., Experientia, 6:66 (1950).
394. Yamamoto, N., and Anderson, T., Genomic masking and recombination between serologically unrelated phages P22 and P221., Virology, 14:430 (1961).
395. Zarnitz, M., and Weidel, W., Über die Rezoptorsubstanz für den Phagen T5. VI. Mitt. Die Thermodynamik der Kontaktbilding zwischen Phagen und Rezeptor sowie deren mögliche Bedeutung als morphogenetischer Modellmechanismus., Z. Naturforsch., 18b:276 (1963).
396. Zinder, M., Valentine, R., Roger, M., and Stoeckenius, W., f1, a rod-shaped male-specific bacteriophage that contains DNA., Virology, 20:638 (1963).

Index

MIX
Papier aus verantwortungsvollen Quellen
Paper from responsible sources
FSC® C105338

If you have any concerns about our products,
you can contact us on
ProductSafety@springernature.com

In case Publisher is established outside the EU,
the EU authorized representative is:
Springer Nature Customer Service Center GmbH
Europaplatz 3, 69115 Heidelberg, Germany

Printed by Libri Plureos GmbH
in Hamburg, Germany